Quick Reference to Speech-Language Pathology

Sally G. Pore, M.Ed, CCC-SP, MS
Owner, Capital Research & Writing Services
Concord, New Hampshire

Kathlyn L. Reed, PhD, OTR, MLIS, AHIP
Visiting Professor
School of Occupational Therapy
Texas Woman's University - Houston Center
Houston, Texas

AN ASPEN PUBLICATION
Aspen Publishers, Inc.
Gaithersburg, Maryland
1999

Library of Congress Cataloging-in-Publication Data

Pore, Sally G.
Quick reference to speech-language pathology / Sally G. Pore, Kathlyn L. Reed.
p. cm.
Includes bibliographical references and index.
ISBN 0-8342-1278-1
1. Speech disorders—Handbooks, manuals, etc. 2. Language disorders—
Handbooks, manuals, etc. I. Reed, Kathlyn L. II. Title.
[DNLM: 1. Speech Disorders handbooks. 2. Language Disorders handbooks.
3. Speech-Language Pathology handbooks. WL 39 P835q 1999]
RC423.P665 1999
616.85'5—dc21
DNLM/DLC
for Library of Congress
98-54628
CIP

Orders: (800) 638-8437
Customer Service: (800) 234-1660

About Aspen Publishers • For more than 35 years, Aspen has been a leading professional
publisher in a variety of disciplines. Aspen's vast information resources are available in both
print and electronic formats. We are committed to providing the highest quality information
available in the most appropriate format for our customers. Visit Aspen's Internet site for more
information resources, directories, articles, and a searchable version of Aspen's full catalog,
including the most recent publications: **http://www.aspenpublishers.com**
Aspen Publishers, Inc. • The hallmark of quality in publishing
Member of the worldwide Wolters Kluwer group.

Editorial Services: Ruth Bloom
Library of Congress Catalog Card Number: 98-54628
ISBN: 0-8342-1278-1

Printed in the United States of America

1 2 3 4 5

This book is dedicated to our fathers,
William H. Pore
and
Herbert C. Reed,
and to the memory of our mothers,
Anne D. Pore
and
Ruth Krehbiel Reed

Table of Contents

Acknowledgments

We would like to thank all those who helped often but quietly behind the scenes. Particular thanks are due to staff members at the Concord Public Library who so patiently, and even enthusiastically, processed all of the interlibrary loan requests: thanks to Bobbie, Mary Ann, Pat, Peg, Robyn, and Sandi who took the requests; to Donna who processed them and got the materials for me; and to Marie and Patty who made sure the materials got into my hands.

Thanks to Sheila Gorman and Tom Mead at the Dana Library at Dartmouth Medical School and to Peggy Sleeth and her staff at the Matthews-Fuller Health Sciences Library at Dartmouth-Hitchcock Memorial Hospital for their interest and assistance on numerous occasions.

Thanks to Jean Rubé-Ranier and the other members of the speech department at Crotched Mountain Rehabilitation Center who read the original proposal and said, "Do it. We need this book." Thanks, too, for their comments and suggestions for the Table on Augmentative and Alternative Communication.

Thanks to Arthur Stavros for his usual on-the-mark style and editing suggestions.

We also wish to thank Mary Anne Langdon, Senior Developmental Editor; Amy Martin, Acquisitions Editor; and Nick Radhuber, Production Editor, at Aspen Publishers, Inc., for their patience, expertise, and assistance in publishing this text.

Introduction

The purpose of this book is to provide a quick reference to those disorders, syndromes, and conditions seen among clients served by speech-language pathologists. It was written primarily as a source of information regarding those conditions for a diverse group of professionals, including clinicians, students of speech-language pathology, researchers, and educators, and lay people also will find the text informative and helpful in better understanding the nature of these disorders.

The book is organized by a classification of syndromes and conditions rather than by type of communication disorder. This allows clinicians preparing for a new admission to make a quick comparison between a stated diagnosis and information in the book relating to the diagnosis. It also recognizes that many conditions require intervention for more than one type of communication disorder.

The intent of this book is to provide more than a quick reference to specific disorders. It was written also to provide a summation of the present state of knowledge and practice regarding each condition. To that end, no sources used in researching the book were published earlier than 1992. Appendix F, however, contains a bibliography of the writings of several well-known practitioners in the field over the years. We provided it with the hope that readers, in referring to these sources, will gain some perspective on the history of the profession and its practices.

We sought to include in the book as many relevant conditions as possible. Most often the primary factor in excluding any particular one was a lack of published information regarding that condition and/or speech and language implications of the disorder. Whenever possible we included disorders mentioned in the literature. In some instances, this led to the inclusion of syndromes for which literally only a handful of cases have been identified. These are included because as clinicians we may be called on to provide services to someone with such a diagnosis and because it is hoped that their inclusion will generate increased interest and subsequent research and reporting within the field. Some of the diagnoses that were considered for the book, but were not included because of insufficient published information, include Charcot-Marie-Tooth disease, Floating-Harbor syndrome, Gerstmann's syndrome, multiple system atrophy, tuberous sclerosis, Turner's syndrome, and Werdnig-Hoffman disease.

Each disorder in the book follows the format given below:

1. *Disorder*: The name of the disorder, followed by an abbreviation and/or any alternative names by which the disorder is commonly known.

2. *Description*: A brief description of the overall characteristics of the disorder, based on *The Merck Manual, 16th edition,* and/or information found in the cited references.

3. *Etiology*: A review of what is known regarding the cause of the disorder, based on *The Merck Manual, 16th edition,* and/or information found in the cited references.

4. *Speech and Language Difficulties*: A listing of speech and language characteristics associated with the condition.

5. *Associated and Other Difficulties*: A listing of other symptoms and characteristics associated with the condition.

6. *Assessment*: Included in this section are specific assessment instruments mentioned in the literature, with the following exception: tests that are not readily available are excluded. This has led to the exclusion of a few old "standards" that are now out of print, as well as the exclusion of tests and assessment instruments that were mentioned by name in the literature but for which no clear reference or publisher could be located. Appendix H lists all tests mentioned in the text, in alphabetical order, with descriptive information and the name of the publisher. Addresses and phone numbers of publishers are provided in Appendix I. Due to frequent fluctuations, pricing information is not included. Appendix G lists specific references for those assessment instruments that are not commercially available. In addition to specific instruments, the assessment section lists general areas to be evaluated, based on the acknowledged areas of speech and language difficulty.

7. *Intervention Techniques*: Specific techniques mentioned in the literature are covered, as well as general intervention techniques based on the acknowledged areas of speech and language difficulty.

8. *Results of Recent Studies*: This section summarizes those studies that fall within the time frame covered in the book and have been read by at least one of the authors. Not included are the results of studies referred to by other authors. Readers are encouraged to consult the sources given at the end of each chapter for references to additional studies. Also, generally excluded from this section are studies that report on a single case.

9. *Prognosis*: Information on the prognosis for the condition as a whole is discussed in this section. Despite recent calls within the field for specific outcomes data regarding speech and language interventions, very little published information is currently available regarding therapy outcomes for specific conditions.

10. *References*: The final section is a list of the cited references. In addition, Appendix E provides a list of more general readings on the subject of augmentative and alternative communication (AAC) and on the assessment and treatment of dysphagia. In the time period covered by the material in this book, 1992 to 1998, the technique of facilitated communication was strongly advocated by some authorities within the field while being denounced by others. Appendix D provides a list of readings on the topic.

Chapter 1

Developmental Disorders

- Adult developmental disabilities
- Attention deficit disorder (ADD) and attention deficit hyperactivity disorder (ADHD)
- Central auditory processing disorders (CAPD)
- Cerebral palsy (CP)
- CHARGE association
- Child abuse and neglect
- Developmental apraxia of speech (DAS) and developmental verbal dyspraxia (DVD)
- Developmental language disorders (DLD) and developmental receptive language disorders (DRLD)
- Down syndrome (DS)
- Fetal alcohol syndrome (FAS)
- FG syndrome
- Landau-Kleffner syndrome (LKS) (acquired epileptic aphasia)
- Learning disabilities (LD)—adults
- Learning disabilities (LD)—children and adolescent
- Mental retardation (MR)—children and adolescents
- Prenatal cocaine exposure (PCE)
- Specific language impairment (SLI)

Adult Developmental Disabilities

DESCRIPTION

Federal legislation defines a developmental disability as "a severe, chronic disability of a person 5 years of age or older, which is attributable to a mental or physical impairment or combination of mental and physical impairments, and is manifested before the person attains age 22." It is likely to continue indefinitely and results in substantial functional limitations in three or more areas of major life activity: (1) self-care, (2) receptive and expressive language, (3) learning, (4) mobility, (5) self-direction, (6) capacity for independent living, and (7) economic self-sufficiency. It also reflects the person's need for "a combination and sequence of special, interdisciplinary, or generic care, treatment, or other services that are of lifelong or extended duration and are individually planned and coordinated." (Accardo and Whitman, 1996)

ETIOLOGY

(See Autism; Mental Retardation—Children and Adolescents; Cerebral Palsy)

SPEECH AND LANGUAGE DIFFICULTIES

- Use of pronouns "he" or "she" on first mention in a conversation without supplying a referent.
- Difficulty with pragmatics.
- Lack of strategies for repair of conversational breakdown.
- May be nonverbal.

(See also Autism; Mental Retardation—Children and Adolescents; Cerebral Palsy)

ASSOCIATED AND OTHER DIFFICULTIES

- Hearing and visual deficits are common.

(See also Autism; Mental Retardation—Children and Adolescents; Cerebral Palsy)

ASSESSMENT

- Rule hearing loss in or out.
- Be sure client does not understand or speak only a foreign language.
- Assess pragmatic skills in a variety of real-life situations applicable to each client.

(See also Autism; Mental Retardation—Children and Adolescents; Cerebral Palsy)

INTERVENTION TECHNIQUES

- NOTE: The use of facilitated communication to enhance the communication skills of persons with mental retardation and other developmental disabilities has been reported in the literature. The reader should be aware that use of this technique is controversial. References on the use of facilitated communication may be found in Appendix D.
- Create situations that empower clients to make choices for themselves. (Domingo, 1994)
- Work with clients in group settings. Address functional communication skills. (Trace, 1996)
- Help clients learn behavioral and language expectations in different settings, e.g., in a library, at a ballgame, and in a restaurant.
- Learn and then teach to clients the vocabulary and mores in any given setting.
- Establish communications books for clients.
- Enlist the aid of a co-worker in integrating a client into the milieu of a work setting.

RESULTS OF RECENT STUDIES

- When observed in two settings, the day-to-day activities of a day habilitation program and a less formal setting, adults with mental retardation evidenced somewhat more control of the speaking situation in the less formal setting. (Domingo, 1994)
- In one study of two severely disabled clients, interaction with co-workers increased with the introduction of communication books. (Storey and Provost, 1996)
- Mothers with mental retardation received home-based training in the areas of praising their child, providing imitation/expansion of the child's

utterances, and physical affection. Following the period of training, when compared with a control group, mothers in the training group showed significant increases in responsive and reinforcing interactions with their children. In addition, children from the targeted group showed significant increases in language development skills and spoke their first words significantly earlier. (Feldman, et al., 1993)

PROGNOSIS

(See Description above)

REFERENCES

Accardo PJ, BY Whitman. *Dictionary of Developmental Disabilities Terminology.* Baltimore: Paul H. Brookes Publishing Co. 1996:87.

Domingo R. The expression of pragmatic intentions in adults with mental retardation during instructional discourse. In: Bloom RL, LK Obler, S De Santi, JS Ehrlich, eds. *Discourse Analysis and Applications: Studies in Adult Clinical Populations.* Hillsdale, NJ: Lawrence Erlbaum Associates. 1994:111–30.

Feldman MA, B Sparks, L Case. Effectiveness of home-based early intervention on the language development of children of mothers with mental retardation. *Research in Developmental Disabilities.* 1993;14(5):387–408.

McLean LK, NC Brady, JE McLean. Reported communication abilities of individuals with severe mental retardation. *American Journal on Mental Retardation.* 1996;100(6):580–91.

Storey K, O Provost. The effect of communication skills instruction on the integration of workers with severe disabilities in supported employment settings. *Education and Training in Mental Retardation and Developmental Disabilities.* 1996;31(2):123–41.

Trace R. For adults with MR program is essential link to functional communication. *Advance for Speech-Language Pathologists & Audiologists.* 1996;6(6):6–7.

Zarrella S. Quality of life: improving social interactions in DD. *Advance for Speech-Language Pathologists & Audiologists.* 1995;5(11):4,38.

Attention Deficit Disorder (ADD) and Attention Deficit Hyperactivity Disorder (ADHD)

DESCRIPTION

A neurobiological disorder characterized by developmentally inappropriate levels of inattention, impulsivity, and, in some cases, hyperactivity. ADD may exist with or without hyperactivity. ADD affects 5% to 10% of school-aged children and is seen 10 times more frequently in males than in females. Onset is usually before the age of 4 years and nearly always before 7 years. Age of referral is generally between 8 and 10 years.

ETIOLOGY

Etiology is unknown. Theories of biochemical, sensory and motor, physiologic, and behavioral origin have been postulated. The condition is more prevalent among children of mothers who smoked or used drugs during their pregnancies.

SPEECH AND LANGUAGE DIFFICULTIES

- Poor oral motor skills, as evidenced by open-mouth posture and poor tongue control.
- Difficulty understanding when and how to use strategies, even when those strategies can be verbalized by the client.
- Difficulty understanding verbal, nonverbal, and situational cues.
- Difficulty understanding social roles.
- Poor sequencing skills.
- Difficulty maintaining topic of conversation.
- Poor pragmatic skills, including blurting out responses, difficulty attending to any information that is presented, interrupting others, difficulty with turn-taking, and difficulty with maintaining topics.
- Difficulty developing self-regulatory behavior and language.
- Difficulty organizing, planning, monitoring, and evaluating actions and responses.
- Inefficient problem-solving strategies and memory retrieval strategies.

ASSOCIATED AND OTHER DIFFICULTIES

- Inattention.
- Impulsivity.
- Hyperactivity.
- Restlessness.
- Distractibility.
- Difficulty following instructions.
- Difficulty sustaining attention.
- Difficulty playing or working quietly.
- Difficulty with turn-taking.
- Difficulty with organizational tasks.
- May talk excessively.
- May exhibit excessive motor activity.
- Interrupts others often.
- May exhibit motor incoordination.
- May exhibit perceptual-motor deficits.
- Difficulty with auditory and visual figure-ground perception.
- Difficulty with note-taking in school.
- Anxiety.
- Aggressiveness.
- Low tolerance for frustration.
- Low self-esteem.
- Difficulty learning appropriate social behavior.
- Demonstrates poor peer relationships.
- At risk for developing behavioral problems, such as oppositional defiant disorder.
- May exhibit learning difficulties, especially math and/or reading difficulties, although standardized tests may not document these difficulties. Between 50% and 80% exhibit some learning disabilities, including dyscalculia.
- Demonstrates inconsistent academic or work performance.
- Difficulty anticipating consequences or learning from mistakes.
- Demonstrates pervasive behaviors associated with ADHD; they are seen not only in school or work settings.

ASSESSMENT

- Be aware that scores on standardized language tests often do not reflect deficits common to this population.

- Be prepared to make adjustments: i.e., allow the student to choose where to sit in the testing area, allow for breaks, and be prepared for impulsive pointing responses. (Schoenbrodt and Smith, 1995)
- Administer the *Test of Language Development (Intermediate) Second Edition* (TOLD-I:2) or *Test of Language Development (Primary) Second Edition* (TOLD-P:2) and track the student's pattern of responses.
- Differentiate attention deficits from language and reading deficits. Administer *the Boston Naming Test* (BNT), the *Boston Diagnostic Aphasia Examination,* 2nd ed. (BDAE), the *Nelson Denny Reading Comprehension Test* and the *Gray Oral Reading Test-III* (GORT-III). (Scott, 1998)
- Assess functional abilities in home, school, and social settings.
- When assessing adults presenting as ADHD, establish a childhood onset from multiple sources such as parent report, school records, work histories, and careful questioning of the client. By definition, ADHD is not an adult-onset disorder.
- To aid in establishing ADHD, use the *Diagnostic and Statistical Manual of Mental Disorders*, 4th ed. (DSM-IV), criteria items and rate occurrence as rarely, sometimes, often, or very often.

INTERVENTION TECHNIQUES

- Particularly with younger children, employ multisensory techniques.
- Intervention should be geared at a level where the student can process the information, then gradually increase in complexity. (Norris and Hoffman, 1996)
- Work with school personnel to make accommodations in environment (modifying classroom arrangement, decreasing distractions), materials (high feedback materials, instructional prompts and cues), method of instruction (allow excess energy to be channeled), criteria and requirements (adjust task length commensurate with attention span, shorten homework assignments), and altered curriculum (focus on prerequisite skills and social skills). (Maag and Reid, 1996)
- Provide frequent repetition of rules and expectations.
- Help the student to feel empowered by focusing on meaningful tasks and on interaction strategies.
- Teach problem-solving skills, including identification of the problem, developing alternative strategies for solving a problem, evaluating consequences, and evaluating outcomes. (Schoenbrodt and Smith, 1995)
- Teach scripts for a variety of situations.

Diagnostic Criteria for Attention Deficit Hyperactivity Disorder

A. Either (1) or (2):

(1) Six (or more) of the following symptoms of **inattention** have persisted for at least 6 months to a degree that is maladaptive and inconsistent with developmental level:

Inattention
(a) often fails to give close attention to details or makes careless mistakes in schoolwork, work, or other activities
(b) often has difficulty sustaining attention in tasks or play activities
(c) often does not seem to listen when spoken to directly
(d) often does not follow through on instructions and fails to finish schoolwork, chores, or duties in the workplace (not due to oppositional behavior or failure to understand instructions)
(e) often has difficulty understanding tasks and activities
(f) often avoids, dislikes, or is reluctant to engage in activities that require sustained mental effort (such as schoolwork or homework)
(g) often loses things necessary for tasks or activities (e.g., toys, school assignments, pencils, books, or tools)
(h) is often easily distracted by extraneous stimuli
(i) is often forgetful in daily activities

(2) Six (or more) of the following symptoms of **hyperactivity–impulsivity** have persisted for at least 6 months to a degree that is maladaptive and inconsistent with developmental level:

Hyperactivity
(a) often fidgets with hands or feet or squirms in seat
(b) often leaves seat in classroom or in other situations in which remaining seated is expected
(c) often runs about or climbs excessively in situations in which it is inappropriate (in adolescents or adults, may be limited to subjective feelings of restlessness)

continues

(d) often has difficulty playing or engaging in leisure activities quietly

(e) is often "on the go" or often acts as if "driven by a motor"

(f) often talks excessively

Impulsivity

(g) often blurts out answers before questions have been completed

(h) often has difficulty awaiting turn

(i) often interrupts or intrudes on others (e.g., butts into conversations or games)

B. Some hyperactive-impulsive or inattentive symptoms that caused impairment were present before age 7 years.

C. Some impairment from the symptoms is present in two or more settings.

D. There must be clear evidence of clinically significant impairment in social, academic, or occupational functioning.

E. The symptoms do not occur exclusively during the course of a pervasive developmental disorder, schizophrenia, or other psychotic disorder and are not better accounted for by another mental disorder (e.g., mood disorder, anxiety disorder, dissociative disorder, or a personality disorder).

Source: Reprinted with permission from the *Diagnostic and Statistical Manual of Mental Disorders,* Fourth Edition. Copyright 1994 American Psychiatric Association.

- Address note-taking skills, test-taking skills, and study skills.
- Work with vocabulary needed in the classroom at any given time.
- Teach memory strategies.
- Help the client with organizational strategies, i.e., using calendars, "to do" lists, and filing systems to reduce clutter.
- Address pragmatic skills through role-playing.
- Encourage students to use tape recorders to tape class lectures and assignments.

- Provide oral motor therapy.
- Provide generous encouragement.
- Provide tangible reinforcements.

RESULTS OF RECENT STUDIES

- The handwriting of boys with ADHD who were taking Ritalin was compared with the handwriting of a group of normally developing boys. Frequent difficulties of the boys with ADHD, both on and off the medication, included inability to stay on the baseline, crossovers, mark-overs, confusion of uppercase and lowercase letters, disproportionate letter size, and inappropriate spacing within and between words. Ritalin had a positive effect on speed of writing and on individual letter formation, but not on overall organization and layout on the page. (Marmer, 1995)

PROGNOSIS

ADD and ADHD persist into adolescence and adulthood. Adjustment is often better in work situations than in academic environments, although instability in employment and lower job performance ratings often are noted. Adults with ADD and ADHD show increased likelihood for oppositional defiant behavior, conduct disorder, and substance use/abuse.

REFERENCES

Baker L, DP Cantwell. Attention deficit disorder and speech/language disorders. *Comprehensive Mental Health Care.* 1992;2(1):3–16.

Blum NJ, M Mercugilano. Attention deficit/hyperactivity disorder. In: Batshaw ML, ed. *Children with Disabilities,* 4th ed. Baltimore: Paul H. Brookes Publishing Co. 1997:449–70.

Czesak-Duffy BA. Oral-motor strategies benefit students with ADD. *Advance for Speech-Language Pathologists & Audiologists.* 1995;5(27):15.

Czesak-Duffy BA. Multisensory model for the primary ADD population. *Advance for Speech-Language Pathologists & Audiologists.* 1996;6(12):8.

Damico SK, MB Armstrong. Intervention strategies for students with ADHD: creating a holistic approach. *Seminars in Speech and Language.* 1996;17(1):21–35.

Gross-Tsur V, O Manor, RS Shalev. Developmental dyscalculia, gender, and the brain. *Archives of Disease in Childhood.* 1993;68:510–2.

Heyer JL. The responsibilities of speech-language pathologists toward children with ADHD. *Seminars in Speech and Language.* 1995;16(4):275–88.

Iskowitz M. Addressing all aspects of ADHD. *Advance for Speech-Language Pathologists & Audiologists.* 1997;7(33):4,9.

Maag JW, R Reid. Treatment of attention deficit hyperactivity disorder: a multi-modal model for schools. *Seminars in Speech and Language.* 1996;17(1):37–57.

Marmer L. Handwriting issues for students with ADHD. *Advance for Speech-Language Pathologists & Audiologists.* 1995;5(43):18.

Murphy K. Adults with attention deficit hyperactivity disorder: assessment and treatment considerations. *Seminars in Speech and Language.* 1996;17(3):245–53.

Norris JA, PR Hoffman. Attaining, sustaining, and focusing attention: intervention for children with ADHD. *Seminars in Speech and Language.* 1996;17(1):59–71.

Ricchini W. Promoting a positive self-image in children with ADHD. *Advance for Speech-Language Pathologists & Audiologists.* 1997;7(33):8.

Schoenbrodt L, RA Smith. *Communication Disorders and Interventions in Low Incidence Pediatric Populations.* San Diego, Calif.: Singular Publishing Co. 1995:19–40.

Scott A. Language and ADD. *Advance for Speech-Language Pathologists & Audiologists.* 1998;8(29):10–11.

Trace R. Making the connection between ADD and language learning and use. *Advance for Speech-Language Pathologists & Audiologists.* 1993;3(4):8–9,15.

Trace R. Managing attention deficits: changing perspectives on medication and behavior. *Advance for Speech-Language Pathologists & Audiologists.* 1996;6(12): 6–7.

Westby CE, SK Cutler. Language and ADHD: understanding the bases and treatment of self-regulatory deficits. *Topics in Language Disorders.* 1994;14(4):58–76.

Central Auditory Processing Disorders (CAPD)

DESCRIPTION

Deficits in the processing of audible signals that cannot be attributed to peripheral hearing loss or intellectual impairment. Adults may acquire CAPDs as a result of conditions such as cerebrovascular accident or multiple sclerosis.

ETIOLOGY

Specific etiology is unknown.

SPEECH AND LANGUAGE DIFFICULTIES

• Failure to babble or babble not evolving into more complex vocalizations.
• Reduced ability to attend selectively to auditory stimuli.
• Difficulty incorporating information received auditorially into language, memory, and learning functions.
• Responses to sound are inconsistent.
• Articulation deficits.
• Difficulty following directions.
• Difficulty with auditory decoding.
• Expressive language deficits.
• Cluttering.

ASSOCIATED AND OTHER DIFFICULTIES

• May have aversion to noise.
• Distractibility.
• Poor behavior in noisy situations.
• Difficulty with reading, spelling, or writing.
• Difficulty with sequencing tasks.
• Disorganization.
• Forgetfulness.
• Memory deficits.
• Inconsistent responses.
• CAPD may coexist with attention deficit hyperactivity disorder.

ASSESSMENT

• Work with interdisciplinary team, especially audiologists, in diagnosis of CAPD.
• Administer *Clinical Evaluation of Language Fundamentals, Revised* (CELF-R).
• Administer *Test of Nonverbal Intelligence* (TONI).
• Administer *Slosson Intelligence Test* (SIT).
• Administer Screening Test for Auditory Processing Disorders (SCAN) (ages 3-11 years) or Screening Test for Auditory Processing Disorders in Adolescents and Adults (SCAN-A) (ages 11-50 years).
• Assess listening and comprehension skills not only in testing environments but in real-life situations as well.

INTERVENTION TECHNIQUES

- Work with parents to develop home strategies, such as reducing background noise, maintaining eye contact when speaking with the child, and using short, simple directions.
- Work with parents to maintain a consistent schedule at home.
- Work with student on "how" to listen.
- Work with classroom teachers and audiologist to consider use of an assistive listening device (ALD) or an FM system.
- Work for consistencies throughout the child's school day, i.e., having all teachers give preferential seating, write out assignments, and review upcoming assignments at the end of the day.
- Provide consultation to classroom teachers. Assist teachers with strategies such as giving only one instruction at a time and using visual aids.
- Make the child part of the team in figuring out successful strategies.
- Work with the student on each of the following areas: attending behavior, awareness, identification, discrimination, memory, sequencing, directions, context, relevance, purpose, conceptualization, critical analysis, feedback, and appreciation. (Bacon, 1992)
- Work with the student on phonemic decoding skills.
- Consider use of cued speech. (Beck, 1998)
- Present material visually.
- Work on desensitization to noise by gradually combining background noise with listening to a story or to directions.
- Instruct the client to repeat instructions before beginning the task.

RESULTS OF RECENT STUDIES

- In a study of 136 persons diagnosed with chronic fatigue syndrome (CFS), 52% exhibited some central auditory dysfunction. Symptoms of vestibular dysfunction were found in 68% of those studied. (Trace, 1995)

PROGNOSIS

No statements regarding prognosis were found in the literature.

REFERENCES

Bacon SE. Speech-language management of central auditory processing disorders. In: Katz J, N Stecker, D Henderson, eds. *Central Auditory Processing: A Transdisciplinary View.* St. Louis, Mo: Mosby Year Book. 1992:199–204.

Beck PH. Sound approach. *Advance for Speech-Language Pathologists & Audiologists.* 1998;8(27):30–31.

Geffner D, J Lucker. Assessment and management of CAPD in ADD. *Advance for Speech-Language Pathologists & Audiologists.* 1994;4(1):5,42.

Gordon N, S Ward. Abnormal response to sound and central auditory processing disorder. *Developmental Medicine and Child Neurology.* 1994;37:645–52.

Harris DP. Central auditory processing disorders in children: are we listening? In: *Hearing Care for Children.* Boston: Allyn and Bacon. 1996:161–79.

Iskowitz M. Establishing link between language, CAPD by exclusion. *Advance for Speech-Language Pathologists & Audiologists.* 1996;6(46):10,19.

Iskowitz M. Strategies for children with CAPD at school and home. *Advance for Speech-Language Pathologists & Audiologists.* 1997;7(26):9.

Koay MET. Speech and speech disorders: implications for central auditory processing. In: Katz J, NA Stecker, D Henderson, eds. *Central Auditory Processing: A Transdisciplinary View.* St. Louis, Mo: Mosby Year Book. 1992:169–76.

Lecomte BJ. Strategies to improve listening skills in students. *Advance for Speech-Language Pathologists & Audiologists.* 1996;6(46):13,21.

Perez E, JR Slate, R Neeley, M McDaniel, T Baggs, K Layton. Validity of the CELF-R, TONI, and SIT for children referred for auditory processing problems. *Journal of Clinical Psychology.* 1995;51(4):540–43.

Riccio CA, GW Hynd, MJ Cohen, J Hall, L Molt. Comorbidity of central auditory processing disorder and attention deficit hyperactivity disorder. *Journal of the American Academy of Child and Adolescent Psychiatry.* 1994;33(6):849–57.

Trace R. Exploring connection between CFS and auditory dysfunction. *Advance for Speech-Language Pathologists & Audiologists.* 1995;5(21):3.

Zarrella S. Category system, test battery enhance diagnosis and management of CAPD. *Advance for Speech-Language Pathologists & Audiologists.* 1995;5(27):6–7.

Cerebral Palsy (CP)

DESCRIPTION

A term used to describe any of several motor disorders resulting from central nervous system (CNS) damage before, during, or immediately after birth. An umbrella term covering a group of nonprogressive, but often changing, motor impairment syndromes secondary to lesions or anomalies of the brain arising in the early stages of its development. Between 0.1% and 0.2% of all children have some form of CP, with the incidence rising to 1% of premature babies. A hallmark of CP is the inability to voluntarily control motor movements.

ETIOLOGY

Although a cause cannot always be determined, common causes include in utero disorders, neonatal jaundice, birth trauma, and neonatal asphyxia. Severe illness or CNS damage in early childhood, as from meningitis or severe dehydration, also may cause CP characteristics. Approximately 70% of those with CP have spastic involvement, characterized by underdevelopment of affected limbs, increased deep tendon reflexes, muscular hypertonicity, and a tendency to develop contractures. A "scissors gait" and toe-walking are characteristics of those with spastic cerebral palsy. Another 20% have athetoid involvement, characterized by slow, writhing, involuntary movements, as well as sudden, jerky movements that increase with emotional tension and attempts at purposeful movements. Dysarthria is generally present and may be severe. Ataxia accounts for 10% of cases of CP and is characterized by weakness, incoordination, and intention tremors. Mixed forms are common.

SPEECH AND LANGUAGE DIFFICULTIES

- Dysarthria.
- Poor overall oral motor skills.
- Difficulty coordinating respiration for speaking.
- Poor ability to control volume.
- Receptive and/or expressive language deficits may be present.
- May be unable to communicate verbally.

ASSOCIATED AND OTHER DIFFICULTIES

- Convulsive seizures occur in about 25% of cases, most often among those with spastic CP.
- Hearing impairment.
- Visual impairments, including retinopathy of prematurity, nystagmus, homonymous hemianopsia, and strabismus.
- Perceptual impairments.
- Mental retardation.
- Learning disabilities.
- Persistent primitive reflexes.
- Scoliosis.
- Short attention span.
- Hyperactivity.
- Dysphagia, often characterized by weak suck, tonic bite reflex, poor coordination of swallowing, hyperactive gag reflex, and tongue thrust.
- Oral sensory defensiveness.
- Deficits in visuospatial and visuoconstructive function among those with hemiplegia, regardless of the side of the lesion.
- Persons with severe CP may experience hypoxemia during oral intake.
- Deprivation of experience of a variety of foods and food textures, possibly resulting in praxic difficulties with oral motor planning.
- Deprivation of experience in developmental activities due to lack of opportunity or lack of motor ability.

ASSESSMENT

- Administer the *Oral Motor/Feeding Rating Scale.*
- Perform thorough oral motor evaluation, including examination of oral reflexes, respiratory function, oral postural control, control of oral secretions, and adequacy of swallow for nutrition.
- Evaluate chewing movements and jaw control for feeding.
- Obtain videofluoroscopic swallowing studies.
- Assess receptive and expressive language skills.
- Assess articulation skills and assess for dysarthria. (See Appendix A.)
- Administer the *Rehabilitation Institute of Chicago Functional Assessment Scale,* 4th ed. (RIC-FAS).
- If appropriate, assess for system of augmentative and alternative communication (AAC).

INTERVENTION TECHNIQES

- Use principles of neurodevelopmental treatment (NDT) to facilitate trunk alignment and support necessary for respiration and oral-motor development. (Zarrella, 1995)
- To prevent or reduce hypoxemia during oral intake, use careful feeding techniques combined with a careful selection of food textures. (Rogers, et al., 1993)
- Work with caregivers and with other team members to design and implement a comprehensive feeding program. Work to ensure proper rate of presentation, proper size of bite or amount of liquid, and proper consistency.
- In preschool settings, work with other disciplines to provide integrated therapy within the classroom. (Scott, 1998b)
- Be aware of the effects on development of poor or inadequate diet. Provide assistance in this area by systematically introducing clients to a variety of foods. (Scott, 1998a).
- Work on articulation skills, breath support and proper phrasing. Emphasize functional speech rather than focusing on drills.
- Work with client on evaluating critically the use of speech and the use of a system of AAC. If this is an issue, ask the client to speak in a variety of situations and evaluate listener's reactions. Help the client to understand and accept that use of a system of AAC does not imply failure.
- Develop systems of AAC.
- Work with classroom teachers to improve and enhance literacy skills. Be aware of common obstacles to literacy learning in this population, i.e., lack of teacher training in methods for promoting literacy in children with severe speech and physical impairments (SSPI), lack of teacher experience in teaching such students, time lost to equipment breakdowns, time lost to absence from classroom activities due to therapies, toileting, etc. (Koppenhaver and Yoder, 1993)
- Encourage full participation in family, school, social, and community activities.
- Be prepared for long-term therapy. However, know when to terminate therapy. Remember that articulation skills will probably never be "normal."
- Terminate therapy when communication skills are functional and additional progress is not being noted. Help the client as well as family members and others to accept this level of proficiency.

(See also Appendix C—Factors in Assessment for Augmentative and Alternative Communication [AAC])

RESULTS OF RECENT STUDIES

- When compared with normal controls and with a group of children with dysarthria secondary to Traumatic Brain Injury (TBI), those with CP performed less well than either of the other groups on all measures—maximum sound prolongation, range of pitch, and maximum repetition rate, indicating inadequate motor development, as well as inadequate control. (Wit, et al., 1994)

PROGNOSIS

CP is a lifelong condition. Although the actual damage to the brain is static and is not progressive, physiological and functional changes do occur over time. To date, a collected body of information regarding these changes is lacking. Statistics indicate that 10% of adults with CP are totally self-supporting; another 40% work in sheltered workshops or supported employment programs; 35% are able to be partially independent at home; and the remaining 15% are dependent on others. (Pellegrino, 1997)

Treatment goals should be aimed at maximizing independence.

REFERENCES

Carlsson G, P Uvebrant, K Hugdahl, J Arvidsson, L Wiklund, L von Wendt. Verbal and non-verbal function of children with right- versus left-hemiplegic cerebral palsy of pre- and perinatal origin. *Developmental Medicine & Child Neurology.* 1994;36(6):503–12.

Koppenhaver DA, DE Yoder. Classroom literacy instruction for children with severe speech and physical impairments (SSPI): what is and what might be. *Topics in Language Disorders.* 1993;13(2):1–15.

Letto M, JL Bedrosian, E Skarakis-Doyle. Application of Vygotskian developmental theory to language acquisition in a young child with cerebral palsy. *AAC: Augmentative and Alternative Communication.* 1994;10(3):51–60.

Murphy J, I Marková, S Collins, E Moodie. AAC systems: obstacles to effective use. *European Journal of Disorders of Communication.* 1996;31(1):31–44.

Murphy J, I Marková, E Moodie, J Scott, and S Boa. Augmentative and alternative communication systems used by people with cerebral palsy in Scotland: demographic survey. *AAC Augmentative and Alternative Communication.* 1995;11(1):26–36.

Mutch L, E Alberman, B Hagberg, K Kodama, MV Perat. Cerebral palsy epidemiology: where are we now and where are we going? *Developmental Medicine & Child Neurology*. 1992;34(6):547–51.

Pellegrino L. Cerebral palsy. In: Batshaw ML, ed. *Children with Disabilities, 4th Edition*. Baltimore: Paul H. Brookes Publishing Co. 1997:499–528.

Rogers B, M Msall, D Shucard. Hypoxemia during oral feedings in adults with dysphagia and severe neurological conditions. *Dysphagia*. 1993;8(1):43–48.

Scott A. Diet and development. *Advance for Speech-Language Pathologists & Audiologists*. 1998a;8(10):16–17.

Scott A. Integrated therapy: an effective classroom approach for children with severe or multiple disabilities. *Advance for Speech-Language Pathologists & Audiologists*. 1998b;8(10):6–9.

Sheppard JJ. Clinical evaluation and treatment. In: Rosenthal SR, JJ Sheppard, M Lotze, eds. *Dysphagia and the Child with Developmental Disabilities: Medical, Clinical, and Family Interventions*. San Diego, Calif: Singular Publishing Group. 1994:37–75.

Shoemaker A. Ensuring safe intake of food in children with CP. *Advance for Speech-Language Pathologists & Audiologists*. 1997;7(33):7,18.

Smith MM. Speech by any other name: the role of communication aids in interaction. *European Journal of Disorders of Communication*. 1994;29(3):225–40.

Wit J, B Maassen, FJM Gabreels, G Thoonen, et al. Traumatic versus perinatally acquired dysarthria: assessment by means of speech-like maximum performance tasks. *Developmental Medicine & Child Neurology*. 1994;36(3):221–9.

Zarrella S. NDT approach to feeding treats whole child. *Advance for Speech-Language Pathologists & Audiologists*. 1995;5(26):5.

CHARGE Association

DESCRIPTION

A rare disorder resulting from several defects in early fetal development. A minimum of four of the following characteristics must be present for the diagnosis: **c**oloboma of the eye, **h**eart defects, **a**tresia of the choanae, retardation of growth and development, **g**enital hypoplasia in males, **e**ar abnormalities and loss of hearing, and central nervous system abnormalities. The disorder is very rare; only about 200 persons in the United States are affected.

ETIOLOGY

Etiology is unknown. In some cases the disorder is transmitted as an autosomal-recessive trait. Recurrence of some of the abnormalities associated with the disorder have been observed within families.

SPEECH AND LANGUAGE DIFFICULTIES

- Delayed development of receptive and expressive language skills.

(See also Clefts of the Lip and Palate)

ASSOCIATED AND OTHER DIFFICULTIES

- 80% of those affected have cardiac abnormalities.
- Mental impairment and/or central nervous system abnormalities occur in 90% of cases.
- Mixed, progressive hearing loss.
- Cleft lip and palate.
- Feeding difficulties as a result of poor suck and velopharyngeal incompetence.
- Facial weakness and palsy.
- Cranial nerve dysfunctions.
- Tracheoesophageal atresia.
- Growth hormone deficiency.

ASSESSMENT

- Perform hearing screening and refer to audiologist as indicated.
- Assess oral motor skills for eating as well as for the development of speech.
- Perform complete evaluation for dysphagia.

INTERVENTION TECHNIQUES

- Assist parents in the development of oral-motor and feeding skills.

(See also Mental Retardation—Children and Adolescents; Clefts of the Lip and Palate; Hearing Loss—Children and Adolescents)

RESULTS OF RECENT STUDIES

• In a retrospective study, sensorineural hearing loss was present in 9 of 10 patients with facial palsy. Of those without facial nerve paralysis, 3 of 10 exhibited some sensorineural hearing loss. (Edwards, et al., 1995)

PROGNOSIS

A normal life span may be expected if heart problems and choanael atresia can be dealt with adequately.

REFERENCES

Byerly KM, RM Pauli. Cranial nerve abnormalities in CHARGE association. *American Journal of Medical Genetics.* 1993;45:751–7.

Edwards BM, LA Van Riper, PR Kileny. Clinical manifestations of CHARGE Association. *International Journal of Pediatric Otorhinolaryngology.* 1995;33:23–42.

Gilbert P. *The A-Z Reference Book of Syndromes and Inherited Disorders: A Manual for Health, Social and Education Workers.* New York: Chapman & Hall. 1993: 47–50.

Jones KL. *Smiths's Recognizable Patterns of Human Malformation*, 5th ed. Philadelphia: W.B. Saunders Co. 1997:668–70.

Thoene JG, NP Coker, eds. *Physicians' Guide to Rare Diseases.* New York: Dowden Publishing Co. 1995:30.

Child Abuse and Neglect

DESCRIPTION

Abuse and neglect are defined as physical injury, mental harm, sexual abuse, negligent treatment, or maltreatment of a child under age 18 years by a parent or other person responsible for the child's welfare. It is estimated that 1 in every 10 children has been abused or neglected. Approximately 25% of cases occur in children under age 2 years. Males and females are affected in equal numbers. More than 1.5 million children are affected annually. Approximately 70% to 75% of victims of abuse and neglect have some communication disorder. (Trace, 1992) It is expected that children subjected to physical abuse have experienced negative maternal communication and reduced rates of verbal stimulation.

ETIOLOGY

Abuse of children is the result of the breakdown of impulse control in the person responsible for the child's welfare. Factors that have been identified as often leading to abuse include:

1. Parental personality features, including a lack of affection and warmth received as a child.
2. A child who is irritable, demanding, or hyperactive or who has a disability.
3. Inadequate support for the parents.
4. A crisis and its resulting stress.

Neglect generally is seen in families experiencing multiple problems and with poorly organized lifestyles. Maternal depression is often a factor, along with drug or alcohol abuse by one or both parents and desertion by the father. Chronic medical problems of a parent also may be a contributing factor.

SPEECH AND LANGUAGE DIFFICULTIES

- Delayed development of language skills.
- Elective mutism.
- May develop communication anxieties based on the abusing relationship.
- Decreased requests for information.
- Increased use of redundancy and fillers.
- Lack of syntactic complexity.
- Limited expressive vocabulary.
- Difficulty with pragmatics.
- Difficulty using language to express feelings and needs.
- Inability to use abstract language.

- Difficulties at the level of discourse include paucity of information, lack of detail, and content that is often violent and destructive.

ASSOCIATED AND OTHER DIFFICULTIES
- Failure to thrive.
- Delayed development of social skills.
- Difficulty forming relationships with others.
- Irritability.
- Increased distractibility.
- Fearfulness.
- Insomnia.
- Functional dysphagia.
- May be overcompliant.
- Passive.

ASSESSMENT
- Observe for behaviors such as distractibility, withdrawal, limited ability to cope, and anger.
- Conduct in-depth assessment, including receptive and expressive vocabulary, syntax, abstract language, articulation, voice, and fluency.
- Use storytelling to assess narrative and discourse.
- Evaluate pragmatic skills and ability to interact with and make requests of others.
- Be aware that the child may be overly concerned about his or her performance and feedback from the evaluator.

INTERVENTION TECHNIQUES
- In preschool years, focus attention on improving interaction patterns between the child and the parents or other caregivers.
- Provide therapy to counteract limited stimulation, limited activity, and negativism.
- Advise teachers that seemingly oppositional behavior may in fact reflect a lack of adequate language skills.
- Teach language to convey emotion. Use role-playing.
- Address pragmatic skills and help the child learn appropriate ways of interacting with both peers and adults.

- To treat functional dysphagia, work with others in designing and implementing a multimodal approach including behavioral, family, and play therapy. (Atkins, et al., 1994)
- When presented with cases of elective mutism in children, suspect abuse or neglect and make appropriate referrals. (MacGregor, et al., 1994)

RESULTS OF RECENT STUDIES

- In one case of functional dysphagia, a prescription of alprazolam before meals produced rapid improvement when used in conjunction with behavioral, family, and play therapy. (Atkins, et al., 1994)
- In a study comparing adolescents who had been abused as young children with a group of adolescents who had not been abused, the following language characteristics were found: Those who had been abused used less self-related language, had a poorer level of syntax, and used somewhat more self-repetitions. Significant differences were not found between the two groups in vocabulary usage, language comprehension, or ability to offer minimal support. (McFadyen and Kitson, 1996)

PROGNOSIS

As many as 20% of physically abused children sustain permanent injuries, and about 1,200 deaths from abuse and neglect occur annually.

REFERENCES

Atkins DL, MS Lundy, AJ Pumariega. A multimodal approach to functional dysphagia. *Journal of the American Academy of Child & Adolescent Psychiatry.* 1994;33(7): 1012–6.

Katz KB. Communication problems in maltreated children: a tutorial. *Journal of Childhood Communication Disorders.* 1992;14(2):147–63.

MacGregor R, A Pullar, D Cundall. Silent at school—elective mutism and abuse. *Archives of Disease in Childhood.* 1994;70(6):540–1.

McFadyen RG, WJH Kitson. Language comprehension and expression among adolescents who have experienced childhood physical abuse. *Journal of Child Psychology & Psychiatry & Allied Disciplines.* 1996;37(5):551–62.

Schoenbrodt L, RA Smith. *Communication Disorders and Interventions in Low-Incidence Pediatric Populations.* San Diego, Calif: Singular Publishing Co. 1995:93–111.

Trace R. In search of the link between child abuse and communication disorders. *Advance for Speech-Language Pathologists & Audiologists.* 1992;2(16):7.

Developmental Apraxia of Speech (DAS) and Developmental Verbal Dyspraxia (DVD)

DESCRIPTION

Apraxia is the inability to execute purposeful learned acts, despite the willingness and the physical ability to do so.

ETIOLOGY

It is thought to be caused by a lesion in the neural pathways that retain memories of learned movement patterns.

SPEECH AND LANGUAGE DIFFICULTIES

- Audible or visual "groping" mannerisms while attempting to produce a target sound or word.
- Articulation error patterns typical of early speech development.
- Additional error patterns not typical of early speech development, such as difficulties with syllable structure, vocal tract coordination, and continuing difficulty with novel and complex utterances.
- Inconsistent errors.
- Substitutions are more common than distortions or omissions.
- May have more difficulty with consonant clusters than with individual consonant sounds.
- Vowel production errors.
- Voicing errors.
- Difficulty with phrasing.
- Difficulty varying intonation to convey meaning.
- Difficulty controlling volume levels of speech.
- May alternate between hyponasality and hypernasality.

- Long pauses, slow rate, and prolongations may be efforts to "buy time" rather than dysfluencies.
- Omission of grammatical morphemes; may persist and be evident in written expression in later years.
- Speech production abilities lag significantly behind comprehension abilities and nonverbal skills.
- Slow progress in therapy.
- Apraxia may coexist with dysarthria.

ASSOCIATION AND OTHER DIFFICULTIES

- May have underdeveloped play skills.
- Difficulty learning general rules about motor actions.
- Difficulty using perceptual cues.
- Difficulty organizing and using information from the senses.
- Difficulty with motor planning in other areas.
- Difficulty with problem solving.
- Difficulty analyzing task requirements.
- Low self-esteem may develop.

ASSESSMENT

- Exclude other possible diagnoses by confirming normal hearing, normal IQ and receptive language within normal limits, absence of muscle weakness, and absence of organic conditions.
- Assess, through caregivers' reports, early speech and language history. Indicators of DAS include poor coordination of sucking response, little or no babbling, excessive drooling, natural gesture system, evidence of frustration by age 2 years, and family members acting as interpreters. (Velleman and Strand, 1994)
- Refer for complete audiological assessment.
- Observe play skills and note difficulty with sequences of pretend play.
- Assess child's communication environment, i.e., communication behaviors of caregivers.
- Assess social behaviors of the child relative to communication.
- Assess ability to attend, remember, associate, discriminate, organize, reason, and problem-solve.
- For children with expressive vocabularies of 200 or more words, analyze both free speech samples and single-word utterances.

- Administer *Screening Test for Developmental Apraxia of Speech.*
- Administer *Developmental Articulatory Dyspraxia: A Diagnostic Procedure.*
- Administer *Bankson-Bernthal Test of Phonology* (BBTOP).
- Administer *Assessment Link Between Phonology and Articulation* (ALPHA).
- Administer *Phonological Assessment of Child Speech* (PACS).
- Administer *Procedures for the Phonological Analysis of Children's Language.*
- Administer *Natural Process Analysis* (NPA).
- Observe for increasingly distorted syllables and/or significant decrease in rate on tests of diadochokinetic rate.
- Assess spontaneous performance in less formal settings.
- If augmentative and alternative communication (AAC) is being considered, assess motor planning skills.

INTERVENTION TECHNIQUES

- Goal should be improvement of motor planning skills rather than drill on particular sounds or words.
- Assign meaning to syllable productions as soon as possible.
- Work toward imitation of sounds, words, and motor sequences, while realizing the child may be hesitant to attempt imitation activities.
- Avoid using a mirror, particularly in the early stages of therapy. (Blacklin and Crais, 1997)
- Work on several target phonemes simultaneously.
- Use cueing strategies, such as holding up one finger for each syllable. (Blacklin and Crais, 1997)
- Use melodic intonation therapy (MIT).
- Use pacing boards.
- With very young children, encourage a broader repertoire of sounds through play activities.
- Balance the goal of establishing a functional core vocabulary with that of addressing overall motor planning strategies.
- Use paired auditory and visual stimuli.
- Practice target sounds as many times as possible during a treatment session in different contexts.
- Decrease rate to allow for proprioceptive monitoring.

- Incorporate tactile-kinesthetic cues into therapy (Iskowitz, 1998).
- Schedule frequent therapy sessions.
- Consider a break from therapy for older children who have been receiving therapy for several years.
- Teach older children to advocate for needed accommodations, e.g., informing teachers of need for additional time to formulate verbal answers.
- Recognize that for some, normal or easy speech production may never be an achievable goal, and teach compensatory strategies.

RESULTS OF RECENT STUDIES

- Compared with a group of normally developing controls, children ages 5 through 7 years with DAS showed a marked inability to produce or to recognize rhyming words. (Marion, et al., 1993)
- Compared with a group of control subjects, children with DAS showed reduced tongue strength and reduced tongue-strength endurance on tests using objective instrumentation. (Murdoch, et al., 1995)

PROGNOSIS

While for some the speech disorder resolves over time with treatment, for others articulation difficulties remain despite maturation and treatment.

REFERENCES

Blacklin J, ER Crais. A treatment protocol for young children at risk for severe expressive output disorders. *Seminars in Speech and Language.* 1997;18(3):213–37.

Hodge MM. Assessment of children with developmental apraxia of speech: a rationale. *Clinics in Communication Disorders.* 1994;4(2):91–101.

Hodge MM, HR Hancock. Assessment of children with developmental apraxia of speech: a procedure. *Clinics in Communication Disorders.* 1994;4(2):102–18.

Iskowitz M. Enhancing treatment for severe speech disorders. *Advance for Speech-Language Pathologists & Audiologists.* 1998;8(12):24–26.

Marion MJ, HM Sussman, TP Marquardt. The perception and production of rhyme in normal and developmentally apraxic children. *Journal of Communication Disorders.* 1993;26:129–60.

McConnell NL. Integrated, multisensory approach to apraxia. *Advance for Speech-Language Pathologists & Audiologists.* 1995;5(4):9.

Murdoch BE, MD Attard, AE Ozanne, PD Stokes. Impaired tongue strength and endurance in developmental verbal dyspraxia: a physiological analysis. *European Journal of Disorders of Communication.* 1995;30:51–64.

Strand EA. Treatment of motor speech disorders in children. *Seminars in Speech and Language.* 1995;16(2):126–39.

Velleman SL, K Strand. Developmental verbal apraxia. In: Bernthal JE, NW Bankson, eds. *Child Phonology: Characteristics, Assessment, and Intervention with Special Populations.* New York: Thieme Medical Publishers, Inc. 1994:110–39.

Zarrella S. Managing apraxia: helping patients overcome frustration with functional communication. *Advance for Speech-Language Pathologists & Audiologists.* 1995;5(4): 12–13.

Developmental Language Disorders (DLD) and Developmental Receptive Language Disorders (DRLD)

DESCRIPTION

Failure to develop language in the absence of other common causes such as hearing impairment, mental impairment, motor impairment, or severe personality disorder.

ETIOLOGY

Etiology is unknown.

SPEECH AND LANGUAGE DIFFICULTIES

- Impaired verbal comprehension skills relative to nonverbal intellectual skills.
- Absence of words by age 18 months and absence of meaningful two-word phrases by age 2 years.
- Echolalia.
- Poor speech intelligibility.
- Word-finding difficulties.

- Requires frequent repetition of directions and may need gestures to follow directions.
- Executive function skills may be impaired.

ASSOCIATED AND OTHER DIFFICULTIES
- Tendency toward development of learning disabilities.
- Impaired short-term memory skills.
- Delayed development of play skills.
- Poor social interaction with peers.
- Poor school performance.

ASSESSMENT
- Assess receptive and expressive language skills in depth.
- Administer the *Neuro Psychological Investigation for Children* (NEPSY).
- Assess articulation skills and overall phonology.

INTERVENTION TECHNIQUES
- Encourage enrollment in an early intervention program and provide language development activities within the program.
- Work with parents, caregivers, and teachers to provide language development activities.

RESULTS OF RECENT STUDIES
- One proposed classification of DLD is as follows:
  1. Global Subtype—widespread deficiencies in both receptive and naming skills.
  2. Specific Dyspraxia Subtype—specific expressive phonological deficits without receptive deficits.
  3. Specific Comprehension Subtype—some impairment of comprehension of complex verbal instructions and/or concepts.
  4. Specific Dysnomia Subtype—specific impairments in name retrieval. (Korkman and Häkkinen-Rihu, 1994)
- In a study of short-term memory for tone sequences, adolescents and young adults with DRLD exhibited deficits that were not exhibited by a similar group diagnosed with autism. (Lincoln, et al., 1992)

• In a study of the development of executive function in school-aged children, those with DLD performed better than those with ADHD on only one task—mazes. On other executive tasks, i.e., visual search, verbal fluency, abstract reasoning, and flexibility of thought, results differentiated those with ADHD from normal controls but did not differentiate those with ADHD from those with DLD.

PROGNOSIS

No statements regarding prognosis were found in the literature.

REFERENCES

Korkman M, P Häkkinen-Rihu. A new classification of developmental language disorders (DLD). *Brain and Language.* 1994;47:96–116.

Lincoln AJ, P Dickstein, E Courchesne, R Elmasian, P Tallal. Auditory processing abilities in non-retarded adolescents and young adults with developmental language disorder and autism. *Brain and Language.* 1992;43:613–22.

Roncagliolo M, J Benitez, M Pérez. Auditory brainstem responses of children with Developmental Language Disorders. *Developmental Medicine and Child Neurology.* 1994; 36:26–33.

Weyandt LL, WG Willis. Executive functions in school-aged children: potential efficacy of tasks in discriminating clinical groups. *Developmental Neuropsychology.* 1994;10(1): 27–38.

Willig S. General indicators of developmental language disorders. (Let's Talk, No. 70, Developmental Language Disorders.) *ASHA* (Summer). 1998:43–44.

Down Syndrome (DS)

DESCRIPTION

DS is the most common cause of mental retardation. Overall incidence is 1 in 700 live births, with incidence rising significantly in infants born to mothers over age 40 years. Among this group incidence is 1 in 40.

ETIOLOGY

Three types of chromosomal abnormalities cause DS. The most common is trisomy 21, which accounts for 95% of cases. Translocation Down syndrome, accounting for 4% of cases, is caused by the attachment of the long arm of an extra number 21 chromosome to chromosome number 14, number 21, or number 22. Mosaic trisomy, accounting for 1% of cases, involves some but not all cells having the defect. (Roizen, 1997)

SPEECH AND LANGUAGE DIFFICULTIES

- Large protruding tongue and open mouth.
- High, narrow palatal vault.
- Diminished control of tongue and lip movements.
- Articulation deficits. Many of the articulation errors of adolescents and adults with DS are similar to errors made by normally developing children at 2 or 3 years of age.
- Articulation errors may be inconsistent.
- Articulation errors may persist partially because differing productions are accepted as long as meaning is understood. (Dodd, et al., 1994)
- Communication skills are generally below overall projected cognitive ability.
- Receptive language skills are often disproportionally better than expressive skills.
- Plateau of language skills at approximately 3-year-old level.

ASSOCIATED AND OTHER DIFFICULTIES

- Hypotonicity.
- Delayed physical and mental development.
- Congenital heart disease is present in about 35% of cases.
- Congenital hypothyroidism may occur.
- Visual impairments, including strabismus, nystagmus, blepharitis (inflammation of the eyelids), tear duct obstruction, and ptosis.
- Hearing loss is prevalent.
- Approximately 75% of children have otitis media.
- Sensory impairments show an increase with increasing age.
- Sleep apnea may occur.
- Tendency toward obesity beginning in later childhood.

- Hip dislocation.
- Flat feet.
- Instability of patella.
- Periodontal disease, involving gingivitis and loss of alveolar bone. Loss occurs early and progresses rapidly.
- Malocclusions.
- Dental anomalies, including missing teeth, microdontia, and fused teeth.
- Seizures may occur.
- Deterioration of cognitive skills during adolescence may indicate unrecognized hypothyroidism.

ASSESSMENT

- Children as well as adults should be referred to an audiologist to determine any hearing loss.
- Administer language-development scales, such as the *Hawaii Early Learning Profile.*
- Assess early language and vocabulary development annually using the *MacArthur Communicative Development Inventories* (CDI).

INTERVENTION TECHNIQUES

- Be aware that insertion of tympanotomy tubes may not always lead to resumption of normal levels of hearing. (See Selikowitz, 1993, under Results of Recent Studies below)
- To facilitate oral-motor development and prevent tongue protrusion, have infant feed from a position in which the ears are higher than the mouth. Present nipple below the mouth, facilitating tongue retraction and development of stronger suckle. (Rosenfeld-Johnson, 1997)
- Be aware of the effects on development of poor or inadequate diet. Provide assistance in this area by systematically introducing clients to a variety of foods. (Scott, 1998a).
- To maximize auditory skills, and subsequent language development, consider a strong auditory therapy program, without sign language, during the first year of life. (Pappas, et al., 1994)
- Be aware of the complexity of factors affecting articulation development in this population—i.e., hypotonicity, difficulty with motor coordina-

tion, sequencing, and timing. Address each of these areas and be aware that improved articulation proficiency may continue beyond the normal age expectations. (Kumin, et al., 1994)

- With young children, make therapy play-based and use total communication.
- Incorporate into therapy everyday routines used at home.
- Caregivers may be trained to provide modeling and feedback to their child in the area of phonological development. (Dodd, et al., 1994)
- Consider early use of augmentative and alternative communication (AAC).
- Recognize that early use of AAC may foster development of natural speech. (Scott, 1998b)
- Inform caregivers that receptive language skills may decline in persons over age 40 years.

RESULTS OF RECENT STUDIES

- Twenty-four children with DS between the ages of 6 and 15 years, and a control group of 21 normally developing children, underwent bilateral myringotomies. When tested 6 to 9 weeks following surgery, 40% of ears in the DS group continued to have hearing loss compared with 9% of ears in the control group. (Selikowitz, 1993)
- Young children with DS (ages 21 to 47 months) are observed to make use of both declarative/referential and imperative/instrumental pointing in much the same ways as do normally developing children at a younger chronological age. Children with DS make even greater use of visual checking with the communicative partner than do normally developing children. (Franco and Wishart, 1995)
- In a study of language structure and complexity, adolescents with DS were matched with normally developing children with similar mean length of utterances (MLUs). Chronological age of the normally developing children was 30 to 32 months. Results showed few differences in expressive language structure and complexity between the two groups. (Fowler, et al., 1994)
- In a study comparing adults with DS with a group of adults with mental retardation of unknown origin, significant differences were found in the ability to use auxiliary verbs. Those with DS performed significantly

worse on 7 of 10 items probing the use of auxiliary verbs. (Sabsay and Kernan, 1993)

- In a study of the use of sign language by young children with DS, more than twice as many words were signed as spoken at 17 months; by 26 months, spoken vocabularies increased dramatically and sign vocabulary size remained about the same. For the most part, oral vocabularies and signed vocabularies were made up of different words. (Miller, 1992)
- Studies have shown that for persons over age 40 years, there is a decline in receptive skills, while levels of expressive skills are maintained. (Cooper and Collacott, 1995)

PROGNOSIS

Those with heart disease have a decreased life expectancy. There is some susceptibility to acute leukemia. Those without heart disease survive to adulthood, but the aging process is accelerated. Evidence of dementia is common in adults after age 40 years. Currently, 70% of persons with DS survive beyond the age of 30 years.

REFERENCES

Cooper SA, Collacott RA. The effect of age on language in people with Down's syndrome. *Journal of Intellectual Disability Research.* 1995;39(Pt. 3):197–200.

Dodd B, P McCormack, G Woodyatt. Evaluation of an intervention program: relation between children's phonology and parents' communicative behavior. *American Journal on Mental Retardation.* 1994;98(5):632–45.

Fowler AE, R Gelman, LR Gleitman. The course of language learning in children with Down syndrome. In: Tager-Flusberg H, ed. *Constraints on Language Acquisition: Studies of Atypical Children.* Hillsdale, NJ: Lawrence Erblaum Associates. 1994:91–140.

Franco F, JG Wishart. Use of pointing and other gestures by young children with Down syndrome. *American Journal on Mental Retardation.* 1995;100(2):160–82.

Kumin L, C Councill, M Goodman. A longitudinal study of the emergence of phonemes in children with Down syndrome. *Journal of Communication Disorders.* 1994;27(4):293–303.

Kumin L, C Councill, M Goodman, D Chapman. Down syndrome: comprehensive intervention for children. *Advance for Speech-Language Pathologists & Audiologists.* 1996;6(40):4–9.

Messer DJ. *The Development of Communication: From Social Interaction to Language.* New York: John Wiley & Sons. 1994:265–73.

Miller JF. Development of speech and language in children with Down syndrome. In: Lott IT, EE McCoy, eds. *Down Syndrome: Advances in Medical Care.* New York: Wiley-Liss. 1992:39–50.

Pappas DG, C Flexer, L Shackelford. Otological and habilitative management of children with Down syndrome. *Laryngoscope.* 1994;104(9):1065–70.

Roizen NJ. Down syndrome. In: Batshaw ML, ed. *Children with Disabilities,* 4th ed. Baltimore: Paul H. Brookes Publishing Co. 1997:361–76.

Rosenfeld-Johnson S, D Manning. Preventing oral-motor problems in Down Syndrome. *Advance for Speech-Language Pathologists & Audiologists.* 1997;7(31):20.

Sabsay S, KT Kernan. On the nature of language impairment in Down syndrome. *Topics in Language Disorders.* 1993;13(3):20–35.

Scott A. Diet and development. *Advance for Speech-Language Pathologists & Audiologists.* 1998a;8(10):16–17.

Scott A. Improving natural speech. *Advance for Speech-Language Pathologists & Audiologists.* 1998b;8(7):9.

Scott GS, TL Layton. Epidemiologic principles in studies of infectious disease outcomes: pediatric HIV as a model. *Journal of Communication Disorders.* 1997;30:303–24.

Selikowitz M. Short-term efficacy of tympanotomy tubes for secretory otitis media in children with Down syndrome. *Developmental Medicine and Child Neurology.* 1993;35(6): 511–5.

Van Borsel J. Articulation in Down's syndrome adolescents and adults. *European Journal of Disorders of Communication.* 1996;31(4):415–44.

van Schrojenstein Lantman-de Valk HMJ, MJ Haveman, MA Maaskant, AGH Kessels, HFJ Urlings, F Sturmans. The need for assessment of sensory functioning in ageing people with mental handicap. *Journal of Intellectual Disability Research.* 1994;38(Pt. 3):289–98.

Fetal Alcohol Syndrome (FAS)

DESCRIPTION

FAS affects about 1 in 750 live births and is the leading cause of mental retardation in the United States. Each year, 10,000 new cases are reported. Characteristics include smaller-than-normal length, low birthweight, microcephaly, failure to thrive, in addition to mental retardation. Incidence is higher among Native Americans and Alaskan Americans.

ETIOLOGY

The most common cause of FAS is maternal use of alcohol during pregnancy.

SPEECH AND LANGUAGE DIFFICULTIES

- May have cleft lip and/or cleft palate. (See Clefts of the Lip and Palate)
- Delayed speech development and receptive and expressive language development.
- Articulation deficits.
- May exhibit fluency disorder.
- May exhibit breathiness, hoarseness, increased or decreased intensity, or monotone voice quality.
- Difficulty with syntactically and semantically complex sentences.
- Difficulty understanding abstract concepts.
- Difficulty understanding cause and effect.
- Difficulty with pragmatics, i.e., turn-taking rules generally are respected, but content of responses is inappropriate to the topic.

ASSOCIATED AND OTHER DIFFICULTIES

- Central nervous system (CNS) dysfunction.
- Mental retardation may be severe.
- Weak sucking ability and other feeding difficulties in infants.
- High incidence of middle ear disease and sensorineural hearing loss.
- High incidence of chronic otitis media.
- Short stature.
- Cardiac defects.
- Kidney defects.
- Club foot.
- Hip dislocation.
- Joint contractures.
- Dental malalignment and malocclusions.

- Eustachian tube dysfunction.
- Irritability in infancy.
- Hyperactivity in childhood.
- Impulsivity.
- Restlessness.
- Frequent temper tantrums.
- Attention disorders.
- Learning deficits.
- Memory deficits.
- Poor judgment skills.
- Academic performance may deteriorate in later grades as demands increase and become more complex.
- Poor eye-hand coordination.
- Difficulty recognizing social cues.
- Overly friendly.
- Excessive demands for affection and physical contact.
- May exhibit fearlessness.

ASSESSMENT

- Assess for hearing loss and refer to audiologist as appropriate.
- Administer *Test of Language Development (TOLD)*.
- Assess articulation skills and oral-motor skills.
- Assess pragmatic skills in a variety of settings.

INTERVENTION TECHNIQUES

- Provide direct therapy to address receptive, expressive, and pragmatic deficits.
- Assist caregivers and others in providing structure in a child's environment.
- Focus intervention on development of pragmatic and social skills. Work on language needed in specific situations.
- Address pragmatics through role-playing in a group setting.

(See Clefts of the Lip and Palate)

RESULTS OF RECENT STUDIES

No recent studies regarding communication skills were found in the literature.

PROGNOSIS

No statement of prognosis was found in the literature.

REFERENCES

Abkarian G. Communication effects of prenatal alcohol exposure. *Journal of Communication Disorders.* 1992;25:21–240.

Researchers link OM to both FAS and PRSP. *Advance for Speech-Language Pathologists & Audiologists.* 1997;7(40):17.

Gelman J. Study reveals hearing disorders in children with FAS. *Advance for Speech-Language Pathologists & Audiologists.* 1995;5(41):11.

Jones KL. *Smiths's Recognizable Patterns of Human Malformation,* 5th ed. Philadelphia: W.B. Saunders Co. 1997:555–8.

Maxwell LA, J Geschwint-Rabin. Substance abuse risk factors and childhood language disorders. In: Smith MD, JS Damico, eds. *Childhood Language Disorders.* New York: Thieme Medical Publishers, Inc. 1996:255-71.

Thoene JG, NP Coker, eds. *Physicians' Guide to Rare Diseases.* New York: Dowden Publishing Co. 1995:67.

Trace R. Fetal alcohol syndrome: better surveillance needed to enhance treatment and education programs. *Advance for Speech-Language Pathologists & Audiologists.* 1993; 3(13):10-11.

FG Syndrome

DESCRIPTION

A rare disorder. Only males are affected.

ETIOLOGY

An X-linked recessive inherited disorder.

SPEECH AND LANGUAGE DIFFICULTIES

- May have cleft lip/cleft palate.
- May have high-pitched voice.

ASSOCIATED AND OTHER DIFFICULTIES

- Seizures.
- Impaired intellectual development.
- Delayed motor development.
- May have sensorineural hearing loss.
- Hypotonia.
- Strabismus.
- Hyperactive.
- Short attention span.
- Short stature.
- Postnatal onset of macrocephaly.
- Multiple joint contractures.
- Cardiac anomalies.
- Gastrointestinal abnormalities.
- Generally affable, but with frequent tantrums when frustrated.

ASSESSMENT

- Perform hearing screening and refer to audiologist as indicated.
- Administer *Birth to Three Screening Test of Learning and Language Development.*
- Administer *Preschool Language Scale–3* (PLS-3).
- Assess articulation skills.
- Assess oral–motor skills.

INTERVENTION TECHNIQUES

- Provide suggestions to parents and other team members on ways to maximize communication skills.

(See also Clefts of the Lip and Palate)
(See also Hearing Loss—Children and Adolescents)

RESULTS OF RECENT STUDIES

No recent studies regarding communication skills were found in the literature.

PROGNOSIS

Death occurs prior to 2 years of age in a third of the cases. Those who survive early childhood have a normal life expectancy. Survivors generally have affable personalities with adequate social adjustment despite severe intellectual impairment.

REFERENCES

Jones KL. *Smith's Recognizable Patterns of Human Malformation,* 5th ed. Philadelphia: W.B. Saunders Co. 1997:280.

McCardle P, B Wilson. Language and development in FG syndrome with callosal agenesis. *Journal of Communication Disorders.* 1993;26:83–100.

Thoene JG, NP Coker, eds. *Physicians' Guide to Rare Diseases.* New York: Dowden Publishing Co. 1995:69–70.

Landau-Kleffner Syndrome (LKS) (Acquired Epileptic Aphasia)

DESCRIPTION

"An acquired aphasia in association with an abnormal electroencephalograph (EEG) demonstrating spikes, sharp waves, or spike-and-wave discharges that are usually bilateral and occur predominantly over the temporal and parietal regions." (Tuchman, 1994) Up to 25% of affected persons may not have seizures. Males are twice as likely as females to be affected. The syndrome is characterized by deterioration in previously normally developing receptive and expressive language skills. Nonlinguistic cognitive abilities generally remain intact. Symptoms generally appear between the ages of 3 and 8 years.

ETIOLOGY

Etiology is uncertain. In all cases, EEGs are abnormal and resemble those of persons with epilepsy. EEGs show "continuous spike-wave discharge in slow wave sleep" (CSWS).

SPEECH AND LANGUAGE DIFFICULTIES

- Gradual or rapid onset of aphasia in a previously normally developing child. (Mouridsen, 1995)
- Perseveration of words or phrases.
- Paraphasias.
- Neologisms.
- Disorders of syntax.
- May experience auditory agnosia.
- Deficits in both receptive and expressive language skills.
- Deficits in expressive skills may begin as misarticulations and progress to decreased length of sentences and decreased overall verbal expression.
- May become mute.
- Poor social communication skills.
- Language skills may fluctuate over the course of the illness.
- Previously acquired written language skills may be preserved.
- Reading comprehension is generally superior to verbal comprehension.
- Orofacial apraxia.

ASSOCIATED AND OTHER DIFFICULTIES

- 75% experience seizures that may subside before adulthood.
- Deficits in auditory comprehension may suggest peripheral hearing loss, but auditory evoked potential testing reveals normal peripheral hearing.
- Hyperkinesis.
- Outbursts of rage.
- Aggressiveness.
- Attention deficits.
- Distractibility.
- Movement disorders, such as dystonia or apraxia.

ASSESSMENT

- Obtain a thorough history of early speech and language development, as evidence indicates that speech and language development prior to onset of first symptoms may not be completely normal. (Soprano, et al., 1994)
- Assess language skills with instruments such as the *Peabody Picture Vocabulary Test-Revised* (PPVT-R) and the *Test for Auditory Comprehension of Language-Revised* (TACL-R).

INTERVENTION TECHNIQUES

- Consider use of an FM system.
- Consider use of total communication.

RESULTS OF RECENT STUDIES

- Periods of relapse in language skills may coincide with periods of increased EEG abnormalities, particularly in the temporal region. (Lanzi, et al., 1994)
- Surgery to eliminate epileptogenic discharge from the perisylvian region in one hemisphere resulted in reacquisition of speech in 11 of 14 children. (Morrell, et al., 1995)

PROGNOSIS

Outcomes are variable, but for many of those affected, severe language disorders persist. The earlier the age of onset, the worse the prognosis is for recovering language.

REFERENCES

Ballaban-Gil K. Language disorders and epilepsy. In: Pedley TA, BS Meldrum, eds. *Recent Advances in Epilepsy*. New York: Churchill Livingstone. 1995:205–8.

Eslava-Cobos J, L Mejia. Landau-Kleffner syndrome: much more than aphasia and epilepsy. *Brain and Language*. 1997;57:215–24.

Lanzi G, P Veggiotti, S Conte, E Partesana, C Resi. A correlated fluctuation of language and EEG abnormalities in a case of the Landau-Kleffner syndrome. *Brain & Development*. 1994;16(4):329–44.

Morrell F, WW Whisler, MC Smith, TJ Hoeppner, L de Toledo-Morrell, SJC Pierre-Louis, AM Kanner, JM Buelow, R Rostamovic, D Bergen, M Chez, H Hasegawa. Landau-Kleffner syndrome: treatment with subpial intracortical transection. *Brain.* 1995;118: 1529–46.

Mouridsen SE. The Landau-Kleffner syndrome: a review. *European Child and Adolescent Psychiatry.* 1995;4(4):223–8.

Soprano AM, EF Garcia, R Caraballo, N Fejerman. Acquired epileptic aphasia: neuropsychologic follow-up of 12 patients. *Pediatric Neurology.* 1994;11(3):230–4.

Tharpe AM, BJ Olson. Landau-Kleffner syndrome: acquired epileptic-aphasia in children. *Journal of the American Academy of Audiology.* 1994;5:146–50.

Thoene JG, NP Coker, eds. *Physicians' Guide to Rare Diseases.* New York: Dowden Publishing Co. 1995:321.

Tuchman RF. Epilepsy, language, and behavior: clinical models in childhood. *Journal of Child Neurology.* 1994;9(1):95–102.

Learning Disabilities (LD)—Adults

DESCRIPTION
(See Learning Disabilities—Children and Adolescents)

ETIOLOGY
(See Learning Disabilities—Children and Adolescents)

SPEECH AND LANGUAGE DIFFICULTIES
- Ongoing difficulties in word recognition, reading comprehension, and written composition.
- Difficulty with phonemic decoding.
- Word-finding difficulties.
- Difficulty writing complex factual material.
- Syntax errors and reduced syntactic complexity.
- Difficulties with organization of oral text.
- Difficulty with abstract concepts.

ASSOCIATED AND OTHER DIFFICULTIES

- Poor self-concept.
- Low self-esteem.
- Difficulty with social acceptance and adjustment.
- Attention deficits.
- Decreased reading efficiency.
- Difficulty retaining information that is read.
- Deficits in conceptual thinking and problem-solving.
- Difficulty with generalization.
- Difficulty integrating previously learned material into new situations.
- Inconsistency in performance.

ASSESSMENT

- Assessment should be geared to the concerns and goals of the individual.
- Assessment should be transdisciplinary and include a neuropsychologist, a vocational specialist, and an adult learning specialist.
- Assess in a variety of settings and contexts: comprehension of oral and written language; semantics, production, and formulation; pragmatics; executive function; and self-regulation. (Kleinman and Bashir, 1996)
- Administer the Word Attack subtest from the *Woodcock Reading Mastery Test, Revised.*
- Assess spelling skills.

INTERVENTION TECHNIQUES

- Help clients develop improved organizational skills.
- Use multisensory approach to address weak areas.
- Address deficits in pragmatic skills.

(See also Learning Disabilities—Children and Adolescents)

RESULTS OF RECENT STUDIES

- When compared with learning disabled (LD) adolescents in another study, adults with LD exhibited fewer deficits in storytelling discourse. When compared with non-LD adults, those with LD produced stories of overall shorter length, with shorter episode lengths, and use of less sophisticated linguistic markers connecting episodes. (Roth and Spekman, 1994)

PROGNOSIS

Most adults with isolated learning disabilities are able to gain the academic skills necessary for everyday functioning. (Church, et al., 1997)

REFERENCES

Church RP, MEB Lewis, ML Batshaw. Learning disabilities. In: Batshaw ML, ed. *Children with Disabilities,* 4th ed. Baltimore: Paul H. Brookes Publishing Co. 1997:471–97.

Crane R. Improving self-esteem, skills of adult dyslexics. *Advance for Speech-Pathologists & Audiologists.* 1996;6(46):5,24.

Kleinman SN, AS Bashir. Adults with language-learning disabilities: new challenges and changing perspectives. *Seminars in Speech and Language.* 1996;17(3):201–15.

Roth FP, NJ Spekman. Oral story production in adults with learning disabilities. *Discourse Analysis and Applications: Studies in Adult Clinical Populations.* Hillsdale, NJ: Lawrence Erlbaum Associates. 1994:131–47.

Learning Disabilities (LD)—Children and Adolescents

DESCRIPTION

The definition of LD is established by federal law as part of the "Education of All Handicapped Children Act" (Public Law 94-192) and states the following: "Specific learning disabilities mean a disorder in the psychological processes involved in understanding or using language, spoken or written, which may manifest in an imperfect ability to listen, think, speak, read, write, spell, or do mathematical calculation. Exclusion from this group is based upon organic deficits including visual, hearing, motor handicap, retardation, emotion disturbance, or environmental, cultural, or economic disadvantage." (Welsh, et al., 1996)

The National Joint Committee on Learning Disabilities has proposed the following amended definition: "Learning disability is a generic term that refers to a heterogeneous group of disorders manifested by significant difficulties in the acquisition and use of listening, speaking, reading, writing, reasoning, or mathematical abilities. These disorders are intrinsic to the individual and are presumed to be due to a dysfunction of the central nervous system. Even though a learning disability may occur concomitantly with other disabling conditions (e.g., sensory impairment, mental retardation, social and emotional disturbance) or environmental influences (e.g., cultural differences, insufficient/inappropriate instruction), it is not the direct result of those conditions or influences." (Hammill, 1990, reported in Church, et al., 1997)

Prevalence is estimated at 4% to 5% of school-aged children. Groups at risk for learning disabilities include children who are born prematurely, those with childhood cancer, those with metabolic disorders, and those with a history of otitis media.

ETIOLOGY

Magnetic resonance imaging (MRI) studies have shown that in most individuals, the temporal bank within the planum is longer than the parietal bank in both hemispheres. In individuals with dyslexia, the temporal bank is longer on the left while the parietal bank is longer on the right. (Advance, 1992)

Recent research suggests that in persons with LD, the left nucleus of the thalamus may have fewer of the large neurons that help process rapid sounds. (Trace, 1994)

SPEECH AND LANGUAGE DIFFICULTIES

- Central auditory processing disorder also may be present.
- Difficulty following directions.
- Difficulty with phonological processing.
- Difficulty understanding and generating rhyme.
- Difficulty articulating multisyllable words.
- Difficulty with pragmatic skills.
- Difficulty understanding abstract concepts.
- Difficulty processing auditory and/or visual material.
- Slowed rate of vocabulary and concepts acquisition.
- Difficulty understanding multiple meanings of words.
- Difficulty understanding jokes and humor. This may lead to inappropriate, hostile responses.

ASSOCIATED AND OTHER DIFFICULTIES

- May coexist with attention deficit hyperactivity disorder (ADD or ADHD).
- Dysgraphia may be present and may take one of several forms: for example, oral spelling may or may not be preserved, and the ability to copy written text may vary depending on type of dysgraphia. Types of dysgraphia include dyslexic dysgraphia, dysgraphia due to motor clumsiness, and dysgraphia due to defect in understanding of space. (Deuel, 1995)
- Difficulty sustaining attention, particularly in an environment with competing noise.
- Impulsive.
- Impairments in executive function, i.e., the ability to inhibit or defer a response, formulate a strategic, sequential plan of action, and store information in memory for future use. (Church, et al., 1997)
- May be socially isolated.
- Poor self-esteem.
- Depression.
- Conduct disorder.
- Chronic frustration/anxiety.
- Learned helplessness—a learned inability to make one's own decisions or to employ strategies, stemming from long-term reliance on others.

ASSESSMENT

- Administer *California Verbal Learning Test—Children's Version.*
- Administer the *Clinical Evaluation of Language Fundamentals, Revised* (CELF-R).
- Evaluate overall language skills and pragmatic skills in real-life environments of the student.
- Evaluate narrative and expository writing skills by evaluating students' work produced for classroom assignments.
- To evaluate a child's use of language to communicate in the contexts of play, reading, graphics, exploration, and classroom schema, use the *Functional Outcome Measures for LLD Children.* (Iskowitz, 1998b)
- Evaluate organization and planning skills.
- Become familiar with the expectations of any given classroom teacher, and evaluate a student's work against those expectations.

INTERVENTION TECHNIQUES

- Don't assume that young children know what books are for or how to handle them. Introduce children to books and the library, and show parents how to engage their children with picture books. (Iskowitz, 1998a)
- Work in collaboration with classroom teachers and special educators. Design services around classroom needs rather than pull-out therapy.
- Work in collaboration with classroom teachers to establish expectations and accommodations for each student. (Scott, 1998)
- Establish a language-based homework lab. (Iskowitz, 1997)
- Be aware of the challenges faced by culturally and linguistically diverse (CLD) students who are also learning disabled. Strategies for intervention include working with students to learn the vocabulary of the classroom and of the curriculum; helping students to develop higher-level thinking skills; using a term in English paired with the same term in the student's native language; reminding teachers to give instructions more than once and to clarify instructions; becoming aware of differences in pragmatic skills between cultures; and helping students to learn pragmatics appropriate to the culture they are in. (Roseberry-McKibbin and Brice, 1997)
- Teach phonics through a storytelling approach involving each letter of the alphabet. (Weiss-Kapp, 1998)
- Work with classroom teachers to present abstract concepts in concrete ways, i.e., through role-playing, auditory and visual presentations, etc. (Trace, 1996b)
- Provide consultation to teachers to eliminate distracting, competing noise in the classroom.
- Work with students on organizational skills.
- Work with students on discourse and narrative skills.
- Work with students on pragmatic skills.
- Use multisensory language instruction. (Trace, 1996c)
- Teach students how to study.
- Using students' textbooks, teach students to be alert to key words and phrases, including *as a result, in summary, first, second*, and *problems encountered*. (Wallach and Butler, 1995)
- Rather than providing tutoring for specific classroom lessons, use a classroom curriculum to teach generalization of language principles.
- Teach general strategies for reading maps, charts, graphs, and tables.

RESULTS OF RECENT STUDIES

• In one study, two groups of children with LD between the ages of 3 1/2 and 6 years were seen individually for one session with the goal of teaching the concepts of big/little. In one group the teacher used signing for "big" and "little," paired with verbal expression. In the other group, no signing was used. In the group in which signing was used, children used a significantly greater number of appropriate vocalizations, used more signs, exhibited more instances of eye contact, and used eye contact for longer duration. (Hurd, 1995)

PROGNOSIS

Outcome is dependent on a number of coexisting factors, i.e., severity of the disability, overall IQ score, presence or absence of ADHD or other comorbid condition, the child's motivation, and the family support system. Often some deterioration in academic achievement is seen in later grades as schedules and assignments become more complex and demanding. (Church, et al., 1997)

REFERENCES

Ackerman PT, RA Dykman. Phonological processes, confrontational naming, and immediate memory in dyslexia. *Journal of Learning Disabilities.* 1993;26(9):597–609.

Changes in brain structure may be linked to dyslexia. *Advance for Speech-Language Pathologists & Audiologists.* 1992;2(23):9.

Church RP, MEB Lewis, ML Batshaw. Learning disabilities. In: Batshaw ML, ed. *Children with Disabilities,* 4th ed. Baltimore: Paul H. Brookes Publishing Co. 1997: 471–97.

Crane R. Metacognitive strategies: empowering college students with LD. *Advance for Speech-Language Pathologists & Audiologists.* 1996;6(50):9.

Deuel RK. Developmental dysgraphia and motor skills disorders. *Journal of Child Neurology.* 1995;10[Suppl 1]:S6–8.

Hurd A. The influence of signing on adult/child interaction in a teaching context. *Child Language Teaching and Therapy.* 1995;11(3):319–30.

Iskowitz M. Closing the language gap: collaborative service delivery for children with LLD. *Advance for Speech-Language Pathologists & Audiologists.* 1997;7(31):6,46.

Iskowitz M. Language-based homework lab for pre-adolescents. *Advance for Speech-Language Pathologists & Audiologists.* 1997;7(31):8–9.

Iskowitz M. A literacy-based summer program makes language come alive. *Advance for Speech-Language Pathologists & Audiologists.* 1998a;8(27):7–9.

Iskowitz M. Pediatric outcomes: a new test allows clinicians to observe language in a functional context. *Advance for Speech-Language Pathologists & Audiologists.* 1998b; 8(27):14–16.

Nass R. Advances in learning disabilities. *Current Opinion in Neurology.* 1994;7:179–86.

Roseberry-McKibbin C, A Brice. Strategies for LLD. *Advance for Speech-Language Pathologists & Audiologists.* 1997;7(48):26–28.

Scott A. Teaming with teachers: classroom collaboration benefits students with LLD. *Advance for Speech-Language Pathologists & Audiologists.* 1998;8(27):24–25.

Trace R. Researchers: dyslexia may be caused by flawed brain circuitry. *Advance for Speech-Language Pathologists & Audiologists.* 1994;4(27):5,38.

Trace R. Early identification and management of LLD facilitates academic achievement. *Advance for Speech-Language Pathologists & Audiologists.* 1996a;6(17):8–9.

Trace R. Helping students with LLD succeed in regular classrooms. *Advance for Speech-Language Pathologists & Audiologists.* 1996b;6(4):6.

Trace R. Multisensory approaches improve language skills. *Advance for Speech-Language Pathologists & Audiologists.* 1996c;6(17):11,42.

Upham DA, VH Trumbull. *Making the Grade: Reflections on Being Learning Disabled.* Portsmouth, NH: Heinemann. 1997.

Wallach GP, KG Butler. Language learning disabilities: moving in from the edge. *Topics in Language Disorders.* 1995;16(1):1–26.

Weiss-Kapp S. Reading by the rules: teaching rule-governed systematic phonics through storytelling. *Advance for Speech-Language Pathologists & Audiologists.* 1998;8(4): 22,29.

Welsh LW, JJ Welsh, MP Healy. Learning disabilities and central auditory dysfunction. *Annals of Otology, Rhinology & Laryngology.* 1996;105:117–22.

Zarrella S. Studying humor comprehension in children with LD. *Advance for Speech-Language Pathologists & Audiologists.* 1995;5(5):6.

Mental Retardation (MR)— Children and Adolescents

DESCRIPTION

Subaverage intellectual ability present from birth or early infancy. Approximately 3% of the overall population is mentally retarded. Approximately 3.6 births out of every 1,000 live births are children who will develop an IQ below 50. Mental retardation may occur as an isolated disability or may co-occur with associated impairments. These associated impairments include cerebral palsy, visual impairments, seizure disorder, pervasive developmental disorder, and attention deficit hyperactivity disorder.

ETIOLOGY

A variety of factors, singularly or in combination, may cause mental retardation. These include genetic factors, congenital infection, chromosomal abnormalities, genetic metabolic disorders, genetic neurologic disorders, drug or alcohol use by the mother during pregnancy, prenatal malnutrition, and perinatal complications.

SPEECH AND LANGUAGE DIFFICULTIES

- Delayed/deviant development of receptive and expressive language skills.
- May be nonverbal, but overall communication skills may be more highly developed.
- Difficulty establishing referents as speakers.
- Limited use of conversational repair techniques.

ASSOCIATED AND OTHER DIFFICULTIES

- Delayed development of gross motor skills.
- Delayed development of fine motor skills.
- Hearing impairment may be present.
- Visual impairment may be present.
- May have difficulty interacting with peers.

ASSESSMENT

- Administer *Bayley Scales of Infant Development.*
- Administer *Denver II.*
- Administer *Receptive-Expressive Emergent Language Test,* 2nd ed. (REEL-2).
- Assess natural communication repertoires.
- Assess articulation skills and overall intelligibility.

- When assessing conversational skills, be aware that for persons with mental retardation, any given skill may be more problematic in the speaker role than it is in the role of listener. (Abbeduto and Rosenberg, 1992)

INTERVENTION TECHNIQUES

- When developing augmented communication systems, provide training in receptive understanding, as well as expressive use of symbols.
- Provide instructions to caregivers and teachers in use of the augmentative and alternative communication (AAC) system and work together to teach its use in natural settings. (Romski and Sevcik, 1992)
- Encourage enrollment in language-based early intervention and preschool settings, and provide modeling of language development activities within those settings.
- Provide parents and caregivers with information and modeling regarding the development of communication skills.

RESULTS OF RECENT STUDIES

- Acquisition of signing skills was studied in 34 children over a period of 4 years. At the beginning of the study, the children ranged in chronological age from 29 months to 9 years and in mental age from 4 months to 21 months. At the end of 4 years, 20 of the 34 children used no signs independently, and 19 did not even imitate signs. Six of the 34 children used two-word combinations, but none used more than two different combinations. Nine used some spoken words, but none used more than three different words. The author makes the following points: signs are not used consistently throughout the day, reducing the redundancy necessary for learning; signs are more abstract than a picture-based system and so may be more difficult for this population to learn; and sign usage limits the number of communication partners. (Kahn, 1996)

PROGNOSIS

Life expectancy varies, depending on etiology. Generally, the greater the degree of intellectual impairment and the greater the immobility, the shorter the life expectancy. Similarly, vocational and independent living expectations are widely variable. Some will need only intermittent support, will achieve functional literacy, and will achieve some degree of social and economic independence. Others will require limited support and may work in supported employment settings. They may live with family members or in supervised settings. Still others will require extensive supports. Persons in this group often have associated impairments that further limit their chances for independent functioning. (Batshaw and Shapiro, 1997)

REFERENCES

Abbeduto L, S Rosenberg. Linguistic communication in persons with mental retardation. In: Warren SF, J Reichle, eds. *Causes and Effects in Communication and Language Intervention.* Baltimore: Paul H. Brookes Publishing Co. 1992:331–59.

Batshaw ML, BK Shapiro. Mental retardation. In: Batshaw ML, ed. *Children with Disabilities,* 4th ed. Baltimore: Paul H. Brookes Publishing Co. 1997:335–59.

Kahn JV. Cognitive skills and sign language knowledge of children with severe and profound mental retardation. *Education and Training in Mental Retardation and Developmental Disabilities.* 1996;31(2):162–8.

Romski MA, RA Sevcik. Developing augmented language in children with severe mental retardation. In: Warren SF, J Reichle, eds. *Causes and Effects in Communication and Language Intervention.* Baltimore: Paul H. Brookes Publishing Co. 1992:113–30.

Romski MA, RA Sevcik, B Robinson, R Bakeman. Adult-directed communications of youth with mental retardation using the System for Augmenting Language. *Journal of Speech and Hearing Research.* 1994;37(3):17–28.

Sevcik RA, MA Romski, RV Watkins, KP Deffebach. Adult partner-augmented communication input to youth with mental retardation using the System for Augmenting Language (SAL). *Journal of Speech and Hearing Research.* 1994;38(4):902–12.

Wilkinson KM, MA Romski, RA Sevcik. Emergence of visual-graphic symbol combinations by youth with moderate or severe mental retardation. *Journal of Speech and Hearing Research.* 1994;37(4):883–95.

Prenatal Cocaine Exposure (PCE)

DESCRIPTION

Infants born to addicted mothers have low birthweight, reduced body length and head circumference, lowered Apgar scores, and a characteristic high-pitched cry. Following birth, infants may show withdrawal symptoms, characterized by irritability and fussiness. Symptoms don't appear until 7 to 10 days after birth.

ETIOLOGY

The unborn child is affected by cocaine crossing the placenta, leading to neurologic damage.

SPEECH AND LANGUAGE DIFFICULTIES

• Receptive language deficits.
• Severe delays in development of expressive skills in young children.
• Difficulty with pragmatic skills, particularly in areas of eye contact and turn-taking.
• Older children have difficulty with abstract concepts, multiple meanings of words, and temporal/spatial concepts.

ASSOCIATED AND OTHER DIFFICULTIES

• Abnormal sleep and feeding patterns; decreased time spent in sleep.
• Irritability.
• Easily overloaded by environmental stimuli.
• Hyperactive Moro reflex.
• High potential for cardiorespiratory abnormalities.
• Retardation of growth.
• Low muscle tone.
• Attention deficits.
• Decreased problem-solving skills.
• Rapid mood swings.

- Impulsivity.
- Distractibility.
- Reduced attention span.

ASSESSMENT

- Administer the *Bayley Scales of Infant Development*.
- To assess development of receptive vocabulary, administer the *Peabody Picture Vocabulary Test, Revised* (PPVT-R).
- Administer the *Sequenced Inventory of Communication Development, Revised* (SICD-R).
- Administer the *Preschool Language Assessment Instrument* (PLAI).
- Administer the *Expressive One-Word Picture Vocabulary Test, Revised* (EOWPVT-R).
- Administer the *Goldman-Fristoe Test of Articulation*.
- Administer the *Receptive-Expressive Emergent Language Scale* (REEL).
- Administer the *Preschool Language Scale* (PLS).
- Administer the *Assessment of Children's Language Comprehension* (ACLC).
- Administer the *Prutting Pragmatic Protocol* (PPP).
- Administer the *Test of Problem Solving* (TOPS).
- Be aware that the structured environment of standardized testing may mask attention and organizational deficits.

INTERVENTION TECHNIQUES

- Involve child and parent/caregiver in programs designed to provide comprehensive developmental activities.
- Provide therapy in small groups to address pragmatic skills.

RESULTS OF RECENT STUDIES

- In a study comparing preschool children at high risk for PCE and those at low risk, no significant differences were found in receptive language skills as measured by the PPVT-R, in an autism screening assessment, or in overall levels of engagement. Children in the high-risk group engaged in more passive attending activities than those in the low-risk group. (Rotholz, et al., 1995)

- In a study comparing the language skills of 5 cocaine-exposed (C-E) 2-year-old children with a similar group of non–cocaine-exposed (N-E) children, the greatest differences noted were in the area of discourse-pragmatics. C-E subjects produced significantly fewer utterances containing novel propositional information. (Mentis and Lundgren, 1995)

PROGNOSIS

Long-term prognosis is unknown. In one study, of those children whose mothers received intervention during their pregnancy, 60% showed no deficits at 2 to 3 years of age.

REFERENCES

Crites LS, KL Fischer, M McNeish-Stengel , CJ Siegel. Working with families of drug-exposed children: three model programs. In: Rossetti LM, ed. San Diego, Calif: Singular Publishing Group. *Developmental Problems of Drug-Exposed Infants.* 1992:13–23.

Gibbons M. Forecast for cocaine-exposed children 'less gloomy.' *Advance for Speech-Language Pathologists & Audiologists.* 1992;2(21):15.

Johnson JM, JA Seikel, CL Madison, S Foose, KD Rinard. Standardized test performance of children with a history of prenatal exposure to multiple drugs/cocaine. *Journal of Communication Disorders.* 1997;30:45–73.

Maxwell LA, J Geschwint-Rabin. Substance abuse risk factors and childhood language disorders. In: Smith MD, JS Damico, eds. *Childhood Language Disorders.* New York: Thieme Medical Publishers, Inc. 1996:235–42.

Mentis M, K Lundgren. Effects of prenatal exposure to cocaine and associated risk factors on language development. *Journal of Speech and Hearing Research.* 1995;38(6): 1303–18.

Rivers KO, DL Hedrick. Language and behavioral concerns for drug-exposed infants and toddlers. In: Rossetti LM, ed. *Developmental Problems of Drug-Exposed Infants.* San Diego, Calif: Singular Publishing Group, Inc. 1992:63–73.

Rotholz DA. P Snyder, G Peters. A behavioral comparison of preschool children at high and low risk from prenatal cocaine exposure. *Education and Treatment of Children.* 1995;18(1):1–18.

Specific Language Impairment (SLI)

DESCRIPTION

Unexpected and unexplained language impairment despite normal motor, sensory, and nonverbal cognitive skills. (Tomblin, et al., 1997) Significant expressive language deficits in the absence of intellectual, sensory, motor, neurological, or emotional problems. (Craig, 1996)

Subtypes within the general category of SLI have been proposed. These include semantic-pragmatic SLI and grammatical SLI. SLI is more prevalent in males.

ETIOLOGY

At this time etiology is unknown. There is some evidence of abnormalities of cortical development and some evidence of a familial characteristic to the impairment.

SPEECH AND LANGUAGE DIFFICULTIES

- Language is acquired at a slower rate and over a longer period of time.
- Use of grammatical rules remains immature for age. Difficulty with some forms of grammar may persist into adulthood.
- Phoneme, vocabulary, and morpheme repertoires are smaller than those of chronological peers.
- Although children with SLI acquire grammatical rules in the same order as do other children, they do so at a slower rate. Thus, such rules are still being acquired as mean length of utterances (MLUs) are increasing, resulting in deviant utterance patterns. (Kamhi, 1996)
- Difficulty using past tense and third person singular markers.
- Difficulty using auxiliary verbs.
- Difficulty acquiring vocabulary, particularly verbs.
- Auditory processing deficits.
- Short-term memory deficits.
- Older children may exhibit deficits in comprehension of metaphors and abstract concepts.
- Difficulty with cognitive processing.

- Unresponsive or inept at responding to communicative approaches of others.
- Difficulty with pragmatic skills.
- May have significant articulation deficits.

ASSOCIATED AND OTHER DIFFICULTIES

- Deficient symbolic, adaptive, and integrative play skills.
- Increased likelihood of difficulty with reading and other academic skills.
- Nonverbal cognitive deficits may also be present.
- Difficulty interacting socially with peers.

ASSESSMENT

- Administer *Communication and Symbolic Behavior Scale* (CSBS).
- Administer *MacArthur Communication Development Inventories* (CDI).
- Administer *Preverbal Assessment Intervention Profile* (PAIP).
- Administer sentence imitation subtest of the *Test of Language Development 2, Primary* (TOLD2-P).
- Administer the elaborated sentences subtest of the *Carrow Elicited Language Inventory* (CELI).
- Assess communication skills in the child's natural environment.
- From a language sample, calculate the number of different words (NDW) used. (Watkins, et al., 1995)

INTERVENTION TECHNIQUES

- Begin intervention as early as possible.
- Intervention should target pragmatic skills, as well as grammatical skills.
- Employ visual aids to assist learning.
- Intervention should include not only the child with SLI but also others with whom the child interacts.
- With each child, consider as possible methods of treatment imitation, modeling, focused stimulation, milieu teaching, conversational recasting, and expansion. (Leonard, 1998)
- Assist the child in becoming more responsive to the conversational bids of others.

- Evaluate the child's interactions with peers and identify any utterances that may be meaningful to the child but confusing to others. Model other ways to convey the same meaning. (Goldstein and Gallagher, 1992)
- Teach scripts for frequently occurring social interactions.

RESULTS OF RECENT STUDIES

- SLI may be, at least partially, a timing disorder, whereby children have difficulty retrieving information from memory and then organizing and formulating it efficiently. Faced with time constraints, such as turn-taking, children with SLI may learn to take short-cuts by omitting some grammatical endings. (Trace, 1996)
- In one study, grammatical targets were acquired more rapidly, both by SLI children and by normally developing children, under conditions of conversational recasting than under requests for imitation. (Nelson, et al., 1996)

PROGNOSIS

SLI is a long-term impairment, persisting into adulthood. Studies have shown, however, that treatment does effect gains and that such gains are generally maintained and generalized. (Leonard, 1998)

REFERENCES

Craig HK. Specific language impairment: a changing role for normal developmental language theories during the 1990s. In: Smith MD, JS Damico, eds. *Childhood Language.* New York: Thieme Medical Publishers, Inc. 1996:141–56.

Goldstein H, TM Gallagher. Strategies for promoting the social communicative competence of young children with specific language impairment. In: Odom SL, SR McConnell, MA McEvoy, eds. *Social Competence of Young Children with Disabilities.* Baltimore: Paul H. Brookes Publishing Co. 1992:189–213.

Kamhi AG. Linguistic and cognitive aspects of specific language impairment. In: Smith MD, JS Damico, eds. *Childhood Language Disorders.* New York: Thieme Medical Publishers, Inc. 1996:97–116.

Leonard LB. *Children with Specific Language Impairment.* Cambridge, Mass: The MIT Press, A Bradford Book. 1998.

Lockwood SL. Early speech and language indicators for later learning problems: recognizing a language organization disorder. *Infants and Young Children.* 1994;7(2):43–52.

Nelson KE, SM Camarata, J Webb, L Butkovsky, M Camarata. Effects of imitative and conversational recasting treatment on the acquisition of grammar in children with specific language impairment and younger language-normal children. *Journal of Speech and Hearing Research.* 1996;39(4):850–9.

Tomblin JB, NL Records, X Zhang. A system for the diagnosis of specific language impairment in kindergarten children. *Journal of Speech & Hearing Research.* 1996;39(6): 1284–94.

Tomblin JB, E Smith, X Zhang. Epidemiology of specific language impairment: prenatal and perinatal risk factors. *Journal of Communication Disorders.* 1997;30:325–44.

Trace R. Children with SLI need to learn how to learn. *Advance for Speech-Language Pathologists & Audiologists.* 1996;6(25):6–7.

van der Lely HKJ, L Stollwerck. A grammatical specific language impairment in children: an autosomal dominant inheritance? *Brain and Language.* 1996;52(3):484–504.

Watkins RV, ML Rice, eds. *Specific Language Impairments in Children.* Baltimore: Paul H. Brookes Publishing Co. 1994.

Watkins RV, DJ Kelly, HM Harbers, W Hollis. Measuring children's lexical diversity: differentiating typical and impaired language learners. *Journal of Speech and Hearing Research.* 1995;38(6):1349–55.

Chapter 2

Inherited and Congenital Disorders or Abnormalities

- Alport syndrome
- Angelman syndrome
- Clefts of the lip and palate
- Cornelia de Lange syndrome (CdLS)
- Cri-du-chat syndrome
- Fragile X syndrome
- Galactosemia
- Goldenhar syndrome
- Hydrocephalus and MASA syndrome
- Klinefelter syndrome (KS)
- Moebius syndrome
- Pierre Robin syndrome
- Rett syndrome (RS)
- Spina bifida
- Tourette syndrome (Gilles de la Tourette's syndrome) (TS)
- Treacher Collins syndrome
- Usher syndrome
- Waardenburg syndrome

Alport Syndrome

DESCRIPTION

This genetic disorder, also known as hereditary nephritis, is characterized by renal function impairments, frequent sensorineural hearing loss, and occasional ocular abnormalities. There are six forms of Alport syndrome, three of which present as juvenile forms. Approximately 1 in 50,000 Americans carries the gene for Alport syndrome, although not all develop the syndrome. Males are affected more frequently and more severely.

ETIOLOGY

Alport syndrome may present as a dominant X-linked inheritance, or it may occur through gene mutation. Specific etiology is unknown.

SPEECH AND LANGUAGE DIFFICULTIES

• Progressive deterioration of articulation skills.

ASSOCIATED AND OTHER DIFFICULTIES

• Sensorineural hearing loss.
• Chronic renal failure, which may lead to abnormalities of bone formation.
• Cataracts.
• Myopia.

ASSESSMENT

• Assess articulation skills and assess repeatedly over time.

(See also Hearing Impairment—Children and Adolescents)

INTERVENTION TECHNIQUES

• Consider use of a system of augmentative and alternative communication (AAC) as intelligibility decreases.

(See also Hearing Impairment—Children and Adolescents.

RESULTS OF RECENT STUDIES

No recent studies regarding communication skills were found in the literature.

PROGNOSIS

Males generally succumb to renal failure by the fifth decade of life; females have greater potential for a normal life span.

REFERENCES

Magalini SI, SC Magalini. *Dictionary of Medical Syndromes,* 4th ed. Philadelphia: Lippincott-Raven Publishers. 1997:33.

Thoene JG, NP Coker, eds. *Physicians' Guide to Rare Diseases.* New York: Dowden Publishing Co. 1995:692–3.

Angelman Syndrome

DESCRIPTION

Characteristics include severe congenital mental retardation, unusual facial features, and muscular abnormalities. Males and females are affected equally. Exact incidence is not known; over 80 cases have been reported.

ETIOLOGY

Complex genetic etiology involving DNA deletion of chromosome number 15; parental origin is maternal.

SPEECH AND LANGUAGE DIFFICULTIES

- Severe speech and language deficits.
- Frequent tongue thrusting.

ASSOCIATED AND OTHER DIFFICULTIES

- Seizures.
- Feeding difficulties; difficulties in sucking.
- Delayed developmental milestones.
- Delays in gross motor skills.
- Ataxia.
- Decreased muscle tone.
- Poor balance.
- Scoliosis.
- Unusual gait, which may lead to later joint deformities.
- Strabismus.
- Severe intellectual impairment.
- Easily precipitated laughter.
- Microcephaly.
- Large mouth and chin.
- Widely spaced or irregularly spaced teeth.
- Abnormal electroencephalogram (EEG).
- Poor sleep patterns.
- Needs assistance with activities of daily living.
- Social interaction deficits.
- Attention deficits.

ASSESSMENT

- Administer *Receptive Expressive Emergent Language Scales*, 2nd ed. *(REEL-2)*.

INTERVENTION TECHNIQUES

- Encourage children to use natural gestures.
- Work to develop simple systems of augmentative and alternative communication (AAC).
- Encourage joint attention and turn-taking skills.

RESULTS OF RECENT STUDIES

No recent studies regarding communication skills were found in the literature.

PROGNOSIS

Seizure activity may stop at around 10 years of age. Mental retardation is not progressive but is severe. Life expectancy is thought to be normal. Independent living is not a realistic goal.

REFERENCES

Gilbert P. *The A-Z Reference Book of Syndromes and Inherited Disorders: A Manual for Health, Social and Education Workers*. New York: Chapman & Hall. 1993: 22–24.

Jolleff N, MM Ryan. Communication development in Angelman syndrome. *Archives of Disease in Childhood*. 1993;69:148–50.

Jones KL. *Smith's Recognizable Patterns of Human Malformation,* 5th ed. Philadelphia: W.B. Saunders Co. 1997:200–1.

Penner KA, J Johnston, BH Faircloth, P Irish, CA Williams. Communication, cognition, and social interaction in the Angelman syndrome. *American Journal of Medical Genetics*. 1993;46:34–39.

Smith A, C Wiles, E Haan, J Mcgill, G Wallace, J Dixon, R Selby, A Colley, R Marks, RJ Trent. Clinical features in 27 patients with Angelman syndrome resulting from DNA deletion. *Journal of Medical Genetics*. 1996;33(2):107–12.

Thoene JG, NP Coker. *Physicians' Guide to Rare Diseases,* 2nd ed. Montvale, NJ: Dowden Publishing Co. 1995:14.

Clefts of the Lip and Palate

DESCRIPTION

Clefts occur in 1 of every 700 to 800 births and may range from a cleft of the soft palate only to clefts involving the soft and hard palates, the alveolar process of the maxilla, and the lip. One system for the classification of clefts, proposed by Veau as reported in Bzoch (1997b), is as follows:

Class I—Cleft of the soft palate only.

Class II—Cleft of the hard and soft palate to the incisive foramen.

Class III—Complete unilateral cleft of the soft and hard palate and of the lip and alveolar ridge on one side.

Class IV—Complete bilateral cleft of the soft and hard palate and/or the lip and alveolar ridge on both sides.

Virtually all children with clefts of the lip and palate require lip repair, palate repair, nasal surgery, myringotomy, tube surgery, and lip and nose revisions. Maxillary bone grafting and pharyngoplasty are also necessary in a large percentage of cases.

ETIOLOGY

Although clefting may occur in isolation, there are now known to be over 400 syndromes in which clefting is a feature. Etiologies vary and may be the result of chromosome disorders, genetic disorders, teratogenic disorders, or mechanical factors.

SPEECH AND LANGUAGE DIFFICULTIES

- Hypernasal voice quality.
- Hyponasality may be present and is generally indicative of a physical obstruction, such as hypertrophied adenoid tissue, a nasal septal deviation, or a pharyngeal flap that is too wide.
- Mixed nasality.
- Nasal emission.
- Nasal substitutions.
- Nasal grimacing.
- Reduced oral breath pressure.
- Articulation errors may be obligatory or compensatory. Obligatory errors, generally distortions, are the direct result of an anatomical defect. They often are self-corrected when the underlying defect is remedied, but are not easily amenable to speech therapy. Compensatory errors, usually substitutions, are errors in learning that affect place and/or manner of articulation. They are corrected by therapy. (Golding-Kushner, 1995)
- Compensatory strategies used during speech production, including increased respiratory effort, alterations in tongue carriage, interruption of air flow by the vocal cords, and nasal grimace.
- Distortions are lateral, interdental, and retroflexed.

- Voice disorders, including hoarseness, breathiness, abnormal pitch, soft voice, and strangled voice quality.
- Hyponasality may occur following pharyngeal flap surgery. It is usually transitory, and it resolves within 6 months.

ASSOCIATED AND OTHER DIFFICULTIES

- Difficulty with feeding, resulting in weight loss, failure to thrive, and irritability.
- Airway obstruction.
- Nasal obstruction may occur secondary to abnormal size and/or shape of nose.
- Irregular interdental spacing and missing teeth.
- Malocclusions.
- Unilateral or bilateral collapse of the maxillary arch.
- Retrognathia or prognathia of the mandible.
- Palatal fistula may be present after palate repair.
- Enlarged pharynx.
- Otitis media.
- Eustachian tube dysfunction.
- Hearing impairment (generally bilateral and conductive, but not necessarily symmetrical).
- Hypotonia.
- Macroglossia is associated with some clefting syndromes.
- Sleep apnea may occur as a complication of pharyngoplasty.

ASSESSMENT

- To assess receptive and expressive language skills in young children, administer *Receptive-Expressive Emergent Language Test*, 2nd ed. (REEL-2).
- Use *MacArthur Communicative Development Inventory* and *Rossetti Infant-Toddler Language Scale* to assess early speech and language development.
- To evaluate early language development, assess interactions between caregivers and young children.
- Perform examination of oromoter/speech mechanism.
- Assess effects of dental and occlusion disorders on the development of speech.

- Administer *Clinical Assessment of Oropharyngeal Motor Development in Young Children.*
- Evaluate articulation skills and analyze error patterns, and evaluate and distinguish phonologic process errors from developmental articulation errors.
- Administer *Bankson-Berthal Test of Phonology* (BBTOP) and/or *Goldman-Fristoe Test of Articulation—Revised* (GFTA).
- Administer the *Iowa Pressure Articulation Test.*
- Administer *Bzoch Error Pattern Diagnostic Articulation Tests.*
- Assess resonance.
- Assess language skills.
- Observe and assess phenotypic features affecting speech, including size and shape of nose and presence of nasal obstruction; lip closure and movement; dental abnormalities and malocclusions; and size, shape, and position of maxilla.
- Observe hard palate for presence of unrepaired cleft, fistula following surgery, or maxillary collapse.
- Observe for nasal grimacing—generally an indication of inadequate valving.
- Assess parameters of cleft palate speech using *Great Ormond Street Speech Assessment* (GOS.SPASS). (See Sell, et al. 1994, for form and explanation)
- Observe for signs of velopharyngeal insufficiency, including hypernasality, audible nasal emission, weakness of plosives, and compensatory articulations. (Haapanen, 1994)
- Videofluoroscopic studies with computer-assisted edge enhancement and contrast-enhancement image processing may be used to assess velopharyngeal (VP) movement, velar lift, and lateral pharyngeal wall movement. (Coffey, et al., 1993).
- Use multiview videofluoroscopy and nasopharyngoscopy to assess VP function.

INTERVENTION TECHNIQUES

- Assist in instructing parents of newborns in feeding techniques: feed the infant in an upright position; limit feeding time to 20 to 30 minutes; use nipples designed for premature babies and make cross-cuts in the nipples, allowing milk to dribble out slowly; position the bottle underneath a shelf of bone rather than directly into the cleft; and use plastic bottles, making it easier to squeeze additional drops of milk into the mouth even when the baby has stopped sucking. Specially designed feeding devices and feeding plates are generally not necessary. (Sidoti and Shprintzen, 1995)

- Provide education to parents of very young children regarding the role of hard and soft palates in normal speech acquisition, restrictions imposed on early babbling by unrepaired clefts, and avoidance of positive reinforcement of consonant constrictions that involve backed glottal and pharyngeal place features. (D'Antonio and Scherer, 1995)
- Provide models of interaction for parents and caregivers of young children.
- Develop and monitor speech and language stimulation programs for children ages 12 to 30 months.
- To facilitate communication and language development, consider use of a temporary system of augmentative and alternative communication (AAC) for those children whose speech is unintelligible.
- For children with concomitant language impairments, provide small-group therapy.
- Work to eliminate glottal stops and to eliminate pharyngeal/laryngeal fricatives and nasal snorting.
- For persistent resonance problems following surgical repair of the cleft, consider use of continuous positive airway pressure (CPAP). (Trace, 1995)
- Employ auditory training and use of a nasal mirror to help the client become aware of nasal distortion.
- Demonstrate VP closure or inconsistent closure through use of video-fluoroscopy.
- If nasal emission cannot be eliminated, decrease the perception of nasality by instructing the client to speak with a larger mouth opening.
- For remediation of tongue placement in articulation, consider use of visual feedback through the use of electropalatograph (EPG). (Michi, et al., 1993)
- For treatment of hypernasality, exercises such as blowing, massage, icing, sucking, gagging, and cheek puffing are generally ineffective. (Golding-Kushner, 1995)
- When adequate VP function has been confirmed, employ techniques of voice therapy, i.e., increasing volume and using clear phonation, to treat cases of aspirate voice quality. (Bzoch, 1997a)

- Employ standard voice therapy techniques (identifying stressful speaking situations, training for relaxed phonation) for management of hoarse voice quality.
- Speech bulbs and palatal lifts may be used as permanent obturators, on a temporary basis prior to surgery or as a therapeutic technique to reduce velopharyngeal incompetence (VPI). The purpose of speech bulbs is to effect VP closure. Therapy should focus on eliminating compensatory articulation errors. (Golding-Kushner, et al., 1995)
- Make frequent use of a tape recorder to document performance prior to therapy, during therapy, and at the end of therapy; as a tool in auditory training with the client, and to document progress or lack of progress.
- Recognize that in some cases a plateau will be reached and little if any further progress will be realized. Guard against continuing therapy beyond the time when progress can be documented.

RESULTS OF RECENT STUDIES

- To reduce or eliminate occurrences of otitis media (OM), parents are taught to stimulate contractions of the velar muscles of the soft palate many times a day. In one study of 280 children, after 4 1/2 years, 264 children had no OM, 15 children had occasional OM, and 1 child had chronic OM. Hearing levels were 6 to 10 dB in the majority of children and 25 to 30 dB in those with occasional OM. (Trujillo, 1994)
- Following surgical repair of the palate, both VPI and compensatory articulation (CA) disorders may remain. At a later time, surgical correction of VPI is made with a pharyngeal flap. In a study assessing the timing of this procedure, results indicated that surgical correction of VPI does not have a significant influence on the CA disorder. Speech therapy is generally needed to address the CA, and whether the surgical correction of VPI is accomplished early or later during the course of therapy does not have a significant influence on the amount of therapy needed. (Pamplona, et al., 1996)
- Videofluoroscopic studies with computer image processing show no correlation between severity of hypernasality and soft palate and pharyngeal movement. Some correlation was found between degree of lateral pharyngeal wall excursion and velar lift and increased hypernasality. (Coffey, et al., 1993)
- Hypertrophic tonsils may serve as obturators in clients for whom the VP flap is too low, too narrow, or both. In such instances, tonsil removal is

not desirable. If tonsillectomy is necessary due to obstructive sleep apnea, lateral augmentation of the VP flap should be considered. (Finkelstein, et al., 1994)

- Tonsillectomy and velopharyngoplasty may be performed simultaneously. (Eufinger and Eggeling, 1994)
- In a study conducted in Finland, children who had undergone the Cronin modification as the primary repair were more likely to have normal resonance than were those who had a Veau-Kilner pushback procedure. The two groups did not differ in number or severity of articulation errors related to VPI. (Haapanen, 1995)

PROGNOSIS

Eighty percent of children born with nonsyndromic cleft palate, and who undergo palatal repair by 18 months of age, develop adequate speech without the need for therapy. For others, the course of therapy may be of several years duration.

REFERENCES

Bzoch KR. Clinical assessment, evaluation, and management of 11 categorical aspects of cleft palate speech disorders. In: Bzoch KR, ed. *Communication Disorders Related to Cleft Lip and Palate*, 4th ed. Austin, Tex: Pro-Ed. 1997a:261–311.

Bzoch KR. Introduction to the study of communication disorders in cleft palate and related craniofacial anomalies. In: Bzoch KR, ed. *Communication Disorders Related to Cleft Lip and Palate,* 4th ed. Austin, Tex: Pro-Ed. 1997b:3–44.

Coffey JP, D Hamilton, M Fitzsimons, PJ Freyne. Image processing of videofluoroscopy of patients with velopharyngeal insufficiency and hypernasal speech. *Clinical Radiology.* 1993;48:260–63.

D'Antonio LL, NJ Scherer. The evaluation of speech disorders associated with clefting. In: Shprintzen RJ, J Bardach, eds. *Cleft Palate Speech Management: A Multidisciplinary Approach.* St. Louis, Mo: Mosby. 1995:176–220.

Eufinger H, V Eggeling. Should velopharyngoplasty and tonsillectomy in the cleft palate child be performed simultaneously? *Journal of Oral & Maxillofacial Surgery.* 1994;52(9):927–30.

Finkelstein Y, A Nachmani, D Ophir. The functional role of the tonsils in speech. *Archives of Otolaryngology — Head & Neck Surgery.* 1994;120:846–51.

Girolametto L. The evaluation and remediation of language impairment. In: Shprintzen RJ, J Bardach, eds. *Cleft Palate Speech Management: A Multidisciplinary Approach.* St. Louis, Mo: Mosby. 1995:167–75.

Golding-Kushner KJ. Treatment of articulation and resonance disorders associated with cleft palate and VPI. In: Shprintzen RJ, J Bardach, eds. *Cleft Palate Speech Management: A Multidisciplinary Approach.* St. Louis, Mo: Mosby. 1995:327–51.

Golding-Kushner KJ, G Cisneros, E LeBlanc. Speech bulbs. In: Shprintzen RJ, J Bardach, eds. *Cleft Palate Speech Management: A Multidisciplinary Approach.* St. Louis, Mo: Mosby. 1995:352–63.

Haapanen M-L. Cleft type and speech proficiency. *Folia Phoniatrica et Logopaedica.* 1994;46:57–63.

Haapanen M-L. Effect of method of cleft palate repair on the quality of speech at the age of 6 years. *Scandinavian Journal of Plastic & Reconstructive Surgery & Hand Surgery.* 1995;29:245–50.

Harding A, P Grunwell. Characteristics of cleft palate speech. *European Journal of Disorders of Communication.* 1996;31(4):331–57.

Lohmander-Agerskov A, E Söderpalm. Evaluation of speech after completed late closure of the hard palate. *Folia Phoniatrica.* 1993;45(1):26-30.

Lohmander-Agerskov A, E Söderpalm, H Friede, E Persson , J Lilja. Pre-speech in children with cleft lip and palate or cleft palate only: phonetic analysis related to morphologic and functional factors. *Cleft Palate-Craniofacial Journal.* 1994;31(4):271–9.

Michi K, Y Yamashita, S Imai, N Suzuki, H Yoshida. Role of visual feedback treatment for defective "s" sounds in patients with cleft palate. *Journal of Speech and Hearing Research.* 1993;36(2):277–85.

Pamplona M, AY Sunza, M Guerrero, I Mayer, M Garcia-Velasco. Surgical correction of velopharyngeal insufficiency with and without compensatory articulation. *International Journal of Pediatric Otorhinolaryngology.* 1996;34:53-59.

Peterson-Falzone SJ. Speech outcomes in adolescents with cleft lip and palate. *Cleft Palate-Craniofacial Journal.* 1995;32(2):125–8.

Sell D, A Harding, P Grunwell. A screening assessment of cleft palate speech (Great Ormond Street Speech Assessment). *European Journal of Disorders of Communication.* 1994;29(1):1–15.

Sidoti EJ, RJ Shprintzen. Pediatric care and feeding of the newborn with a cleft. In: Shprintzen RJ, J Bardach, eds. *Cleft Palate Speech Management: A Multidisciplinary Approach.* St. Louis, Mo: Mosby. 1995:63–74.

Tanimoto K, G Henningsson, A Isberg, Y Ren. Comparison of tongue position during speech before and after pharyngeal flap surgery in hypernasal speakers. *Cleft Palate-Craniofacial Journal.* 1995;31(4):280–6.

Trace R. Current trends in managing cleft lip and palate. *Advance for Speech-Language Pathology & Audiology.* 1995;5(34):6–7.

Trujillo L. Prevention of conductive hearing loss in cleft palate patients. *Folia Phoniatrica et Logopaedica.* 1994;46(3):123–26.

Van Denmark DR. Speech and voice therapy techniques for school-age and adult patients with remaining cleft palate speech disorders. In: Bzoch KR, ed. *Communicative Disorders Related to Cleft Lip and Palate,* 4th ed. Austin, Tex: Pro-Ed. 1997:493–508.

Witzel MA. Communicative impairment associated with clefting. In: Shprintzen RJ, J Bardach, eds. *Cleft Palate Speech Management: A Multidisciplinary Approach.* St. Louis, Mo: Mosby. 1995:137–66.

Cornelia de Lange Syndrome (CdLS)

DESCRIPTION
Major characteristics of the syndrome include skeletal and facial anomalies, excessive hairiness, and severe mental retardation. Males and females are affected in equal numbers.

ETIOLOGY
A dysmorphogenic disorder characterized by multiple congenital abnormalities. A defect of the gene on the long arm of chromosome number 3 is suspected but not proven.

SPEECH AND LANGUAGE DIFFICULTIES
- Severe speech and language deficits. Most do not develop speech skills, although some develop some form of nonverbal communication.
- Expressive abilities are significantly more impaired than are receptive skills.
- Syntactic development lags disproportionately behind vocabulary development.
- Articulation errors. Consonants are typically distorted or omitted.

ASSOCIATED AND OTHER DIFFICULTIES
- Growth failure and limb reduction.
- Seizures.
- Ocular abnormalities.
- Cleft palate may be present.
- Hearing loss.

- Feeding difficulties.
- Gastrointestinal disorders with reflux.
- Heart defects may be present.
- Aspiration.
- Anemia.
- Overactivity.
- Frequent mood changes.
- Stereotyped behaviors.
- Severe intellectual impairment.
- Self-injurious behaviors.

ASSESSMENT

- Administer *Pre-Verbal Communication Schedule* (PVCS).
- Perform hearing screening and refer to audiologist as indicated.
- Assess for dysphagia.

INTERVENTION TECHNIQUES

- Provide and encourage a communication-rich environment.
- Encourage development of speech as well as forms of nonverbal communication.

RESULTS OF RECENT STUDIES

- Some association has been found between low birth weight (under 5 pounds) and inability to use two-word utterances by age 4 years. Similarly, those with upper limb malformations were significantly less likely to have developed two-word utterances than were those with no upper limb malformation. (Goodban, 1993)
- In one study, self-injurious behaviors were more prominent in older children with severe intellectual impairment and low communication competence. (Sarimski, 1997)

PROGNOSIS

Early death may occur, generally as a result of apnea, aspiration, or cardiac complications. Independent living is not a realistic goal.

REFERENCES

Gilbert P. *The A-Z Reference Book of Syndromes and Inherited Disorders: A Manual for Health, Social and Education Workers.* New York: Chapman & Hall. 1993:58–60.

Goodban MT. Survey of speech and language skills with prognostic indicators in 116 patients with Cornelia de Lange syndrome. *American Journal of Medical Genetics.* 1993;47:1059–63.

Jackson L, AD Kline, MA Barr, S Koch. de Lange syndrome: a clinical review of 310 individuals. *American Journal of Medical Genetics.* 1993;47:940–6.

Jones KL. *Smith's Recognizable Patterns of Human Malformation,* 5th ed. Philadelphia: W.B. Saunders Co. 1997:88–89.

Sarimski K. Communication, social-emotional development, and parenting stress in Cornelia de Lange syndrome. *Journal of Intellectual Disability Research.* 1997;41(Part 1):70–75.

Thoene JG, NP Coker, eds. *Physicians' Guide to Rare Diseases.* New York: Dowden Publishing Co. 1995:49.

Cri-Du-Chat Syndrome

DESCRIPTION

The disorder, also known as cat's cry syndrome, takes its name from the high-pitched, mewing cry that is heard in the immediate newborn period. It lasts several weeks, and then disappears. Incidence is approximately 1 in every 50,000 births.

ETIOLOGY

The syndrome is caused by a partial deletion of the short arm of chromosome number 5.

SPEECH AND LANGUAGE DIFFICULTIES

- Severely deficient speech and language skills.
- Echolalia.

ASSOCIATED AND OTHER DIFFICULTIES

- Low birth weight.
- Short stature.
- Facial asymmetry.
- Microcephaly.
- Strabismus.
- Heart defects.
- Hypotonicity.
- Significantly impaired mental and physical development.
- Myopia.
- Cleft lip and palate.
- Severe respiratory difficulties, especially during infancy.
- Severe feeding difficulties.
- Dental malocclusion.
- Absent kidney and spleen.
- Club foot and flat feet.
- Scoliosis may occur.
- Hypersensitivity to sensory stimuli.
- Self-injurious behaviors.
- Repetitive movements.

ASSESSMENT

- Assess for early feeding difficulties.
- Evaluate receptive and expressive language skills.

(See also Clefts of the Lip and Palate)

INTERVENTION TECHNIQUES

- Assist parents with feeding techniques.
- Provide early intervention to facilitate development of communication skills.
- Provide early exposure to sign language.

(See also Clefts of the Lip and Palate)
(See also Mental Retardation—Children and Adolescents)

RESULTS OF RECENT STUDIES

No recent studies regarding communication skills were found in the literature.

PROGNOSIS

Independent living is generally not a realistic goal. Life span is limited, due to cardiac and/or respiratory problems.

REFERENCES

Cornish KM, J Pigram. Developmental and behavioural characteristics of cri-du-chat syndrome. *Archives of Disease in Childhood.* 1996;75:448–50.

Gilbert P. *The A-Z Reference Book of Syndromes and Inherited Disorders: A Manual for Health, Social and Education Workers.* New York: Chapman & Hall. 1993:61–63.

Jones KL. *Smith's Recognizable Patterns of Human Malformation,* 5th ed. Philadelphia: W.B. Saunders Co. 1997:44.

Thoene JG, NP Coker, eds. *Physicians' Guide to Rare Diseases.* New York: Dowden Publishing Co. 1995:51.

Fragile X Syndrome

DESCRIPTION

Fragile X syndrome, along with Down syndrome, is the most common cause of mental retardation that can be specifically diagnosed. The syndrome is more prevalent in males. Characteristics include a long, narrow face; large, protruding ears and a prominent chin and forehead; hand calluses, flat feet; and hyperextensible joints. While there is a high incidence of mental retardation, some affected males have normal intellectual ability. Incidence is approximately 1 in 1,000 male births and 1 in 2,000 female births. There is increased likelihood of autism among boys with Fragile X. The syndrome may be present in 14% of persons diagnosed with autism.

ETIOLOGY

Cause is a fragile site on the long arm of the X chromosome. In addition to passage of the affected gene from mother to son, passage may also occur from a normal, transmitting male to daughters. A carrier female has a 50% chance of passing the gene to all of her children, while transmitting males pass the gene to all of their daughters. These daughters almost always are of normal intelligence. However, their daughters—granddaughters of normal transmitting males—show a high level of expression of the syndrome. In the third generation, both males and females may have the syndrome. (Santos, 1992)

SPEECH AND LANGUAGE DIFFICULTIES

- Auditory processing disorder.
- In early years, expressive skills may lag considerably behind receptive skills.
- Relative strength in vocabulary; relative weakness in abstract reasoning.
- Rapid rate of speech and uneven rate of speaking, particularly in older boys.
- Excessive volume.
- Breakdown in speech intelligibility in connected passages.
- Whole-word and part-word repetitions.
- Articulation errors.
- Cluttering may occur.
- Echolalia.
- Perseveration.
- Hoarse, breathy voice quality.
- Frequent use of automatic phrases.
- Lack of subject-verb agreement.
- Poor short-term memory responses.
- Marked vocabulary limitations.
- May be nonverbal, depending on degree of retardation.
- Difficulties with pragmatics and topic maintenance, particularly among males.
- Hypersensitivity/hyposensitivity to oral and facial stimulation. Hypersensitivity and hyposensitivity may occur in the same child.

ASSOCIATED AND OTHER DIFFICULTIES

- Approximately 63% of boys with Fragile X syndrome have otitis media.
- Seizures occur in approximately 20% of cases.
- Cardiac problems may be present; mitral valve prolapse occurs in 80% of affected males.
- High-arched palate.
- Increased likelihood of cleft palate.
- May have mild to severe feeding problems, beginning in infancy.
- Strabismus.
- Dental abnormalities.
- Hypotonia.
- Moderate to severe mental retardation in males.
- Mild to severe learning disabilities in females.
- Sensory integration disorder.
- Difficulty with sequential processing.
- Attention deficits, with or without hyperactivity.
- Tactile defensiveness.
- Hand-flapping.
- Hand-biting.
- Poor eye contact; hypersensitivity to gaze.
- High level of social anxiety.
- Delayed motor development.
- Behavioral problems.
- Dyscalculia may be present and is more prevalent among female carriers of Fragile X.

ASSESSMENT

- Be aware that high levels of anxiety, combined with attention difficulties, may affect performance on standardized tests. Assess skills in natural settings as much as possible.
- Assess all areas of language—receptive skills, expressive skills, and pragmatic skills.
- Assess articulation skills.
- Assess oral-motor skills.

INTERVENTION TECHNIQUES

- As a member of a team, provide early intervention services. Instruct parents and caregivers on handling techniques to reduce stress and on feeding techniques.
- Work with young children on oral motor activities geared toward increasing awareness of drooling and management of food bite size.
- Help the child to develop an internal sense of order and structure by providing these externally.
- Advise classroom teachers that presenting material visually may enhance learning.
- Consider use of an auditory trainer.
- Consider early use of sign language and augmentative and alternative communications (AAC).
- Provide language development activities in both individual and group settings.

RESULTS OF RECENT STUDIES

No recent studies regarding communication skills were found in the literature.

PROGNOSIS

Males with mild retardation as children often have moderate to severe mental retardation as adults.

REFERENCES

Dykens EM, RM Hodapp, JF Leckman. *Behavior and Development in Fragile X Syndrome*. Thousand Oaks, Calif: Sage Publications. 1994:50–58.

Gibb C. The most common cause of learning difficulties: a profile of Fragile-X Syndrome and its implications for education. *Educational Research*. 1992;34(3):221–8.

Gross-Tsur V, O Manor, RS Shalev. Developmental dyscalculia, gender, and the brain. *Archives of Disease in Childhood*. 1993;68:510–12.

Santos KE. Fragile X syndrome: an educator's role in identification, prevention, and intervention. *Remedial and Special Education*. 1992;13(2):32-39.

Schoenbrodt L, RA Smith. *Communication Disorders and Interventions in Low Incidence Pediatric Populations*. San Diego, Calif: Singular Publishing Co. 1995:59-91.

Scott GS, TL Layton. Epidemiologic principles in studies of infectious disease outcomes: pediatric HIV as a model. *Journal of Communication Disorders*. 1997;30:303–24.

Smith SE. Cognitive deficits associated with Fragile X syndrome. *Mental Retardation.* 1993;31(5):279–83.

Thoene JG, NP Coker, eds. *Physicians' Guide to Rare Diseases.* New York: Dowden Publishing Co. 1995:125.

Galactosemia

DESCRIPTION

Incidence figures range from 1 in 40,000 births to 1 in 80,000 births. If an affected infant is given milk after birth, anorexia, jaundice, and an enlarged liver develop. Without prompt treatment, mental retardation may occur. Cataracts also may develop. Short stature often results, particularly in females. Avoidance of all milk products must be maintained throughout life.

ETIOLOGY

An inherited autosomal-recessive trait resulting in inborn errors of galactose metabolism characterized by elevated levels of galactose in the blood, which arise from the inability to convert galactose to glucose.

SPEECH AND LANGUAGE DIFFICULTIES

• Verbal dyspraxia is common.

ASSOCIATED AND OTHER DIFFICULTIES

• In infancy, widespread infection in any part of the body is a major concern.
• Intellectual impairment may be present.
• Cataracts may develop.
• Seizures may occur.

- Motor incoordination.
- Ataxia.

ASSESSMENT

- Perform in-depth assessment of articulation and phonology.
- Assess oral-motor skills in depth.

INTERVENTION TECHNIQUES

- Be aware of the high incidence of speech impairment and develop procedures for alerting parents of newborns.
- Increase awareness of oral sensations.
- Work toward development of self-monitoring skills.
- Establish key vocabulary.
- Use rhythm.
- Use visual, visual-auditory, and kinesthetic feedback.

RESULTS OF RECENT STUDIES

No recent studies regarding communication skills were found in the literature.

PROGNOSIS

With prompt treatment, normal physical and intellectual growth may occur, although persons with this condition tend to be underachievers. Some studies report declining IQ with increasing age.

REFERENCES

Gilbert P. *The A-Z Reference Book of Syndromes and Inherited Disorders: A Manual for Health, Social and Education Workers.* New York: Chapman & Hall. 1993:99–101.

Nelson D. Verbal dyspraxia in children with galactosemia. *European Journal of Pediatrics.* 1995;154(Suppl 2):6–57.

Schweitzer S, Y Shin, C Jakobs, J Brodehl. Long-term outcome in 134 patients with galactosaemia. *European Journal of Pediatrics.* 1993;152:36–43.

Goldenhar Syndrome

DESCRIPTION

This syndrome, which occurs in about 1 in 45,000 births, is characterized by varying combinations of several anomalies, including malar, maxillary, and mandibular hypoplasia; absent or closed nares; frontal bossing; microtia; middle ear anomalies; deafness; anomalies of the tongue and soft palate; and hemivertebra. Often, although not always, these anomalies are asymmetric and unilateral.

ETIOLOGY

Cause is unknown and patterns of inheritance seem to vary.

SPEECH AND LANGUAGE DIFFICULTIES

- Articulation deficits as a result of cleft lip and palate and as a result of hearing loss.

(See also Clefts of the Lip and Palate; Hearing Loss—Children and adolescents)

ASSOCIATED AND OTHER DIFFICULTIES

- Cleft lip and cleft palate.
- Dysphagia.
- Outer and middle ear anomalies affecting one or both ears.
- Eustachian tube may be malformed.
- Conductive hearing loss.
- Gastrointestinal anomalies.
- Pulmonary anomalies.
- Renal anomalies.
- Visual problems occur in about one-third of cases.
- Strabismus.
- Scoliosis may develop.
- Intellectual impairment may be present.
- Emotional problems may develop as a result of severe deformities.

ASSESSMENT

- Assess for dysphagia.
- Assess oral-motor function, keeping in mind that this area may be very sensitive and anxiety-provoking for the child.
- Refer for audiological assessment.
- Assess articulation skills.

(See also Clefts of the Lip and Palate; Hearing Loss—Children and adolescents)

INTERVENTION TECHNIQUES

- Through tactics of play, exploration, and pleasurable sensory experiences, work to decrease oral hypersensitivity.
- Work with parents to establish and implement a feeding program.

(See also Clefts of the Lip and Palate; Hearing Loss—Children and adolescents)

RESULTS OF RECENT STUDIES

No recent studies regarding communication skills were found in the literature.

PROGNOSIS

Life span is normal unless heart defects are severe.

REFERENCES

Gilbert P. *The A-Z Reference Book of Syndromes and Inherited Disorders: A Manual for Health, Social and Education Workers*. New York: Chapman & Hall. 1993:105–8.

Jones KL. *Smith's Recognizable Patterns of Human Malformation*, 5th ed. Philadelphia: W.B. Saunders Co. 1997:642–4.

Perlman AL. The successful treatment of challenging cases. *Clinics in Communication Disorders*. 1993;3(4):37–44.

Thoene JG, NP Coker, eds. *Physicians' Guide to Rare Diseases*. New York: Dowden Publishing Co. 1995:78–79.

Hydrocephalus and MASA Syndrome

DESCRIPTION

Incidence of hereditary hydrocephalus is 1 in 30,000. The condition results in an accumulation of cerebrospinal fluid (CSF), which may be relieved by insertion of a shunt. A similar condition, MASA syndrome (**m**ental retardation, **a**phasia, **s**huffling gait, and **a**dducted thumbs), is believed to be caused by the same X-linked locus. Hydrocephalus which is not X-linked also may occur, and in these cases most survivors have normal intelligence and normal or near-normal muscle tone. Normal pressure hydrocephalus (NPH), characterized by cerebral ventricular dilation with normal lumbar CSF pressure, is a rare cause of dementia in the elderly. Classic characteristics of the syndrome include dementia, urinary incontinence, and apraxia of gait. Shunting may improve function.

ETIOLOGY

The most common form of hereditary hydrocephalus is X-linked and recessive. Gene localization is on Xq28. The increased volume of CSF may be due to an increased amount of fluid; an obstruction of flow of the fluid; or impaired absorption of the fluid.

SPEECH AND LANGUAGE DIFFICULTIES

- Content-poor language skills despite adequate articulation, fluency, and grammatical skills.
- "Cocktail Party Syndrome" characterized by fluent and well-articulated speech, verbal perseveration, excessive social forms, irrelevant verbosity, and overfamiliarity of manner. (Dennis, et al., 1994)
- Difficulty making inferences.
- Difficulty interpreting metaphors.

ASSOCIATED AND OTHER DIFFICULTIES

- Mental retardation. IQs are highly variable, from "too low to test" to over 70.
- Delayed achievement of motor developmental milestones.

- Spasticity.
- Increased muscle tone.
- Poor fine motor coordination.

ASSESSMENT
- Assess discourse skills.

(See also Spina Bifida)

INTERVENTION TECHNIQUES
(See Spina Bifida)

RESULTS OF RECENT STUDIES
- When compared with normally developing children, those with hydro-cephalus produced discourse that was less cohesive, more verbose, and less concise. (Dennis, et al., 1994)

PROGNOSIS
Those who reach 2 years of age have a 50% chance of reaching adult-hood. Further prognosis is dependent on the underlying cause of the condition.

REFERENCES

Dennis M, MA Barnes. Oral discourse after early-onset hydrocephalus: linguistic ambiguity, figurative language, speech acts, and script-based inferences. *Journal of Pediatric Psychology.* 1993;18(5):639–52.

Dennis M, B Jacennik, MA Barnes. The content of narrative discourse in children and adolescents after early-onset hydrocephalus and in normally developing age peers. *Brain and Language.* 1994;46:129–65.

Kenwrick S, M Jouet, D Donnai. X-linked hydrocephalus and MASA syndrome. *Journal of Medical Genetics.* 1996;33:59–65.

Raftopoulos C, J Deleval, C Chaskis, A Leonard, F Cantraine, F Desnyttere, S Clarysse, J Brotchi. Cognitive recovery in idiopathic pressure hydrocephalus: a prospective study. *Neurosurgery.* 1994;35(3):397–405.

Walton J, ed. *Brain's Diseases of the Nervous System,* 10th ed. New York: Oxford University Press. 1993:147–52.

Klinefelter Syndrome (KS)

DESCRIPTION

Incidence is 1 in 700 live male births. Affected boys tend to be taller than average.

ETIOLOGY

A chromosome anomaly in which affected males receive an extra X chromosome.

SPEECH AND LANGUAGE DIFFICULTIES

- Delayed acquisition of speech.
- Articulation deficits.
- Deficits in language processing including auditory memory and language comprehension.

ASSOCIATED AND OTHER DIFFICULTIES

- Learning disabilities.
- Difficulty acquiring conceptual knowledge.
- Achievement tends to lag further behind age peers as school years progress.

ASSESSMENT

- Assess receptive and expressive language skills.
- Assess articulation skills.

(See also Learning Disabilities—Children and Adolescents)

INTERVENTION TECHNIQUES

- Encourage participation in language-based early intervention and preschool programs, and provide language development activities within the program.

• Provide parents with information regarding language development activities.

(See also Learning Disabilities—Children and Adolescents)

RESULTS OF RECENT STUDIES

No recent studies regarding communication skills were found in the literature.

PROGNOSIS

Life expectancy is normal.

REFERENCES

Magalini SI, SC Magalini. *Dictionary of Medical Syndromes*, 4th ed. Philadelphia: Lippincott-Raven Publishers. 1997:456–7.

Rovet J, C Netley, M Keenan, J Bailey, D Stewart. The psychoeducational profile of boys with Klinefelter syndrome. *Journal of Learning Disabilities*. 1996;29(2):180–96.

Moebius Syndrome

DESCRIPTION

An inherited type of facial paralysis.

(See also Clefts of the Lip and Palate)

ETIOLOGY

A rare genetic disorder causing underdeveloped sixth and seventh cranial nerves and resulting in lifelong facial paralysis. Approximately 1,000 people in the U.S. have the disorder.

SPEECH AND LANGUAGE DIFFICULTIES

- Inability to move the lips.
- High-arched palate.
- Paralysis of soft palate.
- Short or deformed tongue.
- Limited tongue movement.
- Dysarthria.
- Sounds formed with the lips are most affected, due to unilateral or bilateral underdevelopment or paralysis of the seventh cranial nerve. Poor saliva control also affects articulation.

ASSOCIATED AND OTHER DIFFICULTIES

- Inability to smile, frown, or show any emotion on the face.
- Inability to blink or move the eyes laterally.
- Difficulty with feeding and swallowing beginning early with inability to suck.
- Choking; aspiration.
- Fluid secretions of the mouth may be breathed into the lungs, resulting in bronchopneumonia.
- Pneumonia.
- Hearing problems.
- Poor muscle tone, which may result in breathing and respiratory problems.
- Weakness in palatal and tongue muscles also may be present.
- Intellectual impairment occurs in approximately 10% to 15% of cases.
- Club foot.
- Other abnormalities of the feet and hands.
- Congenital dislocation of the hip may occur.
- Mild spastic diplegia.

ASSESSMENT

- Administer *Assessment of Intelligibility of Dysarthric Speakers.*
- Administer *Frenchay Dysarthria Assessment* (FDA).
- Assess respiratory function.

INTERVENTION TECHNIQUES

- Treat dysphagia in early months of life.
- Provide therapy exercises following "smile surgery" in which a segment of the gracilis muscle from the thigh is transplanted to each side of the face (Breske, 1997).
- Consider use of biofeedback.
- Work to improve lip strength and fine motor control.

RESULTS OF RECENT STUDIES

No recent studies regarding communication skills were found in the literature.

PROGNOSIS

Life span is near normal.

REFERENCES

Breske S. Facing the challenges of Moebius Syndrome. *Advance for Speech-Language Pathologists & Audiologists.* 1997;7(1):17.

Gilbert P. *The A-Z Reference Book of Syndromes and Inherited Disorders: A Manual for Health, Social and Education Workers.* New York: Chapman & Hall. 1993:148–50.

Jones KL. *Smith's Recognizable Patterns of Human Malformation*, 5th ed. Philadelphia: W.B. Saunders Co. 1997:230–1.

Murdoch BE, SM Johnson, DG Theodoros. Physiological and perceptual features of dysarthria in Moebius syndrome: directions for treatment. *Pediatric Rehabilitation.* 1997;1(2):83-97.

Thoene JG, NP Coker, eds. *Physicians' Guide to Rare Diseases.* New York: Dowden Publishing Co. 1995:106.

Pierre Robin Syndrome

(See also Clefts of the Lip and Palate)

DESCRIPTION

This condition occurs when, prior to 9 weeks in utero, the tongue becomes posteriorly located, interfering with closure of the posterior palatal shelves and resulting in micrognathia, glossoptosis, and U-shaped cleft of the soft palate.

ETIOLOGY

The syndrome may be the result of autosomal-recessive inheritance or also may be caused by mechanical constraint of the fetus within the womb. Recent research suggests that the condition may appear more frequently in infants born to mothers who take drugs during their pregnancy.

SPEECH AND LANGUAGE DIFFICULTIES

- Hypernasality.

(See also Clefts of the Lip and Palate)

ASSOCIATED AND OTHER DIFFICULTIES

- Placement of the tongue may obstruct normal breathing, resulting in failure to thrive, apnea, and dysphagia.
- Dental abnormalities.
- Pulmonary disturbances.
- Vomiting.
- Sleep disturbances.
- Mental retardation may occur secondary to hypoxia and upper airway obstruction.

ASSESSMENT

(See Clefts of the Lip and Palate)

INTERVENTION TECHNIQUES

- Treat for dysphagia in early life.
- Consider early use of augumentive and alternative communication (AAC) and consider that such use may enhance development of natural speech.

(See also Clefts of the Lip and Palate)

RESULTS OF RECENT STUDIES

- For optimum speech results, clients with Pierre Robin syndrome require a second surgery more often than do those with nonsyndromic cleft palate. (Haapanen, et al., 1996)

PROGNOSIS

Up to 30% of children born with the syndrome may not survive due to complications of airway obstruction. For those who do survive the first few years of life, and who do not have multiple malformation syndrome, the prognosis is very good.

REFERENCES

Gilbert P. *A-Z Reference Book of Syndromes and Inherited Disorders: A Manual for Health, Social and Education Workers*. New York: Chapman & Hall. 1993:165–7.

Haapanen ML, S Laitinen, M Passo, R Ranta. Quality of speech correlated to craniofacial characteristics of cleft palate patients with the Pierre Robin sequence. *Folia Phoniatrica et Logopaedica*. 1996;48:215–22.

Jones KL. *Smith's Recognizable Patterns of Human Malformation*, 5th ed. Philadelphia: W.B. Saunders Co. 1997:234–5.

Lehman JA, JRA Fishman, GS Neiman. Treatment of cleft palate associated with Robin sequence: appraisal of risk factors. *Cleft Palate-Craniofacial Journal*. 1995;32(1):25–29.

Scott A. Improving natural speech. *Advance for Speech-Language Pathologists & Audiologists*. 1998;8(7):9.

Thoene JG, NP Coker, eds. *Physicians' Guide to Rare Diseases*. New York: Dowden Publishing Co. 1995:123.

Rett Syndrome (RS)

DESCRIPTION

A severe neurological disorder that affects only females. Estimates of incidence range from 1 in 10,000 to 1 in 20,000 births. Initial symptoms appear after the first 7 to 18 months of life. Some developmental abilities, such as early expressive language skills and hand use, are acquired early in life but may be lost during regression. A repetitive hand-wringing motion is characteristic.

ETIOLOGY

Rett syndrome is an X-linked dominant genetic disorder; a degenerative disease with progressive encephalopathy.

SPEECH AND LANGUAGE DIFFICULTIES

- Severely disordered speech and language skills. Speech and language skills acquired prior to regression may be—but are not always—preserved.
- Delayed auditory processing.
- Oral dyspraxia.
- Dysarthria.
- Severe expressive deficits may mask somewhat higher comprehension.

ASSOCIATED AND OTHER DIFFICULTIES

- Severe to profound intellectual impairment.
- Epilepsy.
- Dyspraxia.
- Abnormal breathing patterns.
- Severely limited if any functional hand use.
- Visual skills are a relative strength, but clients may need longer than average time for visual processing.
- Feeding problems caused by oral motor dysfunction, oral pharyngeal problems, and/or gastroesophageal reflux. Contributors to feeding prob-

lems include abnormal tongue movements, cervical and upper thoracic spinal alignment, neck and shoulder girdle rigidity, and excessive neck extension.
- Scoliosis.
- Deterioration of fine and gross motor abilities.
- Self-feeding, if attained, may be lost.

ASSESSMENT
- Administer *Clinical Linguistic Auditory Milestone Scale (CLAMS)*.

Diagnostic Criteria for Rett Syndrome

A. All of the following:
    (1) apparently normal prenatal and perinatal development
    (2) apparently normal psychomotor development through the first 5 months after birth
    (3) normal head circumference at birth

B. Onset of all of the following after the period of normal development:
    (1) deceleration of head growth between ages 5 and 48 months
    (2) loss of previously acquired purposeful hand skills between ages 5 and 30 months with the subsequent development of stereotyped hand movements (e.g., hand-wringing or hand washing)
    (3) loss of social engagement early in the course (although often social interaction develops later)
    (4) appearance of poorly coordinated gait or trunk movements
    (5) severely impaired expressive and receptive language development with severe psychomotor retardation

Source: Reprinted with permission from the *Diagnostic and Statistical Manual of Mental Disorders,* Fourth Edition. Copyright 1994 American Psychiatric Association.

- Through observation and parent report, evaluate responses to cause and effect, making choices, following simple commands, and showing recognition of objects and people.
- Evaluate potential for alternative forms of communication.
- Evaluate for dysphagia.

INTERVENTION TECHNIQUES

- Because visual skills are a relative strength, encourage eye gaze for communication.
- Work with others on team to address feeding problems.

RESULTS OF RECENT STUDIES

No recent studies regarding communication skills were found in the literature.

PROGNOSIS

Deterioration continues, and death often occurs by age 40 years.

REFERENCES

Budden SS. Management of Rett syndrome: a ten year experience. *Neuropediatrics.* 1995;26:75–77.

Gilbert P. *The A-Z Reference Book of Syndromes and Inherited Disorders: A Manual for Health, Social and Education Workers.* New York: Chapman & Hall. 1993:179–81.

Smith MD, JS Damico. *Childhood Language Disorders.* New York: Thieme Medical Publishers, Inc. 1996:161–2.

Tams-Little S, G Holdgrafer. Early communication development in children with Rett syndrome. *Brain & Development.* 1996;18:376–8.

Thoene JG, NP Coker, eds. *Physicians' Guide to Rare Diseases.* New York: Dowden Publishing Co. 1995:125.

von Tetzchner S, KH Jacobsen, L Smith, OH Skjeldal, A Heiberg, JF Fagan. Vision, cognition and developmental characteristics of girls and women with Rett syndrome. *Developmental Medicine and Child Neurology.* 1996;38:212–5.

Spina Bifida

(See also Hydrocephalus and MASA Syndrome)

DESCRIPTION

A neural tube defect affecting closure of the vertebral column. The defect is most common in the lumbar, low thoracic, or sacral regions, resulting in varying degrees of paralysis below the affected area. Bladder and rectal functions generally are affected, and kidneys may become damaged. Hydrocephalus also may occur.

Shortly after birth, surgery is performed to close the opening in the back. When hydrocephalus is present, a second surgery is performed to insert a cerebrospinal fluid shunt.

Incidence is approximately 1 in 2,000 live births in the United States. Incidence is higher in Ireland and Wales and is less common in Israel and among Jews in general. Occurrence is three to four times greater among lower socioeconomic groups in all cultures. If one child has spina bifida, there is some increased risk of subsequent siblings having the condition. Eighty percent of those with spina bifida have normal intelligence.

ETIOLOGY

Although an exact etiology is unknown, it is known that the malformation causing spina bifida occurs within 26 days of fertilization. There is an apparent strong link between folic acid deficiency and the development of neural tube defects. Women who have had one child born with a neural tube defect reduce the risk of reccurrence by 70% by taking folic acid. Within the general population, occurrence may be reduced by 50% when supplemental folic acid is taken by women contemplating a pregnancy. (Liptak, 1997)

SPEECH AND LANGUAGE DIFFICULTIES

• "Cocktail party syndrome," in which utterances frequently are not related to the topic; content is superficial, and expressions are overused.
• Deficits in comprehension of abstract vocabulary.

- Use of words and phrases in inappropriate contexts, indicating deficits in comprehension.
- Frequent repetition of a limited number of topics.
- Difficulty maintaining turn-taking exchanges.
- Tendency to dominate conversation.
- Introduction of irrelevant topics.

ASSOCIATED AND OTHER DIFFICULTIES

- Congenitally dislocated hips.
- Club feet.
- Approximately 30% develop seizures.
- Increased incidence of strabismus.
- Arnold-Chiari malformation, a displacement of the posterior portion of the brain into the cervical spinal canal, leading to difficulty swallowing, choking, frequent gagging, breath-holding, apnea, hoarseness, and a tendency to hold the head arched backward.
- Difficulty with bladder and bowel control.
- Paralysis and sensory loss, the extent of which depends on the location of the defect in the spinal cord.
- Loss of sensation may lead to injuries that are not felt and thus not recognized.
- Scoliosis.
- Kyphosis.
- Kyphoscoliosis.
- Skin sores and decubitus ulcers.
- At risk for obesity.
- Allergy to latex is common.
- High incidence of learning disabilities, often with specific deficits in attention, perception, and language.
- Memory deficits.
- Difficulty maintaining attention.
- Difficulty with organizational skills.
- Difficulty isolating relevant from irrelevant stimuli.
- Deficits in figure-ground perception.
- Difficulty with fine motor skills.
- Difficulty with visual-motor skills.
- Difficulty with mathematics.

- Symptoms of a blocked shunt include lethargy, headache, vomiting, and irritability. More subtle signs include a change in personality, decline in school performance, or weakness of the arms and legs. (Liptak, 1997)
- Tendency to be overly friendly and too personal.
- Learned helplessness.

ASSESSMENT

- An in-depth evaluation is essential and should include tests of listening and reading comprehension, knowledge of abstract concepts, narrative, conversational, metalinguistic, and problem-solving skills. (Culatta, 1993a)
- Assess listening comprehension by having the client answer questions about a story that has been read aloud by the examiner. Assess inferential as well as factual understanding. Administer tests such as *Burns/Roe Informal Reading Inventory* or *Diagnostic Reading Scales*.
- Assess ability to produce relevant remarks in relation to specific task demands through administration of the *Preschool Language Assessment Instrument (PLAI)*.
- Assess student's understanding of his or her texts.
- To assess metalinguistic, metaphoric, and problem-solving skills, administer tests such as *Test of Problem Solving (TOPS)*, *Analysis of the Language of Learning (ALL)*, *Ross Test of Higher Cognitive Processes*, *The Language Processing Test* and the *Word Test*.
- Assess comprehension of abstract concepts informally by having the student demonstrate knowledge.
- Assess conversational skills by observing, with different communication partners, the student's ability to maintain exchanges and elaborate on a topic. Observe whether the student frequently repeats the same content, dominates the conversation, changes the topic abruptly or introduces irrelevant statements. (Culatta, 1993b)
- Evaluate narrative skills by staging an unusual experience and having the student relate the experience to someone who was not present. Assess organization, detail, sequence, and inclusion of unusual events.

INTERVENTION TECHNIQUES

- Teach abstract words and concepts by presenting many examples, exaggerating the relevant characteristics, varying the types of examples, pro-

viding explanations, providing reasons for identification and calling attention to real-world examples. (Culatta, 1993a)
- Assist classroom teachers in developing strategies such as ensuring preferential seating, cueing the student to remain on task, and tailoring the complexity of material that is presented.
- Work with students to develop pragmatic skills.

RESULTS OF RECENT STUDIES

- The *PLAI* was used to compare the discourse skills at four levels of abstraction of children with spina bifida and a group of children matched by language-age. While the two groups performed comparably on concrete tasks, and while the performance of both groups showed deterioration as tasks became more abstract, those with spina bifida produced significantly more "no response" and irrelevant responses. (Culatta and Young, 1992)

PROGNOSIS

Prognosis is dependent on the number and severity of abnormalities. Approximately 85% survive to adulthood. One study found that less than 12% had minimal disabilities, average intelligence, community ambulation, and well-managed continence; 52% had moderate disability with borderline intelligence; 37% had severe disability with mental retardation, incontinence, and dependence for most self-help skills. Overall, about 25% were employed. (Hunt, 1990, reported by Liptak, 1997)

REFERENCES

Culatta B. Developing abstract concepts. In: Rowley-Kelly FL, DH Reigel, eds. *Teaching the Student with Spina Bifida.* Baltimore: Paul H. Brookes Publishing Co. 1993a: 125–43.

Culatta B. Intervening for language-learning disabilities. In: Rowley-Kelly FL, DH Reigel, eds. *Teaching the Student with Spina Bifida.* Baltimore: Paul H. Brookes Publishing Co. 1993b:171–191.

Culatta B, C Young. Linguistic performance as a function of abstract task demands in children with spina bifida. *Developmental Medicine and Child Neurology.* 1992;34(5): 434–40.

Liptak GS. Neural tube defects. In: Batshaw ML, ed. *Children with Disabilities*, 4th ed. Baltimore: Paul H. Brookes Publishing Co. 1997:529–52.

Thoene JG, NP Coker, eds. *Physicians' Guide to Rare Diseases.* New York: Dowden Publishing Co. 1995:376–7.

Tourette Syndrome (Gilles de la Tourette's Syndrome) (TS)

DESCRIPTION

TS is the most severe of the tic disorders. Tics are defined as involuntary, rapid, and repetitive movements occurring suddenly and irregularly. Incidence of TS is approximately 5 of every 1,000 persons. Males are more likely to be affected, with the male to female ratio in children 9:1 and in adults 3:1. The condition may be present in approximately 1.6% of the pediatric population. Symptoms generally appear between the ages of 5 and 10 years. Less than 30% of those with TS develop either coprolalia or copropraxia. Stress exacerbates the symptoms of TS. TS is not progressive and not degenerative.

ETIOLOGY

An autosomal-dominant multiple tic disorder that begins in childhood. The disorder begins with simple tics and progresses to multiple, complex movements including vocal and respiratory tics. TS may be a polygenic disorder of the genes involved in the metabolism of dopamine, serotonin, norepinephrine, and other neurotransmitters. (Comings, et al., 1996)

SPEECH AND LANGUAGE DIFFICULTIES

- Approximately 10% have delayed onset of speech.
- Approximately 25% of children have rapid or loud speech.
- Vocal tics may begin as grunting or barking noises and evolve into compulsive utterances.
- Coprolalia (involuntary obscenities).
- Echolalia.

- Imitation of others' accents, pitch changes, and mispronunciations of words.
- May carry on conversations with oneself, assuming different identities.
- Dysfluencies.
- Uneven rhythm while speaking.
- May exhibit poor pragmatic skills.

ASSOCIATED AND OTHER DIFFICULTIES

- Alcohol and drug abuse.
- Depression.
- Inattention.
- Impulsivity.
- Hyperactivity.
- Sleep disorders.
- Conduct disorders.
- Learning disorders.
- Impaired organizational skills.
- Impaired motor skills.
- Anxiety disorders.
- Sexual disorders.
- Copropraxia (involuntary obscene gestures).
- Severe tics may be physically and socially disabling. Common complex tics include touching people or objects, smelling fingers or objects, jumping or skipping, poking or jabbing, punching, kicking, hopping, flapping arms, twirling around, tensing muscle groups, imitating movements of others. (Packer and Gentile, 1994)
- Attention deficit hyperactivity disorder (ADHD).
- Low tolerance for frustration.
- Obsessive compulsive disorder (OCD).
- Aggressiveness.
- Immaturity.
- Withdrawal.

ASSESSMENT

- Assess receptive and expressive language skills.
- Assess pragmatic skills in a variety of situations.

Diagnostic Criteria for Tourette Syndrome

A. Both multiple motor and one or more vocal tics have been present at some time during the illness, although not necessarily concurrently. (A tic is a sudden, rapid, recurrent, nonrhythmic, stereotyped motor movement or vocalization.)

B. The tics occur many times a day (usually in bouts) nearly every day or intermittently throughout a period of more than 1 year, and during the period there was never a tic-free period of more than 3 consecutive months.

C. The disturbance causes marked distress or significant impairment in social, occupational, or other important areas of functioning.

D. The onset is before age 18 years.

E. The disturbance is not due to the direct physiological effects of a substance (e.g., stimulants) or a general medical condition (e.g., Huntington's disease or postviral encephalitis).

Source: Reprinted with permission from the *Diagnostic and Statistical Manual of Mental Disorders,* Fourth Edition. Copyright 1994 American Psychiatric Association.

INTERVENTION TECHNIQUES
- Differentiate dysfluencies from tics, and treat tics as a separate disorder.
- Provide group therapy to address pragmatic skills.

RESULTS OF RECENT STUDIES
- Current studies indicate that coprolalia is less frequent in younger patients with TS than was previously believed. (Goldenberg, et al., 1994)
- The relationship between severity of tics and behavioral problems is not a simple linear one. (Rosenberg, et al., 1995)

- Clients with concurrent TS and Asperger's disorder (AD) generally show developmental brain anomalies from magnetic resonance imaging (MRI). In most clients with TS only, MRI scans are normal. The two groups were not significantly different in the severity of motor or phonic tics or on measures of general intelligence, memory, and language function. Those with TS and AD had histories of more psychiatric hospitalizations, poorer academic achievement, and greater difficulty with complex problem-solving and spatial tests. (Berthier, et al., 1993)

PROGNOSIS

Symptoms generally worsen during the first decade following onset. Then, in about 70% of individuals, severity and frequency of tics decreases in the late teen years. Life expectancy is normal.

REFERENCES

Berthier ML, A Bayes, ES Tolosa. Magnetic resonance imaging in patients with concurrent Tourette's disorder and Asperger's syndrome. *Journal of the American Academy of Child & Adolescent Psychiatry.* 1993;32(3):633–9.

Burd L, C Leech, J Kerbeshian, GG Gascon. A review of the relationship between Gilles de la Tourette syndrome and speech and language. *Journal of Developmental and Physical Disabilities.* 1994;6(3):271–89.

Comings DE, S Wu, C Chiu, R Ring, R Gade, C Ahn, JP MacMurray, G Dietz, D Muhleman. Polygenic inheritance of Tourette syndrome, stuttering, attention deficit hyperactivity, conduct, and oppositional defiant disorder: the additive and subtractive effect of the three dopaminergic genes—DRD2, D beta H, and DAT1. *American Journal of Medical Genetics.* 1996;67(3):264–88.

Goldenberg J, SB Brown, WJ Weiner. Coprolalia in younger patients with Gilles de la Tourette syndrome. *Movement Disorders.* 1994;9(6):622–5.

Packer LE, M Gentile. Tourette Syndrome and child development: school-based treatment. *Advance for Speech-Language Pathologists & Audiologists.* 1994;4(27):8–9.

Rosenberg LA, J Brown, GS Singer. Behavioral problems and severity of tics. *Journal of Clinical Psychology.* 1995;51(6):760–7.

Trace R. Treating communication disorders in patients with Tourette Syndrome. *Advance for Speech-Language Pathologists & Audiologists.* 1994;4(27):12–13.

Walkup JT, LD Scahill, MA Riddle. Disruptive behavior, hyperactivity, and learning disabilities in children with Tourette's syndrome. In: Weiner WJ, AE Lang, eds. *Behavioral Neurology of Movement Disorders.* New York: Raven Press. 1995:259–72.

Treacher Collins Syndrome

(See also Clefts of the Lip and Palate)

DESCRIPTION

A rare genetic disorder characterized by slanted eyes, dysphagia, deafness, and deformities of the maxilla, mandible, and ears. (Thoene and Coker, 1995) Physical characteristics include a long face, slanted eyes, a beaklike nose, a receding chin, and maxillary and mandibular hypoplasia. Intelligence is generally not affected. Incidence is approximately 1 in 50,000 live births, with males and females affected in equal numbers.

ETIOLOGY

The affected gene is the long arm of chromosome number 5 (5q31.3-32).

SPEECH AND LANGUAGE DIFFICULTIES

• Muffled resonance.

(See also Clefts of the Lip and Palate)

ASSOCIATED AND OTHER DIFFICULTIES

• Difficulty with feeding.
• Cleft palate.
• Small or absent external ears.
• Tympanic membrane abnormalities.
• Middle ear cavity may be absent or abnormally small; ossicles may be absent or poorly developed.
• Conductive deafness.
• Respiratory problems.
• Intermittent cyanosis.
• Small pharynx.
• Partial or total absence of lower eyelashes.
• Strabismus.

ASSESSMENT
• In very young children, evaluate feeding skills and oral-motor skills.

(See also Clefts of the Lip and Palate)

INTERVENTION TECHNIQUES
(See Clefts of the Lip and Palate)

RESULTS OF RECENT STUDIES
No recent studies regarding communication skills were found in the literature.

PROGNOSIS
Life expectancy is normal.

REFERENCES

Jones KL. *Smith's Recognizable Patterns of Human Malformation,* 5th ed. Philadelphia: W.B. Saunders Co. 1997:250.

Thoene JG, NP Coker, eds. *Physicians' Guide to Rare Diseases.* New York: Dowden Publishing Co. 1995:147.

Witzel MA. Communicative impairment associated with clefting. In: Shprintzen RJ, J Bardach, eds. *Cleft Palate Speech Management: A Multidisciplinary Approach.* St. Louis, Mo: Mosby. 1996:137–66.

Usher Syndrome

DESCRIPTION
An inherited disorder characterized by night blindness, vision loss, and deafness. There are four forms of the disorder. Usher syndrome type 1 (USH1) is characterized by complete neurosensory deafness at birth,

night-vision problems beginning before age 10 years, and progressive loss of peripheral vision. Usher syndrome type 2 (USH2) is characterized by moderate to severe neurosensory deafness at birth and mild to moderate visual field loss. Usher syndrome type 3 (USH3) generally begins in puberty with progressive hearing loss. Usher syndrome type 4 (USH4) is extremely rare, affects mostly males, and is characterized by hearing loss and progressive visual problems.

Incidence of Usher syndrome is 5 in 100,000 to 10 in 100,000. Incidence of USH1 is higher in persons of French Canadian descent in Canada, Louisiana, and east Texas; in persons of Jewish descent in Berlin, Germany; in Nigerians; and in Argentineans of Spanish descent. Usher syndrome is the leading cause of deaf-blindness in early adulthood.

ETIOLOGY

Inheritance for USH1, USH2, and USH3 is autosomal recessive. USH4 is thought to be inherited as an X-linked recessive trait. The gene for USH2 has been mapped to chromosome 1q41; USH3 has been mapped to chromosome 3q.

SPEECH AND LANGUAGE DIFFICULTIES

- Speech may be absent, severely unintelligible, or moderately to mildly unintelligible, depending on severity and time of onset of the hearing loss.

ASSOCIATED AND OTHER DIFFICULTIES

- Profound sensorineural hearing loss.
- Peripheral vision may begin to become limited later in childhood. Complete blindness may gradually occur. Cataracts may also be present.
- Ataxia.

ASSESSMENT

(See Hearing Loss—Children and Adolescents; Hearing Loss—Adults; Dual-Sensory Impairment)

INTERVENTION TECHNIQUES

• Consider use of sign language and consider tactile sign language if visual defect warrants.

(See also Hearing Loss—Children and Adolescents; Hearing Loss—Adults; Dual-Sensory Impairment)

RESULTS OF RECENT STUDIES

No recent studies regarding communication skills were found in the literature.

PROGNOSIS

A normal life span may be expected, although severe visual and auditory handicaps are generally present by early adulthood.

REFERENCES

Everson JM, ed. *Supporting Young Adults Who Are Deaf-Blind in Their Communities: A Transition Planning Guide for Service Providers, Families, and Friends.* Baltimore: Paul H. Brookes Publishing Co. 1995.

Gilbert P. *The A-Z Reference Book of Syndromes and Inherited Disorders: A Manual for Health, Social and Education Workers.* New York: Chapman & Hall. 1993:218–20.

Thoene JG, NP Coker, eds. *Physicians' Guide to Rare Diseases.* New York: Dowden Publishing Co. 1995:814–5

Waardenburg Syndrome

DESCRIPTION

A hereditary disorder characterized by deafness and abnormalities of the face and hair. Partial albinism is present and is most notably marked by a white forelock and premature graying. Other features are a thin nose and full lips. Clefts of the lip and palate, cardiac anomalies, esophageal atresia, and upper limb defects also may occur. Incidence is 1 in 4,000 live births, with males and females affected equally. Among children who are deaf from birth, 3 in every 100 have Waardenburg syndrome.

ETIOLOGY

The condition is inherited through dominant genes. Mutations on PAX3, a gene on chromosome 2q35-37, have been identified, as have mutations to chromosome 3q12-p14.1.

SPEECH AND LANGUAGE DIFFICULTIES

(See Clefts of the Lip and Palate; Hearing Loss—Children and Adolescents)

ASSOCIATED AND OTHER DIFFICULTIES

• Congenital sensorineural deafness.
• Glaucoma may develop.
• Small nose, which may lead to more frequent upper respiratory infections.

ASSESSMENT

(See Clefts of the Lip and Palate; Hearing Loss—Children and Adolescents)

INTERVENTION TECHNIQUES

(See Clefts of the Lip and Palate; Hearing Loss—Children and Adolescents)

RESULTS OF RECENT STUDIES

No recent studies regarding communication skills were found in the literature.

PROGNOSIS

Life expectancy is normal.

REFERENCES

Gilbert P. *The A-Z Reference Book of Syndromes and Inherited Disorders: A Manual for Health, Social and Education Workers.* New York: Chapman & Hall. 1993:224–6.

Jones KL. *Smith's Recognizable Patterns of Human Malformation,* 5th ed. Philadelphia: W.B. Saunders Co. 1997:248.

Thoene JG, NP Coker, eds. *Physicians' Guide to Rare Diseases.* New York: Dowden Publishing Co. 1995:158.

Wiedemann H-R, J Kunze. *Clinical Syndromes,* 3rd ed. English Translation. London: Times Mirror International, Mosby-Wolfe. 1997:390–1.

Chapter 3

Neurological Disorders

- Acquired childhood aphasia (ACA) and cerebrovascular accidents (CVA) in children
- Alzheimer's disease (AD)
- Amyotrophic lateral sclerosis (ALS)
- Brainstem stroke
- Brain tumors
- Cerebrovascular accidents (CVA) in adults—left hemisphere damage (LHD)
- Cerebrovascular accidents (CVA) in adults—right hemisphere damage (RHD)
- Encephalitis
- Epilepsy
- Friedreich's ataxia (FA)
- Guillain-Barré syndrome (GBS)
- Head injury (HI)—adults
- Head injury (HI)—children and adolescents
- Huntington's disease (HD)
- Motor neuron disease (MND)
- Multi-infarct dementia (MID)
- Multiple sclerosis (MS)
- Muscular dystrophy (MD)
- Myasthenia gravis (MG)
- Neurofibromatosis type 1 (NF1)
- Parkinson's disease (PD)
- Pick's disease
- Postpolio (poliomyelitis) syndrome (PPS)
- Primary progressive aphasia (PPA)
- Progressive supranuclear palsy (PSP)
- Pseudobulbar palsy (PBP)
- Shy-Drager syndrome

Acquired Childhood Aphasia (ACA) and Cerebrovascular Accidents (CVA) in Children

DESCRIPTION

A CVA often is preceded by an apparently mild illness or follows a prolonged seizure. Incidence is about 3,700 cases per year.

(See also Cerebrovascular Accidents [CVA] in Adults—Left Hemisphere Damage)

ETIOLOGY

The CVA may be occlusive or hemorrhagic and may be caused by trauma, metabolic disorders, or neoplasm.

SPEECH AND LANGUAGE DIFFICULTIES

- Mutism immediately post-CVA.
- Dysarthria.
- Aphasia.
- Naming deficits.
- Verbal apraxia.

ASSOCIATED AND OTHER DIFFICULTIES

- Hemiparesis or quadriparesis.
- Visual impairments.
- Learning disabilities.
- Ataxia.
- Drooling may be evident.
- Behavior disorders.

ASSESSMENT

- Administer *Frenchay Dysarthria Assessment* (FDA).
- Evaluate respiratory function for speech.

- Administer *Boston Naming Test* (BNT).
- Administer *McCarthy Scales of Children's Abilities.*

INTERVENTION TECHNIQUES

- Provide augmentative and alternative communication (AAC) as needed, especially immediately following the CVA.
- Provide articulation therapy and therapy to improve breath support and overall intelligibility.

RESULTS OF RECENT STUDIES

- In one study of children who sustained unilateral, focal brain lesions as the result of prenatal or perinatal strokes, a decline in overall IQ, as measured by the Wechsler Intelligence Scale, was noted in subjects with both left hemisphere (LH) and right hemisphere (RH) damage. Within the LH group, verbal and performance abilities were equally affected. Within the RH group, performance abilities were more adversely affected than verbal skills. Across the LH and RH groups, nonverbal abilities were equally affected, while verbal abilities were preserved to a greater extent in the RH group. (Ballantyne, et al., 1994)

PROGNOSIS

Language outcomes are variable. In a group of children assessed 2 years after acute onset of aphasia, outcomes ranged from near-normal language performance to nonfluent aphasias and persistent problems with auditory-verbal comprehension and naming. (Lees, 1997)

Prognosis for normal functioning is improved if the stroke occurs after the age of 2 years and if the stroke is not associated with status epilepticus. (Burg, et al., 1996)

REFERENCES

Ballantyne AO, KM Scarvie, DA Trauner. Verbal and performance IQ patterns in children after perinatal stroke. *Developmental Neuropsychology.* 1994;10(1):39–50.

Burg FD, ER Wald, JR Ingelfinger, RA Polin. *Gellis & Kegan's Current Pediatric Therapy.* Philadelphia: W.B. Saunders Co. 1996;15:111–12.

Casby MW. Acquired childhood language disorders. In: Smith MD, JS Damico, eds. *Childhood Language Disorders*. New York: Thieme Medical Publishers, Inc. 1996: 198–217.

Horton SK, BE Murdoch, DO Theodoros, EC Thompson. Motor speech impairment in a case of childhood basilar artery stroke: treatment directions derived from physiological and perceptual assessment. *Pediatric Rehabilitation*. 1997;1(3):163–77.

Hynd GW, J Leathem, M Semrud-Clikeman, KL Hern, M Wenner. Anomic aphasia in childhood. *Journal of Child Neurology*. 1995;10:289–93.

Lees J. Long-term effects of acquired aphasias in childhood. *Pediatric Rehabilitation*. 1997;1(1):45–49.

Alzheimer's Disease (AD)

DESCRIPTION

AD is the major cause of dementia. It affects 10% of the population by age 65 years and half of all people who live to age 85 years. Alzheimer's presenile generally begins in the fifth and sixth decades, while Alzheimer's senile onset dementia generally begins in the seventh and eighth decades. The two are similar in both clinical and pathologic features. The dementia is progressive and is well advanced in 2 to 3 years. Early symptoms are widely variable but often include memory loss, depression, paranoia, or anxiety. As the disease progresses, there is disintegration of personality and intellect due to impaired insight and judgment and loss of affect.

ETIOLOGY

A degenerative process with a loss of cells from the basal forebrain, cerebral cortex, and other areas of the brain. Acetylcholine-transmitting neurons and their target nerve cells are particularly affected. Worsening of symptoms parallels growth of amyloid deposits in the brain. Laboratory experiments indicate that the formation of amyloid fibers may be accelerated by advanced glycosylation end products (AGEs).

SPEECH AND LANGUAGE DIFFICULTIES

- Communication skills are always disrupted.
- Memory impairment is present and increases over time. Recent memory is impaired sooner than memory for remote events.
- Recognition memory is generally preserved.
- Aphasia may be present.
- Word retrieval problems during conversation are common.
- Semantic paraphasias.
- Marked deficits in confrontational naming.
- Repetitiveness.
- Circumlocutions during discourse.
- Digression from topic.
- Echolalia.
- Use of word intrusions—inappropriate recurrences of words used earlier.
- Jargon and/or unintelligible speech.
- In early stages: occasional repetition of ideas, but topic is preserved, mild word-finding difficulties, imprecise answers to questions.
- In middle stages: more frequent repetitions, revision of ideas, decrease in amount of information conveyed, increase in self-referential comments.
- In late stages: increased repetitions and revisions, further reduction in number of ideas expressed, decreased mean-length of utterance, violations in turn-taking (either excessive talking or failure to initiate speech).

ASSOCIATED AND OTHER DIFFICULTIES

- Progressive memory, orientation, and intellectual deterioration.
- Motor apraxia may be present.
- Spatial disorientation.

ASSESSMENT

- Periodically reassess cognitive status for revision of communication strategies.
- Assess hearing and consider an assistive hearing device if warranted.
- Use a collaborative team approach and integrate information from medical and laboratory studies, neuroimaging and neuropsychological tests, and speech and language tests.

- Assess speech and language skills with formal tests for comprehension of language, pragmatics, syntax, phonology, word learning, and semantics, including lexical comprehension, confrontation naming, and word fluency.
- In addition to formal language skills, assess functional skills in real-life settings.
- Administer *Functional Communication Profile* (FCP).
- Use all or portions of *Boston Diagnostic Aphasia Examination* (BDAE).
- Use *Fuld Object-Memory Evaluation* to test for word intrusions.
- Administer *Mini-Mental State Examination* (MMSE).
- Assess strengths as well as weaknesses and use strengths in programming.
- Assess and address concerns of caregivers.

INTERVENTION TECHNIQUES

- Be aware that many clients with AD also have hearing loss. Fitting these clients with a hearing aid may result in improved behaviors.
- Goal of therapy is to maximize remaining communication function.
- Focus therapy on maximizing and maintaining functional skills.
- Work to stabilize routines and begin early to introduce compensatory strategies that will be used later as the disease progresses.
- Instruct caregivers to give verbal reminders to enhance eating (take another bite, then chew, then swallow).
- Teach caregivers the seven-step FOCUSED program: face-to-face speaking; orient to topic; continue the topic; unstick communication block by supplying a word the client can't remember; structure questions so they can be answered by "yes" or "no," or with a closed set of choices, exchange conversation, keep it going, and do not ask "test" questions; and use direct, short sentences. (Trace, 1996)
- Use nonlanguage cues.
- Use cues and reminders such as colored stickers.
- Use colorful pictures as aids to communication. For example, place bright pictures of different foods on walls of the dining room in a nursing home. Residents may be prompted to point to what they want. (Eisner, 1997)
- Maintain eye contact.
- Reduce environmental distractions and excess stimulation as much as possible when communicating.

- In the early stage of the disease, involve clients in support groups.
- In the middle and late stages of the disease, focus treatment on the caregiver rather than the client.
- Even in the end stages of the disease, clients may have some limited success with conversation. To facilitate this, use attention-arousing signals such as a touch or using the client's name before attempting to communicate; allow sufficient time for the client to join the conversation; allow for long pauses before the client responds; encourage response through repetitions and rephrasing; request clarification when the client's message is unclear, supplement verbal messages with physical contextual cues when addressing the client; use yes or no questions, or questions with the provision of two choices, rather than open-ended questions; provide frequent opportunities for communication but do not expect the client to initiate conversation. (Lamar, et al., 1994)
- Use the Communication Enhancement Model to facilitate interactions between the client and caregivers. (Orange, et al., 1995)

RESULTS OF RECENT STUDIES

- Persons with onset of aphasia early in the course of AD show over time a more rapid decline on *MMSE* scores than do those without early onset of aphasia. (Yesavage, et al., 1993)
- Deficits in language expression are correlated with incidence of total aggression, verbal aggression, and aggression toward objects, while deficits in comprehension are more clearly correlated with physical aggression toward others. (Welsh, et al., 1996)
- When compared with clients with Huntington's disease (HD) and those with progressive supranuclear palsy (PSP), those with AD did just as poorly on tasks of category fluency but were less impaired on tasks of letter fluency. On these tasks, which involve naming as many words as possible beginning with a given letter, the performance of the clients with AD was near normal. This suggests that the poorer performance on category naming is due to a breakdown of semantic knowledge, possibly reflecting temporal neocortical involvement. (Rosser and Hodges, 1994)
- In a study of one-page autobiographies of 25 nuns written at an average age of 22 years, a relationship was found between the degree of linguistic ability (idea density and grammatical complexity) early in life and subsequent diagnosis of AD. Those whose autobiographies showed low

idea density early in life were more likely to exhibit poor cognitive function and AD later in life. (Snowdon, et al., 1996)

- In a recent study, clients with AD were placed in either a music reminiscence group or a verbal reminiscence group that met for 30-minute sessions, twice a week for 10 months. Those in the music group showed significant improvement in recognition memory and a marked decrease in agitation. (Anonymous, 1997)
- As the disease progresses, markedly fewer requests for clarification are made during conversation, indicating decreasing ability to assess comprehension ability and needs. (Hamilton, 1994)
- In a study comparing confrontation naming performance of clients in differing stages of AD, results indicated that the errors of those in the early stages were more likely to be semantic, while the errors of those in later stages were more likely to be no-relationship errors. (Chenery, et al., 1996)
- In a study comparing loss of prosody in clients with AD and in clients with multi-infarct dementia (MID), prosodic loss was found to be more frequent and more severe in those with AD. Differences between the two groups were significant for emotional and intrinsic aprosody; differences were not significant for intellectual or inarticulate aprosody. (Trullen and Pardo, 1996)
- Naming and word recognition skills of women in the early stages of AD are poorer than those of men. From this baseline, however, rates of decline in these skills are similar for women and men. (Pollmann, et al., 1995)
- Use of stuffed animals and other toys has been shown to increase meaningful communication in clients with AD. (Iskowitz, 1998)

PROGNOSIS

AD is the fourth leading cause of death in the United States. The disease is progressive, although the rate of progression is variable. The disease may last from 5 to 20 years. Cause of death is often aspiration pneumonia or infection.

REFERENCES

AGEs more common in brains of Alzheimer's patients. *Advance for Speech-Language Pathologists & Audiologists.* 1994;4(14):17.

Music improves memory in patients with dementia. *Advance for Speech-Language Pathologists & Audiologists.* 1997;7(35):3.

Remediating hearing loss in patients with Alzheimer's. *Advance for Speech-Language Pathologists & Audiologists.* 1997;7(1):5.

Brookshire RH. *An Introduction to Neurogenic Communication Disorders,* 4th ed. St. Louis, Mo: Mosby Year Book. 1992:228.

Chenery HJ, BE Murdoch, JCL Ingram. An investigation of confrontation naming performance in Alzheimer's dementia as a function of disease severity. *Aphasiology.* 1996;10(5):423–41.

Ehrlich JS. Studies of discourse production in adults with Alzheimer's disease. In: Bloom RL, LK Obler, S De Santi, JS Ehrlich, eds. *Discourse Analysis and Applications: Studies in Adult Clinical Populations.* Hillsdale, NJ: Lawrence Erlbaum Associates. 1994:149–60.

Eisner E. If the walls could talk: using visual cues for people with Alzheimer's. *Advance for Speech-Language Pathologists & Audiologists.* 1997;7(6):4.

Glickstein JK. Goal-setting in Alzheimer's care key to success in treatment and reimbursement. *Advance for Speech-Language Pathologists & Audiologists.* 1996;6(32):7,11.

Glickstein JK. *Therapeutic Interventions in Alzheimer's Disease,* 2nd ed. Gaithersburg, Md: Aspen Publishers, Inc. 1997.

Glickstein JK, GK Neustadt. Speech-language interventions in Alzheimer's disease: a functional communication approach. *Clinics in Communication Disorders.* 1993; 3(1):15–30.

Grossman M, M D'Esposito, E Hughes, K Onishi, N Biassou, T White-Devine, KM Robinson. Language comprehension profiles in Alzheimer's disease, multi-infarct dementia, and frontotemporal degeneration. *Neurology.* 1996;47(1):183–9.

Hamilton HE. Requests for clarification as evidence of pragmatic comprehension difficulty: the case of Alzheimer's disease. In: Bloom RL, LK Obler, S De Santi, JS Ehrlich, eds. *Discourse Analysis and Applications: Studies in Adult Clinical Populations.* Hillsdale, NJ: Lawrence Erlbaum Associates. 1994:185–99.

Iskowitz M. Toying with meaningful communication: using recognition to evoke positive fact memory, emotion and action. *Advance for Speech-Language Pathologists & Audiologists.* 1998;8(15):6–9.

Lamar MAC, LK Obler, JE Knoefel, ML Albert. Communication patterns in end-stage Alzheimer's disease pragmatic analyses. In: Bloom RL, LK Obler, S De Santi, JS Ehrlich, eds. *Discourse Analysis and Applications: Studies in Adult Clinical Populations.* Hillsdale, NJ: Lawrence Erlbaum Associates. 1994:217–35.

Orange JB, EB Ryan, SD Meredith, MJ MacLean. Applications of the communication enhancement model for long-term care residents with Alzheimer's disease. *Topics in Language Disorders.* 1995;15(2):20–35.

Pérez Trullen JM, PJ Modrego Pardo. Comparative study of aprosody in Alzheimer's disease and in multi-infarct dementia. *Dementia.* 1996;7:59–62.

Pollman S, M Haupt, A Kurz. Changes of the relative severity of naming, fluency and recall impairment in the course of dementia of the Alzheimer type. *Dementia.* 1995;6:252–7.

Rosser A, JR Hodges. Initial letter and semantic category fluency in Alzheimer's disease, Huntington's disease, and progressive supranuclear palsy. *Journal of Neurology, Neurosurgery & Psychiatry.* 1994;57(11):1389–94.

Scott A. Assessment models for Alzheimer's. *Advance for Speech-Language Pathologists & Audiologists.* 1998;8(15):10–11.

Shoemaker A. Alzheimer's disease: research at Alzheimer's disease centers yields insights into diagnosis and treatment. *Advance for Speech-Language Pathologists & Audiologists.* 1996;6(16):6–7,11.

Snowdon DA, SJ Kemper, JA Mortimer, LH Greiner, DR Wekstein, WR Markesbery. Linguistic ability in early life and cognitive function and Alzheimer's Disease in late life. *Journal of the American Medical Association.* 1996;275(7):528–32.

Trace R. Communication issues in Alzheimer's and dementia. *Advance for Speech-Language Pathologists & Audiologists.* 1994;4(19):12–13.

Trace R. Normal aging vs. dementia: recognizing biologic, neurologic and cognitive changes. *Advance for Speech-Language Pathologists & Audiologists.* 1996;6(16):4,15.

Welsh SW, FM Corrigan, M Scott. Language impairment and aggression in Alzheimer's Disease. *International Journal of Geriatric Psychiatry.* 1996;(11):257–61.

Yesavage JA, JO Brooks III, J Taylor, J Tinklenberg. Development of aphasia, apraxia, and agnosia and decline in Alzheimer's Disease. *American Journal of Psychiatry.* 1993; 150(5):742–7.

Amyotrophic Lateral Sclerosis (ALS)

DESCRIPTION

ALS, better known as Lou Gehrig's disease, is a motor neuron disease characterized by progressive degeneration of corticospinal tracts and/or anterior horn cells and/or bulbar motor nuclei. One classification system is:

1. Bulbar ALS—damage to motor nerve nuclei in the brain stem (19% to 35% of cases). Dysarthria and dysphagia are present in the early stages.
2. Nonbulbar, prebulbar, or spinal ALS—damage to anterior horn cells (37% of cases).
3. Spinal ALS—damage to anterior horn cells and corticospinal tract innervating the limbs. Dysarthria is not present.

Median age of onset of ALS is 55 years, and the incidence is greater in males. Approximately 5,000 new cases are diagnosed in the United States each year. Although the disease is progressive, sensory systems, voluntary eye movements, and urinary sphincters remain unaffected.

ETIOLOGY

The cause is generally unknown; 5% of cases are familial, with an autosomal-dominant inheritance. Some evidence suggests a defect in a gene on chromosome number 21. In some instances, the disease may be the result of an immune system disorder that causes the body to attack calcium gateways in nerve cells.

SPEECH AND LANGUAGE DIFFICULTIES

- Dysarthria.
- Mixed dysarthria (flaccid, spastic).
- Changes in voice quality (wet-hoarse quality, strained-strangled quality, breathiness, harshness, hypernasality).
- Slow rate of speech.
- Low pitch.
- Hypernasality.
- Nasal emission.
- Vowel distortions.
- Weakness of one or both vocal folds.
- Progressively decreasing intelligibility of speech due to decreased range, rate, and strength of articulatory movements of tongue and oropharyngeal musculature.

ASSOCIATED AND OTHER DIFFICULTIES

- Muscular weakness and atrophy.
- Cramps.
- Spasticity.
- Hyperactive deep tendon reflexes.
- Drooling.
- Nasal regurgitation possible, but not a common finding.

- Dysphagia characterized by delayed initiation of pharyngeal swallow, reduced pharyngeal peristalsis, upper esophageal sphincter dysfunction, and esophageal reflux. (Martin, 1994)
- Unilateral or bilateral weakness of the soft palate.
- Weakness, atrophy of the tongue.
- Weakness of the lips.
- Reduced pulmonary function.
- Progressive respiratory insufficiency.
- Feelings of anger, frustration, denial.
- Self-imposed isolation.

ASSESSMENT
- Assess for presence and severity of dysarthria. (See Appendix A)
- Administer *Frenchay Dysarthria Assessment.*
- Assess voice quality (pitch, intensity, quality, resonance, respiration).
- Assess rate of speaking.
- Assess speech intelligibility.
- Assess speech deterioration frequently and long-term.
- Assess diadochokinetic rate.
- Assess velopharyngeal function.
- Assess volume.
- Assess need for and willingness to use AAC.
- Assess cognitive/linguistic skills, sensory/perceptual skills, and motor skills necessary for AAC.
- Provide ongoing assessment of muscles of mastication.
- Assess ability to manage oral secretions.
- Assess for dysphagia.
- Administer *ALS Severity Scale.*
- Use a team approach in assessment, program planning, and recommendations.

INTERVENTION TECHNIQUES
- Remember that the goal of therapy is compensation, not remediation.
- Optimize residual physiologic functions to enhance intelligibility, i.e., instruct in over articulation, breath support, and phrasing. (Mancinelli, 1994)

- Monitor changes in swallowing and recommend textural food changes as indicated. (Mancinelli, 1994)
- Monitor need for alternative nutritional device. (Mancinelli, 1994)
- Instruct client to keep list of which foods he or she can or cannot eat. Monitoring this list will alert one to possible dehydration or nutritional deficits. (Mancinelli, 1994)
- Monitor continuously client's ability and desire to eat, and nutrition and hydration status. (Miller and Groher, 1992)
- Avoid sticky foods and dry, crumbly foods.
- Introduce AAC as needed and provide ongoing support for use of AAC. (Beukelman and Mirenda, 1992; Mancinelli, 1994)
- Work with family members to improve communication dynamics.

RESULTS OF RECENT STUDIES

- Disproportionate tongue impairment may be related to upper motor neuron deficits. (DePaul and Brooks, 1993)
- Muscle weakness is not directly related to speech intelligibility. (DePaul and Brooks, 1993)
- In a study of 10 women, the most disrupted phonetic features related to velopharyngeal valving, lingual function for consonant contrasts of place and manner, and syllable shape. (Kent, et al., 1992)
- Men are more likely to have impairments of voicing in initial syllable position than are women. (Kent, et al., 1992)
- Of the lip, tongue, and jaw, tongue movements are most affected. (Langmore and Lehman, 1994)
- Perceived severity of dysarthria correlated more highly with reduced speed than with reduced strength. (Langmore and Lehman, 1994)
- When instructed to speak at three different rates, dysarthric speakers decreased rate to a smaller extent than did neurologically intact controls. The habitual rate of those with dysarthria was slower. (Turner and Weismer, 1993)
- Voice tremor may be an indication of loss of motor units, which results in intermittent absence of motor unit firing. (Aronson, et al., 1992)
- Four clients with ALS and dementia exhibited different patterns of cognitive impairment, including frontal dementia; aphasic, apraxic, amnesia syndrome; and cognitive decline in association with a blunt affect. All four presented with early dementia progressing rapidly to anarthria. (Cavalleri and De Renzi, 1994)

- In one study, women were more likely than men to present with initial bulbar signs, while men more often presented with spinal signs. In both groups, those with bulbar signs and those with spinal signs, women had earlier onset of dysphagia. Also, in both groups, swallowing ability declined as respiratory capacity declined. (Strand, et al., 1996)

PROGNOSIS

Fifty percent of clients die within 3 years of onset, 20% live 5 years, and 10% live 10 years. In rare instances, patients may survive for 30 years. In recent trials, use of the drug riluzole has prolonged survival rates an average of 3 months. (Kerr, 1996)

REFERENCES

Aronson AE, LO Ramig, WS Winholtz, SR Silber. Rapid voice tremor, or "flutter" in amyotrophic lateral sclerosis. *Annals of Otology, Rhinology & Laryngology.* 1992; 101(6):511–8.

Beukelman DR, P Mirenda. *Augmentative and Alternative Communication: Management of Severe Communication Disorders in Children and Adults.* Baltimore: Paul H. Brookes Publishing Co. 1992:313–6.

Cavalleri F, E De Renzi. Amyotrophic lateral sclerosis with dementia. *Acta Neurologica Scandinavica.* 1994;89(5):391–4.

DePaul R, BR Brooks. Multiple orofacial indices in amyotrophic lateral sclerosis. *Journal of Speech & Hearing Research.* 1993;36(6):1158–67.

Immune disorder may be primary cause of ALS. *Advance for Speech-Language Pathologists & Audiologists.* 1993;3(4):18.

Kent JF, RD Kent, JC Rosenbek, G Weismer, R Martin, R Sufit , BR Brooks. Quantitative description of the dysarthria in women with amyotrophic lateral sclerosis. *Journal of Speech & Hearing Research.* 1992;35(4):723–33.

Kerr T. New ALS drug prolongs survival rate. *Advance for Speech-Language Pathologists & Audiologists.* 1996;6(9):15.

Langmore SE, ME Lehman. Physiologic deficits in the orofacial system underlying dysarthria in amyotrophic lateral sclerosis. *Journal of Speech & Hearing Research.* 1994; 37(1):28–37.

Lazzarotti M. Clinic addresses unique needs of ALS patients. *Advance for Speech-Language Pathologists & Audiologists.* 1994;4(20):8.

Mancinelli JM. Dysphagia and dysarthria: the role of the speech-language pathologist. In: H Mitsumoto, F Norris, eds. *Amyotrophic Lateral Sclerosis: A Comprehensive Guide to Management.* New York: Demos Publications. 1994:63–75.

Martin BJW. Treatment of dysphagia in adults. In: Cherney LR, ed. *Clinical Management of Dysphagia in Adults and Children, Second Edition.* Gaithersburg, Md: Aspen Publishers, Inc. 1994:153–83.

Miller RM, ME Groher. General treatment of neurologic swallowing disorders. In: Groher ME, ed. *Dysphagia Diagnosis and Management,* 2nd ed. Boston: Butterworth-Heinemann. 1992:209–11.

Miller RM, ME Groher, KM Yorkston, TS Rees. Speech, language, swallowing, and auditory rehabilitation. In: DeLisa JA, BM Gans, eds. *Rehabilitation Medicine, Principles and Practice,* 2nd ed. Philadelphia: J.B. Lippincott Co. 1993:201–26.

Mulligan M, J Carpenter, J Riddel, MK Delaney, G Badger, P Krusinski, R Tandan. Intelligibility and the acoustic characteristics of speech in amyotrophic lateral sclerosis (ALS). *Journal of Speech & Hearing Research.* 1994;37(3):496–503.

Riddel J, RJ McCaulay, M Mulligan, R Tandan. Intelligibility and phonetic contrast errors in highly intelligible speakers with amyotrophic lateral sclerosis. *Journal of Speech & Hearing Research.* 1995;38(2):304–14.

Strand EA, EH Buder, KM Yorkston, LO Ramig. Differential phonatory characteristics of four women with amyotrophic lateral sclerosis. *Journal of Voice.* 1994;8(4):327–39.

Strand EA, RM Miller, KM Yorkston, AD Hillel. Management of oral-pharyngeal dysphagia symptoms in amyotrophic lateral sclerosis. *Dysphagia.* 1996;11:129–39.

Turner GS, K Tjaden, G Weismer. The influence of speaking rate on vowel space and speech intelligibility for individuals with amyotrophic lateral sclerosis. *Journal of Speech & Hearing Research.* 1995;38(5):1001–13.

Turner GS, G Weismer. Characteristics of speaking rate in the dysarthria associated with amyotrophic lateral sclerosis. *Journal of Speech & Hearing Research.* 1993;36(6):1134–44.

Brainstem Stroke

DESCRIPTION

There are several syndromes associated with brainstem stroke. Among these are:

- Weber syndrome associated with vascular damage at the base of the midbrain, resulting in ipsilateral, complete oculomotor palsy, contralateral hemiplegia and face and tongue involvement. Mild dysarthria and/or dysphagia may result.

- Avellis syndrome, caused by hemorrhage in the tegmentum of the medulla. Results include ipsilateral paralysis of the soft palate and larynx. Dysarthria, hypernasality, and dysphonia may result.
- Jackson syndrome, possibly also caused by hemorrhage in the tegmentum, results in ipsilateral paralysis of the soft palate and larynx. Speech symptoms include hypernasality, dysphonia, mild articulation distortions, and mild dysphagia.
- Dejerine syndrome involves damage to the fibers of the hypoglossal nerve, with ipsilateral weakness of the tongue, resulting in mild dysarthria and/or dysphagia.
- Wallenberg syndrome is generally caused by arteriosclerotic vascular disease of the posterior inferior cerebellar artery or the vertebral artery resulting in damage to the lateral medulla and sometimes to the inferior surface of the cerebellum. Communication impairments generally include hoarseness, absence of swallow response, and dysphagia.
- Locked-in syndrome is generally due to bilateral pontine infarcts or hemorrhage, resulting in paralysis of all four extremities and of facial muscles, mandibular muscles, and muscles of the tongue, lips, palate, pharynx, larynx, and neck. Over time, some voluntary movement may return.

Persons who have sustained a brainstem stroke generally retain premorbid cognitive and language skills.

ETIOLOGY
(See Description)

SPEECH AND LANGUAGE DIFFICULTIES
- Dysarthria—may range from mild to severe, depending on site of lesion.
- Dysphonia.
- Voice disorders.

ASSOCIATED AND OTHER DIFFICULTIES
- Dysphagia.
- May experience loss of sense of pain and of temperature.
- Ataxia.

ASSESSMENT

- Evaluate dysarthria, including assessment of severity.
- Evaluate for dysphagia.

(See also Voice Disorders)

INTERVENTION TECHNIQUES

- In cases of severe dysarthria, the client may be able to communicate via writing.
- Clients with locked-in syndrome may retain vertical eye movements, which can be used to establish a yes/no communication system.
- Arrange letters of the alphabet in a grid so the client can blink a given number of times to indicate the position of a letter in a row and column.

(See also Voice Disorders)

RESULTS OF RECENT STUDIES

No recent studies regarding communication skills were found in the literature.

PROGNOSIS

Outcome depends partially on the specific syndrome.

REFERENCE

Boyle M. The effects of brain stem stroke on communication and swallowing. *Topics in Stroke Rehabilitation*. 1994;1(2):76–86.

Brain Tumors

DESCRIPTION

Brain tumors may occur at any age but are most common in early adult and mid-life. Severity of effects depends on the size, location, rate of growth, and histologic grade of malignancy of the tumor. Symptoms may include seizures, drowsiness, lethargy, personality changes, impaired mental functions, or psychotic episodes.

ETIOLOGY

Primary intracranial neoplasms are divided into six classes. They are tumors of:

1. the skull
2. the meninges
3. the cranial nerves
4. the neuroglia and ependyma
5. the pituitary or pineal body
6. congenital origin.

Secondary effects of tumors include increased intracranial pressure, cerebral edema, and compression of brain tissue, cranial nerves, and cerebral vessels.

SPEECH AND LANGUAGE DIFFICULTIES

- Cerebellar mutism may result following surgery for posterior fossa tumors in children and, more rarely, in adults.
- Following surgery for posterior fossa tumors in children, speech deficits also may include imprecision of consonant sounds, hypernasality or hyponasality, and a pitch level inappropriately high for age and sex. (Murdoch and Hudson-Tennent, 1994)
- Dysarthria.
- Anomia.
- Crossed aphasia may occur under the following conditions: absence of left-handedness in the client or other family members, localization of

lesion in the right hemisphere, absence of previous neurological lesions, documented aphasic symptomatology, and absence of suspect environmental factors. (Primavera and Bandini, 1993)
• Reduced rate.

ASSOCIATED AND OTHER DIFFICULTIES
• Hearing loss may result from chemotherapy. Loss initially occurs in the high frequencies and may progress to lower frequencies. The loss may be permanent or transient.
• Dysphagia.
• Weight loss.
• Fatigue.
• Depression.
• Emotional instability.
• Insomnia.

ASSESSMENT
• Persons with primary brain tumors (PBTs) with dysphagia often experience swallowing difficulties of greater severity than their complaints and reports would indicate. These clients should routinely receive formal swallowing assessments.
• Assess dysphagia using the *Rehabilitation Institute of Chicago Functional Assessment Scale.*
• Assess dysarthria using *Frenchay Dysarthria Assessment.*
• Assess articulation skills.
• Assess for aphasia.

INTERVENTION TECHNIQUES
• Treat for dysphagia.
• Provide therapy for aphasia as indicated.

RESULTS OF RECENT STUDIES
• In one study, the only children to develop oral pharyngeal apraxia and mutism following surgery were those with midline tumors and a complete inferior split of the vermis. (Dailey, et al., 1995)

- In five cases of postoperative transient mutism in children with posterior fossa tumors, a period of cerebellar dysarthria followed the mutism. Cerebellar mutism, therefore, may be a severe form of dysarthria rather than a cognitive deficit or psychological disturbance. (Van Calenbergh, et al., 1995)
- In a review of 46 cases of mutism following posterior cranial fossa surgery, the mutism was transient in all cases and lasted from 4 days to 4 months. In 35 of the 46 cases, the mutism was followed by dysarthria. (Ersahin, et al., 1996)
- Citing a previously published report by different authors, Cakir and others list the following as possible organic causes of transient cerebellar mutism in children: extensive cerebellar damage, vascular damage due to edema or arterial spasm, disturbances of cerebrospinal fluid circulation, and postoperative meningitis. (Cakir, et al., 1994.)
- Surgery to remove tumors located near or within speech areas is often debated. In a study of 100 such clients, 65% showed improvement in speech postoperatively, while 15% deteriorated in speech function. Specifically, 36 patients had normal speech preoperatively, and of these, 4 developed some degree of dysphasia. Fifty-four were dysphasic prior to surgery. Thirty-five showed significant improvement at 1 year post-surgery, speech deteriorated in 11 clients, and 2 became aphasic. (Tandon, et al., 1993)
- Dysphagia in PBTs is often seen in clients with supratentorial unilateral tumors with surrounding edema. (Newton, et al., 1994)
- In clients with deafness as a result of neurofibromatosis type 2 tumors, implantation of a cochlear implant with transcutaneous signal transmission has, in some cases, resulted in some improvement in speech perception. (Laszig, et al., 1995)
- Following surgery for posterior fossa tumors in children, articulation errors may be a combination of acquired dysarthria and developmental errors. Dysarthria may be a direct result of the surgery or an indirect result of radiation. (Murdoch and Hudson-Tennent, 1994)
- In a study of adults with high-grade glioma, the presence of a communication impairment proved to be a significant factor in length of survival. While the overall mean survival was 9.5 months, the survival of those with speech difficulties was 6 months compared with survival of 10.5 months among those with normal speech and language skills. Reasons for this are unclear. (Thomas, et al., 1995)

- In one study, multiple, noncontiguous language sites were identified in 28% of those with tumors. (Haglund, et al., 1994)
- In persons undergoing surgical resection in the left temporal lobe for excision of gliomas, a clear association has been noted between postoperative language deficits and the distance from the nearest language site to the resection margin. Those with a margin of 2.0 cm had no postoperative language deficits, while those with margins of 1.6 to 2.0 cm had deficits lasting 1 to 7 days, those with margins of 0.71 cm had deficits lasting 8 to 30 days, and those with margins of 0.67 cm had permanent language deficits following surgery. (Haglund, et al., 1994)

PROGNOSIS

In one study, the overall mean survival rates of clients with high-grade glioma was 9.5 months. (Thomas, et al., 1995) Prognosis improves with early diagnosis.

REFERENCES

Cakir Y, D Karakisi, O Kocanaogullari. Cerebellar mutism in an adult: case report. *Surgical Neurology.* 1994;41(4):342–4.

Dailey AT, GM McKhann II, MS Berger. The pathophysiology of oral pharyngeal apraxia and mutism following posterior fossa tumor resection in children. *Journal of Neurosurgery.* 1995;83:467–75.

Ersahin Y, S Mutluer, S Cagli, Y Duman. Cerebellar mutism: report of seven cases and review of the literature. *Neurosurgery.* 1996;38(1):60–66.

Haglund MM, MS Berger, M Shamseldin, E Lettich, GA Ojemann. Cortical localization of temporal lobe language sites in patients with gliomas. *Neurosurgery.* 1994;34(4):567–76.

Laszig R, WP Sollmann, N Marangos. The restoration of hearing in neurofibromatosis type 2. *Journal of Laryngology & Otology.* 1995;109(5):385–9.

Magalini SI, SC Magalini. *Dictionary of Medical Syndromes,* 4th ed. Philadelphia: Lippincott-Raven Publishers. 1997:111.

Mastronardi L, L Ferrante, A Maleci, F Puzzilli, P Lunardi, G Schettini. Crossed aphasia: an update. *Neurosurgical Review.* 1994;17:299–304.

Murdoch BE, LJ Hudson-Tennent. Speech disorders in children treated for posterior fossa tumours: ataxic and developmental features. *European Journal of Disorders of Communication.* 1994;29:379–97.

Newton HB, C Newton, D Pearl, T Davidson. Swallowing assessment in primary brain tumor patients with dysphagia. *Neurology.* 1994;44(10):1927–32.

Primavera A, F Bandini. Crossed aphasia: analysis of a case with special reference to the nature of the lesion. *European Neurology*. 1993;33:30–33.

Sweetow RW, TI Will. Progression of hearing loss following the completion of chemotherapy and radiation therapy: case report. *Journal of the American Academy of Audiology*. 1993;4:360–3.

Tandon P, AK Mahapatra, A Khosla. Operations on gliomas involving speech centres. *Acta Neurochirurgica–Supplementum*. 1993;56:67–71.

Thomas R, AM O'Connor, S Ashley. Speech and language disorders in patients with high grade glioma and its influence of prognosis. *Journal of Neuro-Oncology*. 1995;23: 265–70.

Van Calenbergh F, A Van de Laar, C Plets, J Goffin, P Casaer. Transient cerebellar mutism after posterior fossa surgery in children. *Neurosurgery*. 1995;37(5):894–8.

Cerebrovascular Accidents (CVA) in Adults—Left Hemisphere Damage (LHD)

DESCRIPTION

Cerebrovascular disease is the most prevalent cause of neurologic disability in Western countries. It is the third leading cause of death among older persons. Approximately half of all adults who survive a stroke experience difficulty with communication. This incidence holds true for those sustaining either right or left hemisphere damage. Cerebrovascular injury is an interruption of blood flow and is most often secondary to atherosclerosis, hypertension, or a combination of the two. Types of cerebrovascular disease include cerebral insufficiency due to transient disturbances of blood flow; infarction due to either embolism or thrombosis of the intracranial or extracranial arteries; hemorrhage; and arteriovenous malformation, which may cause symptoms of mass lesion, infarction, or hemorrhage.

ETIOLOGY

A stroke is caused by an infarction of brain tissue and is manifested by neurologic deficits of varying severity. Onset is generally abrupt, and outcome is extremely variable. Resulting deficits are dependent on the site of occlusion. Most commonly involved is the middle cerebral artery, resulting in contralateral hemiplegia, usually severe, with hemianesthesia and hemianopia. Aphasia occurs when the dominant hemisphere is affected. Apraxia or sensory neglect are present when the nondominant hemisphere is affected. Occlusion of the internal carotid artery produces identical symptoms and occasional ocular symptoms. Occlusion of the posterior cerebral artery affects areas in the temporal and occipital lobes, internal capsule, hippocampus, thalamus, mammillary and geniculate bodies, choroid plexus, and upper brainstem, resulting in contralateral hemianopia and hemisensory loss. If the dominant hemisphere is involved, alexia may result.

SPEECH AND LANGUAGE DIFFICULTIES
- Aphasia.
- Apraxia of speech. (See also Developmental Apraxia of Speech [DAS] and Developmental Verbal Dyspraxia [DVA])
- Areas of relative pragmatic strength in discourse include preservation of chronological order of events, turn-taking skills, and ability to select important information. Areas of weakness include topic initiation and specificity and accuracy of information.

RELATED AND OTHER DIFFICULTIES
- Dysphagia (in 13% of clients with unilateral hemisphere damage and in 71% of those with bilateral hemisphere damage).
- Pulmonary complications and pneumonia. Incidence of poststroke pneumonia is significantly higher among those with dysphagia.
- Mood changes.
- Depression.
- Self-imposed isolation.
- Denial.

ASSESSMENT
- Establish protocols in acute settings for all persons diagnosed with stroke and hemiparesis to be evaluated for swallowing difficulties within 8 hours of admission. Establish objective criterion for pass/fail and train nursing staff to administer the screening. (Iskowitz, 1997)

Types of Aphasia

Type of Aphasia	Synonyms	Speech and Language Deficits	Relatively Preserved Skills
Broca's aphasia	Motor aphasia; efferent motor aphasia	Speech and writing are limited to word fragments or telegraphic speech; speech and writing are slow, laborious, and effortful; absence of articles, prepositions, conjunctions, auxiliary verbs and inflectional changes to verbs; dysfluent and agrammatic immediate repetition of phrases; incorrect performance of commands; confusion of actor and object.	Ability to recite overlearned sequences (days of week, months of year, etc.); ability to sing previously learned songs.
Conduction aphasia	Afferent motor aphasia	Impaired immediate repetition of oral phrases as a result of omission of words, phonemic paraphasias, substitution of nonsense words; impaired oral reading; fluent but impaired spontaneous speech; fluent but impaired writing.	Comprehension of oral and written material.

Global aphasia	Impaired comprehension of spoken and written material; dysfluent spontaneous and responsive speech often limited to simple terse or telegraphic words; slow, laborious, and effortful speech and writing; agrammatic speech and writing characterized by absence of articles, prepositions, conjunctions, auxiliary verbs, and inflectional changes in verbs to indicate tense; impaired naming of objects; impaired right-left orientation.	
Mixed transcortical aphasia	Total or near total absence of spontaneous speech and writing; impaired comprehension; tendency toward echolalia; impaired naming of objects that does not improve with cueing.	Repetition of recently heard phrases; ability to complete overlearned phrases; ability to sing previously learned songs.

continues

Type of Aphasia	Synonyms	Speech and Language Deficits	Relatively Preserved Skills
Pure word deafness	Auditory speech agnosia; auditory verbal agnosia	Impaired comprehension of spoken sentences; fluent but impaired immediate repetition of oral phrases; impaired writing to dictation.	Spontaneous speech, writing, reading comprehension, and oral reading.
Transcortical aphasia	Dynamic aphasia	Dysfluent spontaneous and responsive speech and writing, limited to simple, isolated concrete words; speech and writing are slow, laborious, and effortful; some tendency toward echolalia; impaired naming of objects and impaired word finding during conversation that may improve when phonetic cues are provided.	Ability to repeat recently heard phrases; oral reading.
Transcortical sensory aphasia	Acoustic amnestic aphasia	Impaired comprehension of spoken or written material; impaired spontaneous and responsive speech and writing characterized by addition of extra words or phrases, substitution of incorrect	Ability to recite previously learned passages; ability to sing previously learned songs.

speech sounds, word substitutions, substitution of nonspecific words for concrete words; tendency toward echolalia; unawareness of own impaired speech and frustration with others for not comprehending; impaired naming of objects that does not improve with cueing.

| Wernicke aphasia | Sensory aphasia | Impaired comprehension of spoken or written sentences; addition of extra words or phrases to target phrases being read, repeated, or written; substitution of sounds in words; semantically related word substitutions; random word substitutions; speech and writing may be produced at a rapid rate and in a greater than normal amount. |

Source: Data from A.Y. Stringer, *A Guide to Adult Neuropsychological Diagnosis*, pp. 251–285, © 1996, F.A. Davis Company.

- Conduct bedside examination within 24 hours poststroke. Evaluate oromotor function, ability to follow directions and level of alertness.
- Administer *Minnesota Test for Differential Diagnosis of Aphasia.*
- Administer *Boston Diagnostic Aphasia Examination* (BDAE).
- Administer *Boston Naming Test* (BNT).
- Administer *Western Aphasia Battery* (WAB).
- Administer *Porch Index of Communicative Ability* (PICA).
- Administer *The Token Test.*
- Administer *The Reading Comprehension Battery for Aphasia* (RCBA).
- Administer *Communicative Abilities in Daily Living* (CADL).
- Assess for dysphagia.
- Administer *The Burke Dysphagia Screening Test* to identify clients at risk for pneumonia, recurrent upper airway obstruction, and death. (DePippo, et al., 1994)
- With higher functioning clients, elicit a writing sample and analyze errors.
- Assess discourse through analysis of pretherapy and posttherapy narrative. (Scott, 1997)
- Perform discourse analysis by taping conversations between the client and a familiar conversational partner, and use the results to assist in implementing conversational repair strategies. (Perkins, 1995)
- To assess psychosocial adjustment, administer the *Freiburg Questionnaire on Coping with Illness* and/or the *Severity of Psychosocial Change.*

INTERVENTION TECHNIQUES

- Guard against initiating intensive therapy too soon, as client may not be ready to accept therapy. (Namnum, 1995)
- Involve the client in setting the goals of therapy.
- Involve family members in setting goals of therapy and recognize that family members may have the best assessment of the client's functional communication skills.
- Work to reduce auditory comprehension deficits through activities such as matching spoken words to pictures, sequencing items, and following directions.
- Work to establish a system for the client to request clarification.

- Establish and work toward functional short-term goals, based on activities of importance to the client.
- Consider PACE therapy (**promoting a**phasics' **c**ommunicative **e**ffectiveness) based on exchange of new information, equal participation in the roles of communication, free choice of communicative channels, and feedback based on communicative adequacy. (Carlomagno, 1994)
- Use right-brain function to facilitate therapy, e.g., use symbol cards that client can manipulate to form sentences or requests; use Melodic Intonation Therapy (MIT). (Code, 1994)
- To work on auditory comprehension of single words, consider use of the *Auditory Language Comprehension Programme* (ALCP). (Bastiaanse, et al., 1993)
- Gear therapy to maximizing functional communication skills rather than work on linguistic form.
- Be aware of factors that may inhibit or delay return to a normal swallow, i.e., medications (particularly antidepressant medications), long-standing diabetes, prior strokes, and previous transient ischemic attacks (TIAs).
- Be aware that swallowing status may change over days, weeks, and months. Continue to assess for dysphagia even if previous results have been normal.
- Consider trial of dysphagia therapy even if dysphagia has been present for several years. Consider compensatory maneuvers such as a modified Valsalva maneuver, the Mendelsohn maneuver, the Masako maneuver, the head lifting maneuver, oral-motor exercises, and vocal adduction exercises. (Crane, 1997a) Other compensatory strategies include changing volume or viscosity of the bolus and changes in feeding procedures.
- Incorporate techniques of sensory stimulation, i.e., changing the temperature of the bolus that is presented, increasing downward pressure of the spoon on the tongue as food is presented, and presenting a bolus requiring chewing.
- Consult with dietician to ensure proper nutrition when designing the feeding program.
- Consult with physical therapists and occupational therapists to ensure proper positioning and use of assistive devices when designing the feeding program.
- For clients with severe dysphagia that doesn't resolve, consider use of a dental prosthesis, the palatal training appliance (PTA). (Selley, et al., 1995)

- When treating clients with ataxic dysarthria, to improve respiration, emphasize steady, controlled exhalation, gradually increasing in length; to improve articulation, work to optimize precision and rate; to improve prosody, work on proper phrasing. (Morganstein and Smith, 1993)
- To reduce rate, have the client point to the first letter of each word on an alphabet board.
- To treat transient phonatory dyspraxia, introduce use of an electrolarynx; work with voluntary imitation of coughing, throat-clearing, humming; and encourage voluntary production of "a," then continue to other vowels and consonants. (Mueller, 1995)
- Train family members and others in use of redundancy to improve comprehension, combining gestural and oral language to facilitate communication, allowing adequate time for the client to formulate a response, and appropriate rates of auditory presentation. (Miller, et al., 1993)
- Provide training in environmental controls, i.e., controlling the number of speakers, controlling distractions, providing favorable seating. (Miller, et al., 1993)
- Consider use of communication boards for clients with severe apraxia of speech.
- When designing augmentative and alternative communication (AAC) systems, keep in mind that a primary goal is often social closeness and social interaction rather than transfer of information. (Beukelman and Mirenda, 1992)
- Refer clients and spouses to aphasia groups and other support networks.

RESULTS OF RECENT STUDIES

- Discourse is defined as the process of word selection, sentence formation, organization of information, linking sentences with ideas, and deciding what should be said versus what should remain unsaid. Clients with left hemisphere damage preserve these aspects of discourse, although their utterances are less complex than those of able-bodied subjects. (Bloom, 1994)
- Emotional content may improve pragmatic performance. (Bloom, 1994)
- In treating dysphagia during inpatient rehabilitation, client and family instruction regarding diet modification and compensatory swallowing techniques may be as effective for the prevention of medical complications associated with dysphagia as therapist control of diet consistency

and daily rehearsal of compensatory swallowing techniques. (DePippo, et al., 1994)

- Some clients thought to be experiencing sequelae TIAs subsequently were found to have brain tumors. Manifestations that should prompt investigation for tumor include focal jerking or shaking, pure sensory phenomena, loss of consciousness, or isolated aphasia. (Anonymous, 1993)
- Computerized axial tomography (CAT) and magnetic resonance imaging (MRI) scans of lesions in clients who had sustained a CVA, some with resulting apraxia and some without apraxia, were compared. In every case of those with apraxia, the left precentral gyrus of the insula showed damage. In every case not exhibiting apraxia, this area was spared. (Crane, 1997b)

PROGNOSIS

In the days immediately following a stroke, neither its progression nor its ultimate outcome can be predicted. About 20% of clients die in the hospital, and this mortality rate increases with age. Any deficits remaining after 6 months are likely to be permanent, although continued slow improvement is seen in some clients. Recurrence of infarction is common, and each recurrence brings the likelihood of additional neurologic deficit. Indicators of a favorable functional outcome following CVA include stable medical condition, adequate family and social support, and significant functional skills early in the recovery period. (Zorowitz, 1995)

In one large study of aphasia and stroke in Scandinavia, the following results were found: Of those admitted with CVA, 38% demonstrated aphasia on admission, 12% had mild aphasia, 6% had moderate aphasia, and 20% had severe aphasia. Another 6% were classified as dysarthric. Of those with aphasia, 31% died during their hospital stay. Of those who survived, 44% had complete recovery from aphasia at the time of discharge from the hospital; this included 12% of those with severe aphasia, 41% of those with moderate aphasia, and 56% of those with mild aphasia. (Pedersen, 1995)

REFERENCES

Amster WW, JB Amster. Treatment of writing disorders in aphasia. In: Chapey R, ed. *Language Intervention Strategies in Adult Aphasia,* 3rd ed. Baltimore: Williams & Wilkins. 1994:458–66.

Anonymous. Intracranial tumours that mimic transient cerebral ischaemia: lessons from a large multicentre trial. The UK TIA Study Group. *Journal of Neurology, Neurosurgery, & Psychiatry.* 1993;56(5):563–6.

Bastiaanse R, S Nijboer, M Taconis. The Auditory Language Comprehension Programme: a description and case study. *European Journal of Disorders of Communication.* 1993;28:415–33.

Beukelman DR, P Mirenda. *Augmentative and Alternative Communication: Management of Severe Communication Disorders in Children and Adults.* Baltimore: Paul H. Brookes Publishing Co. 1992:331–43.

Bloom RL. Hemispheric responsibility and discourse production: contrasting patients with unilateral left and right hemisphere damage. In: Bloom RL, LK Obler, S De Santi, JS Ehrlich, eds. *Discourse Analysis and Applications: Studies in Adult Clinical Populations.* Hillsdale, NJ: Lawrence Erlbaum Associates. 1994:81–94.

Brookshire RH. *An Introduction to Neurogenic Communication Disorders*, 4th ed. St Louis, Mo: Mosby Year Book. 1992:273–86.

Carlomagno S. *Pragmatic Approaches to Aphasia.* San Diego, Calif: Singular Publishing Group, Inc. 1994.

Code C. Role of the right hemisphere in the treatment of aphasia. In: Chapey R, ed. *Language Intervention Strategies in Adult Aphasia,* 3rd ed. Baltimore: Williams & Wilkins. 1994:380–6.

Crane R. Compensatory maneuvers to recover swallowing function. *Advance for Speech-Language Pathologists & Audiologists.* 1997a;7(13):11.

Crane R. Research hones in on lesion site for apraxia. *Advance for Speech-Language Pathologists & Audiologists.* 1997b;7(11):19.

DePippo KL, MA Holas, MJ Reding. The Burke Dysphagia Screening Test: validation of its use in patients with stroke. *Archives of Physical Medicine & Rehabilitation.* 1994a; 75(12):1284–6.

DePippo KK, MA Holas, MJ Reding, FS Mandel, ML Lesser. Dysphagia therapy following stroke: a controlled trial. *Neurology.* 1994b;44(9):1655–60.

Fuller DP, DB Pugh, WM Landau. Management of communication and swallowing disorders. In: Illis LS, ed. *Neurological Rehabilitation,* 2nd ed. Boston: Blackwell Scientific Publications. 1994:409–27.

Goldsmith T. Pragmatic communication disorders following stroke. *Topics in Stroke Rehabilitation.* 1994;1(2):2–64.

Gottlieb D, M Kipnis, E Sister, Y Vardi, S Brill. Validation of the 50 ml³ drinking test for evaluation of post-stroke dysphagia. *Disability and Rehabilitation.* 1996;18(10):529–32.

Iskowitz M. Stroke and hemiparesis: standing order for speech-language pathology. *Advance for Speech-Language Pathologists & Audiologists.* 1997;7(43):6–7.

Iskowitz M. Psychogenic impact. *Advance for Speech-Language Pathologists & Audiologists.* 1998a;8(24):12–14.

Iskowitz M. Measuring outcomes in the home. *Advance for Speech-Language Pathologists & Audiologists.* 1998b;8(14):12–15.

Logemann JA. Management of dysphagia poststroke. In: Chapey R, ed. *Language Intervention Strategies in Adult Aphasia,* 3rd ed. Baltimore: Williams & Wilkins. 1994: 503–12.

Miller RM, ME Groher, KM Yorkston, TS Rees. Speech, language, swallowing, and auditory rehabilitation. In: DeLisa JA, BM Gans, eds. *Rehabilitation Medicine: Principles and Practice,* 2nd ed. Philadelphia: J.B. Lippincott Co. 1993:201–26.

Morganstein S, MC Smith. Motor-speech disorders and dysphagia. In: Gordon WA, ed. *Advances in Stroke Rehabilitation.* Boston: Andover Medical Publishers. 1993:134–61.

Mueller PB. Transient phonatory dyspraxia: identification and treatment of an obscure condition. *Advance for Speech-Language Pathologists & Audiologists.* 1995;5(30):9,13.

Namnum A. Readiness for therapy: aphasia patient offers insights into rehab process. *Advance for Speech-Language Pathologists & Audiologists.* 1995;5(26):11,38.

Peach RK. Treating the fluent aphasias. *Topics in Stroke Rehabilitation.* 1995;2(1):1–14.

Pedersen PM, HS Jorgensen, H Nakayama, HO Raaschou, TS Olsen. Aphasia in acute stroke: incidence, determinants, and recovery. *Annals of Neurology.* 1995;38(4):659–66.

Perkins L. Applying conversation analysis to aphasia: clinical implications and analytic issues. *European Journal of Disorders of Communication.* 1995;30:382–3.

Ramamurthi B, P Chari. Aphasia in bilinguals. *Acta Neurochirurgica* [Suppl]. 1993;56:59–66.

Scott A. Discourse analysis. *Advance for Speech-Language Pathologists & Audiologists.* 1997;7(48):10–11.

Selley WG, MT Roche, VR Pearce, RE Ellis, FC Flack. Dysphagia following strokes: clinical observations of swallowing rehabilitation employing palatal training appliances. *Dysphagia.* 1995;10(1):32–35.

Smithard DG, PA O'Neill, RE England, CL Park, R Wyatt, DF Martin, J Morris. The natural history of dysphagia following a stroke. *Dysphagia.* 1997;12:188–93.

Stringer AY. *A Guide to Neuropsychological Diagnosis.* Philadelphia: F.A. Davis Co. 1996:251–86.

Weinrich M, D McCall, C Weber, K Thomas, L Thornburg. Training on an iconic system for severe aphasia can improve natural language production. *Aphasiology.* 1995; 9(4):343–64.

Zorowitz RD. Comprehensive stroke rehab enhances patient care. *Advance for Speech-Language Pathologists & Audiologists.* 1995;5(45):17.

Cerebrovascular Accidents (CVA) in Adults—Right Hemisphere Damage (RHD)

DESCRIPTION

(See Cerebrovascular Accidents [CVA] in Adults—Left Hemisphere Damage [LHD])

ETIOLOGY

(See Cerebrovascular Accidents [CVA] in Adults—Left Hemisphere Damage [LHD])

SPEECH AND LANGUAGE DIFFICULTIES

- Speech is often vague and nonspecific.
- Increased use of pronouns without antecedents, indefinite terms, and definite articles.
- May have difficulty interpreting indirect requests.
- May have difficulty interpreting idioms, metaphors, and proverbs.
- May have difficulty appreciating humor.
- Difficulty interpreting facial expressions conveying emotions.
- Difficulty with auditory processing.
- Word-finding difficulties.
- Difficulty with verbal problem-solving.
- Difficulty understanding implied meanings.
- Difficulty understanding subtle humor or irony.
- Difficulty generating words within a category.
- Difficulty with topic initiation and maintenance.
- Difficulty interpreting and using turn-taking signals during conversation.
- Narratives contain less specific information.
- Use of tangential comments; difficulty getting to the point.
- Reading difficulties associated with hemispatial neglect.
- May speak in a monotone.

ASSOCIATED AND OTHER DIFFICULTIES

- Dysphagia.
- Right parietal lobe damage often results in difficulty with complex visuospatial information, impaired recognition of objects in unfamiliar views, and difficulty with spatial orientation. Other deficits associated with right parietal damage include difficulty sustaining attention, hemispatial neglect on the side contralateral to the lesion, unawareness or denial of deficits, and difficulty with orientation and location in space. (Tompkins, 1995)
- Difficulties associated with right temporal lobe damage include deficits in processing music and deficits in nonverbal memory. (Tompkins, 1995)
- Deficits associated with frontal lobe damage include difficulty with planning and problem-solving, decreased behavioral initiation and spontaneity, distractibility, perseveration, and poor memory for order of sequence of events. (Tompkins, 1995)
- Anosognosia or denial of illness.
- May exhibit social disinhibition.
- Poor visual discrimination of complex stimuli.
- Impaired color recognition.
- Facial recognition deficits.
- Visual agnosia.
- Visual neglect, especially on the left side.
- Visual memory deficits.
- Difficulty shifting attention from right to left.
- Difficulty with orientation to place.
- Capgras syndrome—belief that familiar people have been replaced with identical-looking impostors.
- Impulsivity.
- Distractibility.
- Difficulty changing tasks.
- Impaired attention.
- Impaired error recognition.
- Low affect, which may be misinterpreted as disinterest or lack of motivation.
- Pneumonia. Incidence of poststroke pneumonia is significantly higher among those with dysphagia.
- Depression.

ASSESSMENT

- Assess for dysphagia.
- Assess those areas of highest priority based on severity; premorbid educational, vocational, and avocational status; and discharge goals. (Halper and Cherney, 1996)
- As a screening tool, administer *Mini Inventory of Right Brain Injury* (MIRBI).
- Administer *Rehabilitation Institute of Chicago Evaluation of Communication Problems in Right Hemisphere Dysfunction* (RICE).
- Administer *Discourse Comprehension Test.*
- To assess auditory processing abilities, administer the Revised *Token Test.*
- To assess functional reading skills administer *The Behavioural Inattention Test.*
- Numerous other tests are available for the assessment of auditory comprehension, discourse and conversation skills, pragmatics, and cognitive abilities. For a review of these tests, see Chapter 3, Appraisal, Evaluation, and Diagnosis: Objectives and Orientations, in *Right Hemisphere Communication Disorders: Theory and Management.* (Tompkins, 1995). See also Chapter 5, Tests for Evaluating Cognitive-Communicative Skills in Patients with Right Hemisphere Damage, in *Clinical Management of Right Hemisphere Dysfunction.* (Halper, et al., 1996)
- Assess for neglect by presenting cancellation tasks, and by having the client read aloud compound words or sentences presented at visual midline.
- Conduct several treatment sessions to assess potential for success of continued therapy. Positive indicators include evidence of learning, generalization, retention, and a willingness to practice. Negative indicators include persistent denial of deficits and an unwillingness to participate in therapy.

INTERVENTION TECHNIQUES

- Remind family members and others that the goal is communication, not perfection.
- To aid memory, advise clients and caregivers to reduce clutter and keep items in same places in home and work environments.
- Establish eye contact before conveying a message.

- Ask questions during a conversation to ensure comprehension.
- To decrease impulsivity, require statement of a verbal plan before the client begins an activity.
- Address a client's interpretation of speech acts through work on understanding of indirect requests.
- Address need for sensitivity to listener, as well as general social skills.
- Use external aids such as calendars, schedules, and labels to assist with orientation. Teach clients to pay attention to and use these aids.
- Address attention deficits by gradually increasing the number of minutes the client participates appropriately in a conversation.
- Address attention deficits through activities such as detection and/or cancellation of target stimuli. State the number of targeted items, thus encouraging the client to continue searching independently until all items have been located.
- Address difficulties with sustained attention by breaking tasks into shorter segments, scheduling breaks, and using check-off sheets as tasks are completed.
- Use tracking and scanning techniques to increase attention to the left side of printed material, first without and then with competing and distracting stimuli.
- Through use of videotapes and/or group therapy sessions, have client identify examples of correct and incorrect turn-taking and topic maintenance.
- Address appropriate use of pronouns through conversation or by having the client relate a personal experience.
- Address organizational skills by having the client arrange pictures or words into sequence (e.g., increasing units of measure, progression of time, steps to complete an activity, progression of a story line).
- Be aware that swallowing status may change over days, weeks, and months. Continue to assess for dysphagia even if previous results have been normal.

RESULTS OF RECENT STUDIES

- In one study of 11 clients with RHD, approximately half showed some language problems. As part of the study, all clients were asked a series of questions about the effects of their illness on their communication skills. Results showed that client answers to such a questionnaire were not reliable indicators of communication difficulties. There was some tendency for those with poorer communication skills to report no difficulties. (Benton and Bryan, 1996)

- When compared with both normal speakers and speakers with left hemisphere damage, clients with right hemisphere damage exhibit a selective deficit when producing stories with emotional content. Performance decreases when emotional content is involved. (Bloom, 1994)
- When compared with a control group of normal subjects, those with right hemisphere damage secondary to a stroke performed as well on a task of paragraph recall, but showed significant difficulty with list-learning tasks. List-learning requires active attention for cues, as well as generation of a strategy for learning and memory. Implications are that these clients will have difficulty learning new materials "out of context." (Welte, 1993)

PROGNOSIS

- Prognosis is generally more favorable for those clients with smaller, unilateral lesions who have not had previous strokes, who were in good health prior to the stroke, and whose vision and hearing are relatively intact. (Tompkins, 1995)
- Some spontaneous improvement may occur in the days, weeks, or even months following the stroke. Such improvement is highly variable but is often greatest in the first 4 to 6 weeks following an occlusive stroke, while clients with hemorrhagic strokes may show a period of rapid improvement only after several months have elapsed. (Tompkins, 1995)

(See also Cerebrovascular Accidents [CVA] in Adults—Left Hemisphere Damage [LHD])

REFERENCES

Benton E, K Bryan. Right cerebral hemisphere damage: incidence of language problems. *International Journal of Rehabilitation Research*. 1996;19:47–54.

Bloom RL. Hemispheric responsibility and discourse production: contrasting patients with unilateral left and right hemisphere damage. In: Bloom RL, LK Obler, S De Santi, JS Ehrlich, eds. *Discourse Analysis and Applications: Studies in Adult Clinical Populations*. Hillsdale, NJ: Lawrence Erlbaum Associates. 1994:81–93.

Cherney LR, AS Halper. A conceptual framework for the evaluation and treatment of communication problems associated with right hemisphere damage. In: Halper AS, LR Cherney, MS Burns, eds. *Clinical Management of Right Hemisphere Dysfunction*, 2nd ed. Gaithersburg, Md: Aspen Publishers, Inc. 1996:21–29.

Cummings JL, MS Burns. Neurological syndromes associated with right hemisphere damage. In: Halper AS, LR Cherney, MS Burns, eds. *Clinical Management of Right Hemisphere Dysfunction*, 2nd ed. Gaithersburg, Md: Aspen Publishers, Inc. 1996:9–20.

Gottlieb D, M Kipnis, E Sister, Y Vardi, S Brill. Validation of the 50 ml³ drinking test for evaluation of post-stroke dysphagia. *Disability and Rehabilitation.* 1996;18(10):529–32.

Halper AS, LR Cherney. Tests for evaluating cognitive-communicative skills in patients with right hemisphere damage. In: Halper AS, LR Cherney, MS Burns, eds. *Clinical Management of Right Hemisphere Dysfunction*, 2nd ed. Gaithersburg, Md: Aspen Publishers, Inc. 1996:41–55.

Halper AS, LR Cherney, MS Burns. Treatment of cognitive-communicative skills in patients with right hemisphere damage. In Halper AS, LR Cherney, MS Burns, eds. *Clinical Management of Right Hemisphere Dysfunction*, 2nd ed. Gaithersburg, Md: Aspen Publishers, Inc. 1996:57–97.

Meyers PS. Communication disorders associated with right-hemisphere brain damage. In: Chapey R, ed. *Language Intervention Strategies in Adult Aphasia,* 3rd ed. Baltimore: Williams & Wilkins. 1994:513–34.

Ramasubbu R, SH Kennedy. Factors complicating the diagnosis of depression in cerebrovascular disease (Part II): neurological deficits and various assessment methods. *Canadian Journal of Psychiatry.* 1994;39(10):601–7.

Smithard DG, PA O'Neill, RE England, CL Park, R Wyatt, DF Martin, J Morris. The natural history of dysphagia following a stroke. *Dysphagia.* 1997;12:188–93.

Tompkins CA. *Right Hemisphere Communication Disorders: Theory and Management.* San Diego, Calif: Singular Publishing Group, Inc. 1995.

Welte PO. Indices of verbal learning and memory deficits after right hemisphere stroke. *Archives of Physical Medicine & Rehabilitation* 1993;74(6):631–6.

Encephalitis

DESCRIPTION

An acute inflammatory disease of the brain due to direct viral invasion or to hypersensitivity initiated by a virus or other foreign protein. Symptoms may include alteration in consciousness, personality change, seizures, paresis, or cranial nerve abnormalities. Rasmussen encephalitis (RE) is a progressive disorder characterized by increasing unilateral seizures, development of hemiparesis, and declining cognitive abilities.

ETIOLOGY

Primary encephalitis may be caused by the arbovirus, poliovirus, echovirus, or coxsackie virus (herpes simplex, varicella zoster, mumps). Mosquito-borne arboviral encephalitides infect man only during warm weather and include St. Louis encephalitis, Eastern and Western equine encephalitis, and California encephalitis. Secondary encephalitis is generally a complication of viral infection and may follow measles, chickenpox, rubella, or smallpox vaccination.

SPEECH AND LANGUAGE DIFFICULTIES

- Ataxic dysarthria.
- Difficulty with organization of thought.
- Difficulty using cohesive links such as conjunctions.
- Verbal communication skills may deteriorate over time.

ASSOCIATED AND OTHER DIFFICULTIES

- Paresis.
- Personality changes.

ASSESSMENT

- Administer *Peabody Picture Vocabulary Test,* revised (PPVT-R).
- Administer *Test of Language Development,* 2nd ed. (TOLD-2).
- Administer *Test of Adolescent and Adult Language,* 3rd ed. (TOAL-3).
- Administer *Clinical Evaluation of Language Functions,* 3rd ed. (CELF-3).
- Assess for dysarthria. (See Appendix A)
- Obtain a spontaneous speech sample and analyze for mean number of morphemes per utterance (MMU), presence of embedded clauses, and use of an inflectional system. (Caplan, et al., 1996)

INTERVENTION TECHNIQUES

• Work on modifying rate and prosody to improve intelligibility. (Duffy, 1995)
• Teach strategies to enhance organization of thought.

RESULTS OF RECENT STUDIES

• In a study of one female client with herpes encephalitis, knowledge of living things categories was impaired, while knowledge of man-made objects was largely preserved except for recall of their color or identification of their sound. It is argued that while retrieval of the perceptual features of both types of categories may be impaired, this deficit may be compensated for in man-made objects by the similarity between shape and function. (De Renzi and Lucchelli, 1994)

PROGNOSIS

Mortality rates vary with the etiology. Permanent brain dysfunction is more likely to occur in infants. Young children show improvement over a longer period of time than do adults with similar infections. In some cases, desperately ill clients may recover completely.

REFERENCES

Caplan R, S Curtiss, HT Chugani, HV Vinters. Pediatric Rasmussen Encephalitis: social communication, language, PET, and pathology before and after hemispherectomy. *Brain and Cognition.* 1996;32:45–66.

De Renzi E, F Lucchelli. Are semantic systems separately represented in the brain? The case of living category impairment. *Cortex.* 1994;30(1):3–25.

Duffy JR. *Motor Speech Disorders: Substrates, Differential Diagnosis, and Management.* St. Louis, Mo: Mosby. 1995:145–65.

Epilepsy

DESCRIPTION

A recurrent paroxysmal disorder of cerebral function characterized by sudden brief attacks of altered consciousness, motor activity, sensory phenomena, or inappropriate behavior caused by abnormal excessive discharge of cerebral neurons. In about 75% of affected young adults, the epilepsy is idiopathic. That is, there are no obvious causes. Symptoms of idiopathic epilepsy generally appear between the ages of 2 and 14 years.

Seizures may be controlled with drug therapy. Such therapy completely controls grand mal seizures in about 50% of cases and reduces the frequency of seizures in another 35%. With drug therapy, petit mal seizures are controlled in 40% of cases and are reduced in another 35%. Psychomotor seizures are controlled in 35% of cases and are reduced in another 50%. (See accompanying table on types and characteristics of seizures.)

Overuse of medication may cause mental dullness. Progressive mental deterioration is generally related to an underlying neurological condition rather than to effects of the seizures themselves. Seventy percent of noninstitutionalized persons with epilepsy have normal intelligence, 20% show mild intellectual impairment, and 10% show moderate to severe intellectual impairment. In status epilepticus, motor, sensory, or psychic seizures follow one another with no intervening periods of consciousness. The condition may persist for hours or days and may be fatal.

ETIOLOGY

Seizures may occur as the result of any of several cerebral or systemic disorders, including hyperpyrexia, central nervous system (CNS) infections, metabolic disturbances, toxic agents, cerebral hypoxia, cerebral edema, anaphylaxis, cerebral trauma, and cerebral infarct or hemorrhage.

SPEECH AND LANGUAGE DIFFICULTIES

- During and following status epilepticus, dysphasia may develop.
- Following status epilepticus, muteness may occur.

Types and Characteristics of Seizures

Type of Seizure	Characteristics
Partial: Simple partial seizure (formerly called a focal motor or focal sensory seizure)	Stereotyped, sudden sensation or move-ment—the same sudden sensation or movement during every seizure (i.e., sudden feeling of pain, perception of a foul odor, or feeling of nausea). Does not affect consciousness.
Complex partial seizure (formerly called a psychomotor seizure or temporal lobe seizure)	Unusual stereotyped behaviors, such as staring, fumbling with clothes, lip smacking, and automatic hand move-ments, accompanied by a change in or loss of consciousness.
Partial with secondary generalization	May initiate as a partial seizure and progress to include a generalized response.
Generalized: Atonic (formerly called drop attacks)	A sudden loss of muscle tone, usually resulting in a fall. In most cases this also includes a loss of consciousness.
Myoclonic	Generalized jerking of extremities, lasting less than 5 seconds, usually with a brief period of unconsciousness that can go unnoticed. May occur in clusters.
Absence (formerly called petit mal)	Loss of consciousness, usually lasting less than 10 seconds, with no other visible change. May involve eye blinking or lip smacking.

continues

| Generalized tonic-clonic (formerly called grand mal) | Tonic phase involves generalized stiffening of muscles usually lasting less than 1 minute. This is followed by a clonic phase of rapid jerking. The individual is unconscious during both phases and will not remember it afterward. |

Source: Reprinted from K.R. Kuntz, Medical and Nursing Issues, in *Handbook of Developmental Disabilities: Resources for Interdisciplinary Care,* L.A. Kurtz, P.W. Dowrick, S.E. Levy, and M.L. Batshaw, eds., p. 398, © 1996, Aspen Publishers, Inc.

- Children with complex partial seizure disorder and full-scale IQ scores below 100 exhibit more illogical thinking and use fewer pronouns, definitives, definite articles, comparatives, and conjunctions. (Caplan, et al., 1993)
- Word finding difficulties may occur in those with left temporal lobe epilepsy (LTLE).
- Aphasia, frequently mild and transitory, may occur following surgery for the control or elimination of seizures.

ASSOCIATED AND OTHER DIFFICULTIES

- Confusion during or following seizures.
- Incontinence during seizures.
- Developmental dyscalculia is common.
- Following status epilepticus, blindness and/or deafness may occur.

ASSESSMENT

- Following development of dysphasia secondary to seizure activity, administer the *Minnesota Test for Differential Diagnosis of Aphasia (MTDDA)* repeatedly over time to document deficits and subsequent recovery.

- To assess word-finding difficulties, administer the *Boston Naming Test* (BNT).
- With clients undergoing surgery for the control or elimination of seizures, administer tests such as the *BNT* and the *Boston Diagnostic Aphasia Examination* (BDAE) both preoperatively and postoperatively to assess changes in language function.

INTERVENTION TECHNIQUES

- Work with neurosurgeon in mapping language areas of the brain prior to and during surgery. (Zarrella, 1995)
- Address any word-finding difficulties that may occur.
- With children, address language deficits.

RESULTS OF RECENT STUDIES

- Electroencephalographic (EEG) studies show epileptic discharges occurring even when nothing is overtly observable. What can be measured are temporary decreases in performance, such as reaction time, sustained attention, and immediate memory. Left-sided discharges affect verbal tasks; right-sided discharges affect nonverbal tasks. (Deonna, 1993)
- Children and young adults who undergo hemispherectomy often exhibit little loss of language function regardless of the side of the surgery, although different studies have reported somewhat differing results. (Stark, et al., 1995)
- Through a study involving electrical stimulation, the following language areas were defined and confirmed:
  1. anterior language area in the posterior portion of the inferior frontal gyrus immediately in front of the face motor strip, corresponding to Broca's area.
  2. posterior language area in the middle and posterior part of the superior temporal gyrus and the adjacent supramarginal gyrus, corresponding to Wernicke's area.
  3. basal temporal language area (BTLA) at the base of the temporal lobe, mainly in the fusiform gyrus.

Beyond the boundaries of these three language areas, language sites were also detected in the perisylvian cortex of the frontal, temporal, and parietal lobes and in gyri adjacent to the fusiform gyrus in the basal temporal region. Language comprehension deficits occurred as frequently in Broca's area as in Wernicke's area. (Schäffler, et al., 1996)

- In a study of 200 adults with epilepsy and 130 age-matched controls, it was found that males with an earlier onset of seizures and left-handed females with epilepsy were more likely to have dyslexia. The study also found that 45% of females with epilepsy were left-handed, compared with 15% of males. (Schachter, et al., 1993)
- Prior to surgery to excise a limited portion of the cerebral cortex, electrical stimulation is performed to determine specific sites of interference with verbal processes. The following results often occur with electrostimulation of the cortex: involuntary vocalization, inability to speak, inability to continue to write, aphasic disorders, and disturbances of verbal memory. Results during electrostimulation are not always the same as those obtained following actual excision. Some functions that are impaired during electrostimulation remain intact following excision, while some functions that remained intact during electrostimulation may be impaired following excision. (Lebrun and Leleux, 1993)
- Left temporal lobectomy impairs the naming of nonliving things more than the naming of living things, while right temporal lobectomy produces no differential effect. (Tippett, et al., 1996)
- In a study of language fluency, adults with LTLE scored significantly lower on confrontation naming tasks than did those with right temporal lobe epilepsy (RTLE) or primary generalized epilepsy (PGE). (Howell, et al., 1994)
- Anterior temporal lobectomy (ATL) in adults produced the following results: Postoperatively, only those persons with left temporal involvement with no early risk (LT-NER) showed evidence of language decline, and that decline was specifically in confrontation naming. Phonemic and semantic fluency, repetition, comprehension, and reading skills were unaffected. No decline was noted in persons with right temporal involvement or in those with left temporal involvement whose seizures began prior to the age of 2 years. (Saykin, et al., 1995)

PROGNOSIS

A normal lifestyle should be encouraged.

REFERENCES

Caplan R, D Guthrie, WD Shields, WJ Peacock, HV Vinters, S Yudovin. Communication deficits in children undergoing temporal lobectomy. *Journal of the American Academy of Child and Adolescent Psychiatry.* 1993;32(3):604–11.

Deonna T. Annotation: cognitive and behavioral correlates of epileptic activity in children. *Journal of Child Psychology & Psychiatry & Allied Disciplines.* 1993;34(5):611–20.

Gross-Tsur V, O Manor, RS Shalev. Developmental dyscalculia, gender, and the brain. *Archives of Disease in Childhood.* 1993;68:510–2.

Howell RA, MM Saling, DC Bradley, SF Berkovic. Interictal language fluency in temporal lobe epilepsy. *Cortex.* 1994;30:469–78.

Kirshner HS, T Hughes, T Fakhoury, B Abou-Khalil. Aphasia secondary to partial status epilepticus of the basal temporal language area. *Neurology.* 1995;45:1616–8.

Lebrun Y, C Leleux. The effects of electrostimulation and of resective and stereotactic surgery on language and speech. *Acta Neurochirurgica* [Suppl]. 1993;56:40–51.

Murchison JT, RJ Sellar, AJW Steers. Status epilepticus presenting as progressive dysphasia. *Neuroradiology.* 1995;37:438–9.

Saykin AJ, P Stafiniak, LJ Robinson, KA Flannery, RC Gur, MJ O'Connor, MR Sperling. Language before and after temporal lobectomy: specificity of acute changes and relation to early risk factors. *Epilepsia.* 1995;36(1):1071–7.

Schachter SC, AM Galaburda, BJ Ransil. Associations of dyslexia with epilepsy, handedness, and gender. *Annals of the New York Academy of Sciences.* 1993;682:402–3.

Schäffler L, HO Lüders, GJ Beck. Quantitative comparison of language deficits produced by extraoperative electrical stimulation of Broca's, Wernicke's, and basal temporal language areas. *Epilepsia.* 1996;37(5):463–75.

Stark RE, K Bleile, J Brandt, J Freeman, EPG Vining. Speech-language outcomes of hemispherectomy in children and young adults. *Brain and Language.* 1995;51:406–21.

Tippett LJ, G Glosser, MJ Farah. A category-specific naming impairment after temporal lobectomy. *Neuropsychologia.* 1996;34(2):139–46.

van Dongen HR, MCB Loonen, DJ Heerseman, R deGroot. Blind, deaf and mute after a status epilepticus caused by hyperpyrexia from shigellosis—a case report with a four-year follow-up. *Neuropediatrics.* 1993;24:343–5.

Zarrella S. Epilepsy surgery program: unique practice area for speech-language pathology. *Advance for Speech-Language Pathologists & Audiologists.* 1995;5(28):9.

Friedreich's Ataxia (FA)

DESCRIPTION

A hereditary degenerative disorder characterized by progressive ataxia due to degeneration of the cerebellum, brainstem, spinal cord, and peripheral nerves. Symptoms generally appear first between the ages of 5 and 15 years, with unsteadiness of gait generally the first symptom, followed by upper extremity ataxia and dysarthria.

ETIOLOGY

The responsible gene is located on chromosome number 9. Inheritance is autosomal recessive.

SPEECH AND LANGUAGE DIFFICULTIES

- Dysarthria, which is characterized by sudden pitch changes, transient harshness, and disturbances of respiratory and articulatory control.

ASSOCIATED AND OTHER DIFFICULTIES

- Progressive muscle weakness in lower extremities.
- Ataxia of gait.
- Difficulty determining position of limbs in space.
- Scoliosis.
- Loss of sensation of touch, although pain and temperature may be felt normally.
- Nystagmus.
- Eventually, the heart is always involved, becoming enlarged and resulting in breathlessness and palpitations.
- Diabetes may develop.
- Hearing loss may be present.

ASSESSMENT

- Assess for dysarthria.

INTERVENTION TECHNIQUES

- Provide therapy to increase breath support.
- Work to modify rate and prosody to improve intelligibility. (Duffy, 1995)

RESULTS OF RECENT STUDIES

- In a study of speech timing, clients with FA performed slower than a group of normal controls on tasks on rapid repetitive articulation (/pa/, /ta/, /ka/). However, the difference in timing was not found on sentence production tasks. The authors note that "speech timing seems to break down relatively late in cerebellar disease, whereas the mere instruction to perform maximally fast seems to shift ataxic patients below their natural-context performance level." (Ziegler and Wessel, 1996)

PROGNOSIS

FA is a progressive condition. Most of those affected must use a wheelchair by their early 20s. Death often, though not always, occurs by the age of 40 years.

REFERENCES

Duffy JR. *Motor Speech Disorders: Substrates, Differential Diagnosis, and Management.* St. Louis, Mo: Mosby. 1995:145–65.

Gilbert P. *The A-Z Reference Book of Syndromes and Inherited Disorders: A Manual for Health, Social and Education Workers.* New York: Chapman and Hall. 1993:96–98.

Ziegler W, K Wessel. Speech timing in ataxic disorders: sentence production and rapid repetitive articulation. *Neurology.* 1996;47:208–14.

Guillain-Barré Syndrome (GBS)

DESCRIPTION

An acute, usually rapidly progressive form of inflammatory polyneuropathy characterized by muscular weakness and mild distal sensory loss. Incidence is 1 or 2 cases per 100,000 persons.

ETIOLOGY

GBS is suspected to be an autoimmune disorder triggered by a preceding viral infection.

SPEECH AND LANGUAGE DIFFICULTIES

- More than 50% of severe cases have weakness of facial and oropharyngeal muscles.
- Dysarthria.

ASSOCIATED AND OTHER DIFFICULTIES

- Weakness and paralysis of limbs, torso, and face.
- Difficulty with respiration.
- Dysphagia. Oral and pharyngeal dysfunction.

ASSESSMENT

- Perform dysphagia evaluation, including videofluoroscopic studies. Perform initial videofluoroscopic studies during progressive or plateau phase and follow-up studies 4 to 8 weeks after onset of symptoms. (Chen, et al., 1996)
- Assess speech intelligibility.

INTERVENTION TECHNIQUES

- Treat for dysphagia.
- As warranted, provide short-term system of augmentative and alternative communication (AAC).

- To treat flaccid dysarthria, work to increase support for speech breathing.

RESULTS OF RECENT STUDIES

No recent studies regarding communication skills were found in the literature.

PROGNOSIS

Up to 5% of clients die, generally due to respiratory failure; 90% of clients reach their maximal degree of weakness within 2 to 3 weeks of onset. Improvement occurs over a period of months. Residual weakness remains in 30% of adults and a somewhat higher percentage of children. In approximately 10% of cases, relapse occurs after initial improvement.

REFERENCES

Chen MYM, PD Donofrio, MG Frederick, DJ Ott, LA Pikna. Videofluoroscopic evaluation of patients with Guillain-Barré Syndrome. *Dysphagia.* 1996;11:11–13.

Duffy JR. *Motor Speech Disorders: Substrates, Differential Diagnosis, and Management.* St. Louis, Mo: Mosby. 1995:99–127.

Thoene JG, NP Coker, eds. *Physicians Guide to Rare Diseases.* New York: Dowden Publishing Co. 1995:307.

Head Injury (HI)—Adults

(See also Head Injury [HI]—Children and Adolescents)

DESCRIPTION

HI results in more deaths and disabilities than any other neurologic cause prior to the age of 50 years. It is the leading cause of death in men and boys below the age of 35 years.

ETIOLOGY

Damage results from penetration of the skull or from rapid brain acceleration or deceleration. Blood vessels, nerve tissues, and meninges may be sheared, torn, and ruptured resulting in neural damage, intracerebral or extracerebral ischemia or hemorrhage, and cerebral edema.

SPEECH AND LANGUAGE DIFFICULTIES

- Decrease in comprehension.
- Decrease in speech and/or language production.
- Anomia.
- Dysarthria.
- Phonatory apraxia.
- Phonatory weakness.
- Hypernasality.
- Decrease in rate of speaking.
- Minimal pitch and loudness variations.
- Imprecise language.
- Word-retrieval difficulties.
- Difficulty shifting, dividing, and maintaining focus.
- Disinhibited, socially inappropriate language.
- Difficulty with pragmatic skills.
- Difficulty with turn-taking skills.
- Difficulty sustaining and extending a conversation; poor topic maintenance.
- Difficulty with irony, sarcasm, abstract references.
- Difficulty with reasoning and problem-solving.
- Impaired executive functions, including self-awareness, goal-setting, planning and organizing, evaluating, and strategic thinking.
- One or more voice pathologies, including hoarseness, decreased vocal intensity, low pitch, breathiness, and glottal fry.
- Aphasia may be present. Indicators include impaired auditory comprehension, anomia, and confused language.
- Primary language dysfunction associated with closed HI is in area of pragmatics. While "aphasics may communicate better than they talk, closed head injury (CHI) patients appear to talk better than they communicate." (Coelho, et al., 1992)

ASSOCIATED AND OTHER DIFFICULTIES

- Posttraumatic epilepsy with seizures may appear as late as several years after the injury. It is present in about 10% of severe closed head injuries and 40% of injuries caused by penetrating wounds.
- Postconcussion syndrome (PCS) may result following a mild HI. Symptoms may include headache, dizziness, difficulty with concentration, variable amnesia, depression, apathy, anxiety, sleep disturbances, blurred vision, nausea, and irritability. Persistence of PCS may be related to persistence of cognitive deficits.
- Visual problems as a result of the injury, including diplopia (double vision), binocular dysfunction, unstable peripheral vision, poor fixation, and spatial disorientation.
- Indications of frontal lobe damage include poor planning, poor self-analysis, impairment of performance monitoring, and inability to regulate one's behavior to meet desired goals.
- Aggression.
- Agitation.
- Impaired ability to plan, organize, and sequence events.
- Impaired ability to modulate emotions.
- Impaired ability to monitor behavior.
- Impaired problem-solving skills.
- Memory deficits.
- Attention deficits.
- Disinhibition.
- Stimulus-bound behavior.
- Decreased initiation.
- Spasticity.
- Headaches.
- Reduced endurance.
- Hearing loss. Often audiograms show a notch in the 500 to 2,000 Hz range.
- Sensory deficits.
- Disorganized thinking or acting.
- Difficulty learning new information.
- Inefficient retrieval of stored information.
- Impairments in self-awareness, goal-setting, planning, self-initiating, self-inhibiting, self-monitoring, and self-evaluation.

- Dysphagia and associated problems such as delayed triggering of swallow reflex, reduced tongue control, and reduced pharyngeal transit.

ASSESSMENT

- In the acute phase, assess daily time and place orientation, knowledge of team member identities, appropriate responses, associative learning, episodic recall, and correct use of scheduling aids. (Zarella, 1995)
- Be aware of the following limitations of formal testing situations: the quiet environment may disguise problems with attention and concentration; a series of short sessions may disguise problems with endurance, perseverance, and fatigue; clear instructions may disguise problems with initiation, task orientation, or problem-solving. (Ylvisaker and Szekeres, 1994)
- Observe the client in a variety of settings.
- Assess client's self-awareness of deficits and their implications.
- When assessing high-functioning clients, keep in mind that language and cognition are closely related; language disturbance after traumatic brain injury (TBI) is generally not aphasia; high-level and subtle deficits often are present; and information processing deficits are a hallmark of mild TBI. Testing must be sufficiently high level to detect subtle deficits. Begin receptive language assessment at paragraph level and assess recognition and recall skills and comprehension of abstract verbal information. Assess narrative discourse skills from picture description through self-generated narrative. Assess verbal fluency. Assess writing skills at paragraph level and beyond, not letters or single words. Assess information processing including perception, attention, meaning, encoding, and retrieval. (Ellmo, 1995)
- Those with mild injuries may seem to fully recover but may continue to experience deficits. Assessments should take place in the client's natural environments and should involve detailed observations of the client's communication skills and strategies.
- Administer *Rehabilitation Institute of Chicago Functional Assessment Scale* (RIC-FAS).
- Administer *Scales of Cognitive Ability for Traumatic Brain Injury* (SCATBI).
- Administer *Brief Test of Head Injury* (BTHI).
- Administer *Ross Information Processing Assessment-2* (RIPA-2).

- To assess patterns of memory deficit, administer the *California Verbal Learning Test* (CVLT).
- Administer *Multilingual Aphasia Examination* (MAE).
- To assess dysarthria, evaluate all speech-related motor systems (respiration, phonation, resonance, articulation). Involve physical therapists, occupational therapists, physiatrists, and otolaryngologists as appropriate.
- Administer *Frenchay Dysarthria Assessment.*
- To evaluate overall intelligibility, administer *Assessment of Intelligibility of Dysarthric Speakers* (AIDS).
- Assess dysphagia with bedside swallowing evaluation and with videofluorographic evaluation.
- Assessment for augmentative and alternative communication (AAC) should be interdisciplinary and include evaluations of motor skills, cognitive potential for learning a new system, academic skills, visual-perceptual skills, emotional and behavioral factors, potential for recovering speech, and client and family willingness to accept AAC. Be aware that recovery of intelligible speech may occur after a year or more postonset, even with intensive therapy. Therefore, expensive AAC solutions should not be considered until final communication skills status is certain. (Ylvisaker and Urbanczyk, 1994)

INTERVENTION TECHNIQUES

- In early and middle stages of recovery, work with others in client's environment to facilitate structure and order. Use log books and memory books to facilitate memory and orientation.
- In early stages of recovery, establish a consistent yes/no response to be used and asked for by all who come into contact with the client. Guard against different people establishing different response systems with the client, and guard against using reflexive movements (such as eye blinks) as a signal system.
- Particularly in early stages of recovery, keep AAC systems simple and flexible.
- To treat transient phonatory dyspraxia, introduce use of electrolarynx; work with voluntary imitation of coughing, throat-clearing, humming; and encourage voluntary production of "a," then continue to other vowels and consonants. (Mueller, 1995)
- When working with clients with mild TBI, establishing some structure to daily routines helps to reduce stress.

- Work on organizational skills through functional activities such as sorting laundry.
- Use the *Empowerment Rehabilitation Model*, composed of structure, motivation, information, acceptance, and skills. The model also involves interpersonal elements such as self-awareness and social skills, emotional elements such as stress management training, and vocational elements such as problem-solving and setting goals. (Trace, 1994)
- Explain to the client and family the reasons for attending speech therapy. (Alumbaugh, 1994)
- Repeat information as often as necessary, being aware of short-term memory deficits. (Alumbaugh, 1994)
- Present information visually or verbally based on strengths of client.
- Advise others to speak slowly and to use less complex sentences.
- Use a transdisciplinary team approach.
- Recognize that intervention must focus on strategies relevant to the client's environment rather than on isolated drills or exercises. (Ylvisaker and Szekeres, 1994)
- Be aware of triggers to noncompliance, i.e., inconsistent expectations, instructions that are too complex, failing to reinforce desired behaviors. (Carter and Menon, 1997)
- In late-stage intervention, focus on compensatory strategies such as use of external aids to enhance memory and organization.
- Involve the client in the process of devising and implementing strategies.
- Work toward empowering the client, partially by giving the client more decision-making authority in the clinical setting. (Togher, et al., 1996)
- Address organizational skills through activities such as writing narratives, writing descriptions, or giving instructions to others. (Ylvisaker and Szekeres, 1994)
- Consider pharyngoplasty or palatal augmentation in cases of velopharyngeal incompetence and hypernasality. These interventions should be considered only after a minimum of 1 year of intensive speech intervention and may be contraindicated in patients with seizures and those with behavioral intolerances. (Upton and Berger, 1995; Ylvisaker and Urbanczyk, 1994)
- In a case of cluttering secondary to TBI, the following six-step program has been used successfully: increase client's awareness of the disorder, increase focus of attention, increase level of confidence, improve

thought organization, facilitate carryover, community reintegration. (Iskowitz, 1997b)

RESULTS OF RECENT STUDIES

- In some clients with continuing PCS, a return to work aggravated the symptoms accompanied by a decrease in cognitive performance. (Bohnen, et al., 1992)
- Because the majority of head injuries are sustained by young adult males who have not attained high educational levels and who often have a history of risk-taking behavior, when assessing discourse skills of TBI survivors, clinicians should use as comparisons data from populations with similar premorbid educational and vocational backgrounds. (Snow, et al., 1997)

PROGNOSIS

Nearly 50% of clients with severe head injury do not survive. Of those who do survive, most recovery is seen within the first 6 months, although smaller gains may be noted up to 2 years or longer.

REFERENCES

Alumbaugh E. Brain injury: a patient's perspective on treatment. *Advance for Speech-Language Pathologists & Audiologists.* 1994;4(28):18.

Bohnen N, A Twijnstra, J Jolles. Performance in the Stroop color word test in relationship to the persistence of symptoms following mild head injury. *Acta Neurologica Scandinavica.* 1992;85(2):116–21.

Bresk S. Visual deficits impact rehab process. *Advance for Speech-Language Pathologists & Audiologists.* 1995;5(27):16–17.

Carter RE, SK Menon. Compliance training for patients with TBI. *Advance for Speech-Language Pathologists & Audiologists.* 1997;7(28):17.

Coelho CA, BZ Liles, RJ Duffy. Communication and swallowing disorders in traumatic brain injury. *Physical Medicine & Rehabilitation Clinics of North America.* 1992;3(2):371–88.

Crosson B, PV Cooper, RK Lincoln, RM Bauer, CA Velozo. Relationship between verbal memory and language performance after blunt head injury. *The Clinical Neuropsychologist.* 1993;7(3):250–67.

Ellmo W. Assessment issues in mild TBI. *Advance for Speech-Language Pathologists & Audiologists.* 1995;5(33):17.

Gelman J. Communication, behavior problems impede TBI rehab. *Advance for Speech-Language Pathologists & Audiologists.* 1995;5(44):8.

Iskowitz M. Testing in TBI: formal and informal mix needed to meet patient needs. *Advance for Speech-Language Pathologists & Audiologists.* 1996;6(35):6–7,10.

Iskowitz M. Mayo audiologists link notches to head trauma. *Advance for Speech-Language Pathologists & Audiologists.* 1997a;7(35):9,17.

Iskowitz M. Treatment program for neurogenic disfluency: six-step protocol key to achieving fluency. *Advance for Speech-Language Pathologists & Audiologists.* 1997b; 7(35):8,11.

McDonald S. Pragmatic language skills after closed head injury: ability to meet the informational needs of the listener. *Brain & Language.* 1993;44(1):28–46.

Mueller PB. Transient phonatory dyspraxia: identification and treatment of an obscure condition. *Advance for Speech-Language Pathologists & Audiologists.* 1995;5(30):9,13.

Murphy J. Long-term needs of TBI survivors should not be shortchanged. *Advance for Speech-Language Pathologists & Audiologists.* 1995;5(44):11.

Paul-Cohen R. The role of the speech-language pathologist in the treatment of mild brain injury: a community-based approach. In: Mandel S, RT Sataloff, SR Schapiro, eds. *Minor Head Trauma: Assessment, Management, and Rehabilitation.* New York: Springer-Verlag. 1993:261–71.

Shoemaker A. Researching voice pathologies of TBI. *Advance for Speech-Language Pathologists & Audiologists.* 1996;6(35):3.

Snow P, J Douglas, J Ponsford. Conversational assessment following traumatic brain injury: a comparison across two control groups. *Brain Injury.* 1997;11(6):409–29.

Togher L, L Hand, C Code. A new perspective on the relationship between communication impairment and disempowerment following head injury in information exchanges. *Disability and Rehabilitation.* 1996;18(11):559–66.

Trace R. Empowering patients with TBI. *Advance for Speech-Language Pathologists & Audiologists.* 1994;4(28):19.

Upton LG, MK Berger. Use of pharyngoplasty to improve resonance in adult closed-head injury patients: report of cases. *Journal of Oral & Maxillofacial Surgery.* 1995;53(6):717–9.

Ylvisaker M, SF Szekeres. Communication disorders associated with closed head injury. In: Chapey R, ed. *Language Intervention Strategies in Adult Aphasia,* 3rd ed. Baltimore: Williams & Wilkins. 1994:546–68.

Ylvisaker M, B Urbanczyk. Assessment and treatment of speech, swallowing, and communication disorders following traumatic brain injury. In: Finlayson MAJ, SH Garner, eds. *Brain Injury Rehabilitation: Clinical Considerations.* Baltimore: Williams & Wilkins. 1994:157–286.

Zarella S. Medical management of TBI utilizes integrated approach. *Advance for Speech-Language Pathologists & Audiologists.* 1995;5(44):5.

Head Injury (HI)—
Children and Adolescents

(See also Head Injury [HI]—Adults)

DESCRIPTION

HI is the second most common form of trauma for which children are admitted to a hospital. More males than females reportedly sustain HI by a ratio of 2 to 1. The greatest incidences are in children younger than 1 year and those 15 years or older. Causes of head injury include motor vehicle accidents, all-terrain vehicle accidents, abuse, assaults, motorcycle accidents, pedestrian accidents, stabbings, and bicycle accidents. Mild traumatic brain injury (TBI) involves very brief or no loss of consciousness at the time of the injury. Symptoms of dizziness, headache, vomiting, nausea, lethargy, irritability, and difficulty concentrating resolve in 90% of mild injuries within days or weeks of the injury. Moderate TBI is associated with loss of consciousness for up to 24 hours and neurological damage including skull fractures, contusions, hemorrhage, or focal damage. Severe TBI is characterized by coma lasting longer than 24 hours followed by multiple physical, social, emotional, behavioral, cognitive, and communicative problems lasting indefinitely.

Effects of an HI sustained early in life may not become apparent until the child becomes older and is required to use more complex cognitive and self-regulatory skills. Unilateral right hemisphere damage sustained within the first year of life often results in language functions being partially or totally assumed by the right hemisphere. When this occurs, "crowding" of the right hemisphere may result with some compromise of visuospatial skills.

ETIOLOGY

Minor HIs may occur without loss of consciousness and without neurologic signs. Symptoms may include vomiting, pallor, irritability, or lethargy. A concussion is a transient and rapidly reversible state of neurologic dysfunction, with a loss of consciousness, immediately following an HI. Clients may have amnesia for the event and for the time just prior to the event, but no neurologic signs are present. Contusions are focal bruising or tearing of cerebral tissue accompanied by hemorrhage and local edema. The ventral surface of the frontal lobe and inferolateral aspects of the temporal lobes are the most common sites of contusions and result in disturbances of strength and sensation and an increase in intracranial pressure. Epidural hematomas are collections of blood between the dura mater and the skull. Subdural hematomas are collections of blood beneath the dura mater and are usually associated with a significant contusion of the brain. There is generally associated hyperemia and cerebral edema, which results in an altered state of consciousness and signs of intracranial pressure. Surgical intervention is often necessary. Incidence of seizures secondary to the contusion is high. Intraventricular or subarachnoid hemorrhage is generally associated with a severe HI and resulting long-term neurologic signs.

SPEECH AND LANGUAGE DIFFICULTIES
- Imprecise articulation; dysarthria.
- Phonatory weakness.
- Hypernasality.
- Impaired prosody.
- Slow rate of speech.
- Rapid rate of speech with cluttering.
- Impairment in confrontation naming.
- Limited verbal output with incomplete statements.
- Normal amount of verbal output but characterized by repetitions, reformulations, and word substitutions.
- Receptive language deficits.
- Disorganized expression in speech and writing.
- Tendency toward concrete and inflexible thinking.
- Disproportionate difficulty with abstract ideas.
- Tangential speech.
- Difficulties in narrative discourse characterized by repetitions, improper sequencing, dysfluencies, and omission of information.
- Confabulation.
- Deficits may become more evident over time as academic expectations involve higher-level skills and increasing degrees of abstraction.

ASSOCIATED AND OTHER DIFFICULTIES

- Dysphagia.
- Retrograde amnesia.
- Behavior changes.
- Emotional lability.
- Sleep disturbances.
- Easily fatigued.
- Low threshold for frustration.
- Seems unmotivated.
- Demanding of attention.
- Irritability.
- Cognitive impairment.
- Memory deficits.
- Attention deficits.
- Processing deficits.
- Difficulty with abstract reasoning.
- Difficulty adjusting to change.
- Decreased self-esteem.
- Decreased self-control.
- Decreased awareness of social rules.
- Impulsive behavior.
- Socially aggressive behavior.
- Decreased initiation.
- Depression.
- Social withdrawal.
- Difficulty interpreting social and emotional cues.
- Hostility.
- Suicidal thoughts.
- Denial.
- Serious family conflicts.

ASSESSMENT

- In the early stages, administer *Glasgow Coma Scale*.
- Administer *Ranchos Los Amigo Scale of Cognitive Functioning*. (See accompanying exhibit)

- Use *Peabody Picture Vocabulary Test—Revised* repeatedly over time to asses acquisition of new concepts and vocabulary.
- Assess all speech-related motor systems (respiration, phonation, resonance, articulation).
- Assess for dysarthria. (See Appendix A)
- Those with mild injuries may seem to fully recover but may continue to experience deficits. Assessments should take place in the client's natural environments and should involve detailed observations of the client's communication skills and strategies.
- Assess carefully for apraxia versus impairment of higher-level executive functioning and planning.
- Analyze verbal and written narratives for organization, coherence, elaboration, and completeness.
- Analyze observed deficits for interaction of cognitive and linguistic processes, i.e., difficulty with reading or auditory comprehension may be due to poor organizational schemes rather than to linguistic deficits.
- Assess pragmatic skills, particularly in terms of topic (selection, introduction, maintenance, change), turn-taking (initiation, response, contingency, conciseness), lexical selection (specificity, accuracy, cohesion), and stylistic variation (context and partner appropriateness). (Ylvisaker, et al., 1994)
- Mild to moderate articulation problems and symptoms of dysarthria present during early stages of recovery may resolve themselves. Reassess at a later time without initially targeting for therapy.
- Use *Pragmatic Protocol* to assess and document conversational behaviors.
- Assess and compare comprehension with and without distracting interference.
- Use appropriate subtests from *Clinical Evaluation of Language Fundamentals—3rd ed. Edition (CELF-3)*.
- Use "The Cookie Theft" from *Boston Diagnostic Aphasia Examination* to assess expressive organization.
- To assess cognitive-semantic complexity and abstractness, use *The Word Test—Revised (Elementary)*, *The Word Test—Adolescent,* and/or the *Test of Language Competence—Expanded (TLC-E)*.
- Use *Ross Information Processing Assessment—2 (RIPA-2)* to assess verbal reasoning and problem-solving.

- Test in a variety of settings and under a variety of conditions, and note differences: in a quiet environment versus in a cafeteria or shopping mall; with varying amounts of visual distraction on a page. Assess gestural and written responses as well as verbal responses. (Blosser and DePompei, 1994)
- Observe and assess in everyday situations.

INTERVENTION TECHNIQUES

- While clients are in Levels 1, 2, and 3 of a coma, therapists can instruct family members in providing sensory stimulation. At Level 4, characterized by confusion and agitation, therapists may help clients to channel energy by engaging in physical tasks such as pushing a wheelchair, or by pointing to objects. At Level 5, therapists may address areas such as attention, word retrieval, and orientation. (Iskowitz, 1997)
- Make early "yes/no" system clearly different, such as thumbs up/thumbs down, rather than a response such as eye blinks, which may be confused with a naturally occurring response. Be sure all communication partners establish and expect the same system of responses.
- In the early stages of recovery, make any augmentative communication system simple and inexpensive as the client's needs may change rapidly.
- Recognize frustration of client who compares slowness of any augmentative and alternative communication (AAC) device with his/her own previous rate of communicating. (Ylvisaker, et al., 1994)
- When a student first returns to school, consider delivering service in the classroom or through consultation, partially to eliminate confusion in the student's schedule.
- Focus of treatment should be on preparing the client to function in different environments—home, school, community, and work—rather than on the remediation of deficits. (Blosser and DePompei, 1994)
- Retraining of processes such as memory, discrimination, and attention should be accomplished through functional activities. Working on such skills through isolated exercises shows little carryover. (Blosser and DePompei, 1994)
- Work on phonological deficits with vocabulary currently relevant to academic subjects or job environment rather than traditional word lists.
- When working with clients with mild TBI, establishing some structure to daily routines helps to reduce stress.

Cognitive Levels of Coma
(Based on Rancho Los Amigos Cognitive Functioning Scale)

Level I (No response). The person shows no evidence of cognitive response.

Level II (Generalized response). Responses are nonspecific and may include physiological changes, gross body movements, or vocalizations.

Level III (Localized response). The person may follow simple commands, such as "close your eyes" or "squeeze my hand." The person may respond inconsistently or in a delayed manner and may respond to some people but not to others.

Level IV (Confused/agitated). The person responds primarily to the internal rather than the external environment. Gross attention is very brief, and selective attention is usually nonexistent. The person is unaware of present events, lacks short-term recall, and may be reacting to past events.

Level V (Confused/inappropriate/nonagitated). The person appears alert and is able to respond to simple commands fairly consistently but responses to complex commands may be nonpurposeful, random, or fragmented. He or she has gross attention to the environment but is highly distractible and lacks ability to focus attention. Memory is severely impaired. He or she may perform previously learned tasks with structure but is unable to learn new information. Maximum supervision is required to ensure safety.

Level VI (Confused/appropriate). The person follows directions consistently and can perform familiar activities, especially those learned and practiced for many years. New learning is difficult and is not remembered. Attention to tasks is improved for structured tasks but not for unstructured tasks. Past memory is better than recent. The person shows goal-directed behavior but is dependent on the external environment for direction. Moderate supervision is required. The person has vague recognition of some staff members.

Level VII (Automatic/appropriate). The person is oriented and able to function in a structured environment with a dependable routine. Learning new tasks is possible but carryover is poor. Judgment of

continues

safety, insight into his or her condition, problem-solving, and planning skills are still poor. Minimal supervision is still needed for safety reasons.

Level VIII (Purposeful/appropriate). The person is alert, oriented, can plan ahead, remembers the past, learns new tasks, and functions in an unstructured setting. Return to the community is possible, including working. However, some decrease in quality and rate of processing information may be evident, and the ability to reason abstractly may be decreased.

Source: Reprinted from K. Reed, *Quick Reference to Occupational Therapy,* pp. 151–152, © 1991, Aspen Publishers, Inc.

- When establishing treatment plans, respond proactively rather than reactively: identify, anticipate, and respond to difficulties in a timely fashion; design treatment with creativity, flexibility, and ingenuity, including "trying the untried"; and use teamwork and involve as many people as possible in planning and implementing the program. (Blosser and DePompei, 1994)
- Goals should address participation in the learning process; development of work-related skills; development of social skills needed at home, in school, and at work; and development of independent living skills. (Blosser and DePompei, 1994)
- For adolescents at cognitive levels 6 and above, consider groups for 3 to 6 weeks that emphasize independence, social skills, and community integration. (Kerr, 1994)
- Simulate the classroom: have clients take notes from audiocassettes, and assign a research project on a topic of interest. (Zarella, 1995)
- Work for accommodations in students' educational setting, including preferential seating to limit distractions, permission to record lectures, a "study buddy," a tutor, a "reader" to record assignments on tape, advance notification of assignments and projects, and a quiet testing environment with no time limits. (Zarella, 1995)
- Consider vocal fold injection or palatal lift only after at least 1 year recovery time and rigorous therapy. (Ylvisaker, et al., 1994)

- Address areas necessary for success in school: skills necessary for successful student-teacher interactions (following directions, completing assignments, making needs known in an appropriate way) and skills necessary for successful peer interactions (cooperating, sharing, conversing, compromising, disagreeing). (Ylvisaker, et al., 1994)
- Use behavioral techniques with clients in stages of confusion, disorientation, and agitation. These techniques include schedules of reinforcement, redirecting, modeling, prompting, shaping, cueing, fading, practicing, role playing, and scripting. (Ylvisaker, et al., 1994)
- In later stages of recovery, use social-cognition and metacognitive approaches, including developing knowledge of self, knowledge of social rules, social roles, and social routines; developing awareness of social situations; teaching the thinking through of alternative actions; using verbal and visual rehearsal; self-monitoring; self-evaluating; self-rewarding; role-playing; and negotiating goals. (Ylvisaker, et al., 1994)
- Teach strategies to compensate for residual deficits, including using external aids such as printed schedules, memory book, or calculator; overt behaviors such as asking for information to be repeated or counting on fingers; and covert behaviors such as mental rehearsal and deliberate organization. (Ylvisaker, et al., 1994)
- To address deficits in sequencing skills, limit the number of steps in a task; have the student repeat multistep instructions before beginning a task; provide pictures or written sequences as cues; tell the student how many steps are in the task; and number the steps in written directions. (Ylvisaker, et al., 1994)
- Use concrete, visual representation, such as a series of pictures, to aid discourse narrative.
- Involve parents, other family members, teachers, and others in the treatment program.
- Anticipate and program for periods of transition—from rehabilitation setting to home, return to school, school to work, etc.

RESULTS OF RECENT STUDIES

- Several cautions are urged when analyzing test results: Although verbal IQ scores generally recover more quickly and completely than performance scores, keep in mind that, unlike performance IQ tasks, verbal IQ tasks are seldom timed. Language tasks used in aphasia assessments generally do not reflect the complexity of language tasks expected in the classroom; while receptive vocabulary scores may return to preaccident range, deterioration may be seen in subsequent years as the child has difficulty learning new concepts. The skills most disrupted in this population are those of processing social meaning and the ability to process and produce extended discourse. (Ylvisaker, 1993)

- In a study of young children who had sustained unilateral brain injury during or shortly after birth, those with left hemisphere damage (LHD) as well as those with right hemisphere damage (RHD) exhibited normally developing mean length of utterance (MLU) during the first 4 years of life. (Feldman, 1994)
- In a study of 60 children who were unconscious for 90 days or longer, 30 regained some language function. (Kriel, et al., 1995)
- In a study completed by Dennis and Barnes, and reported by Ylvisaker, discourse performance was dissociated from performance on other language tasks. That is, comprehension of metaphor was unrelated to comprehension of literal meaning. Ability to generate multiple meanings was unrelated to naming ability, and ability to make inferences was unrelated to social knowledge. (Ylvisaker, 1993)
- In a study of possible causes of slowed speaking rate among children with TBI, reduced articulatory rate and increased pausing was found to be a factor independent of reduced cognitive-linguistic processing speed. Both factors contributed to slowed speaking rate. (Campbell and Dollaghan, 1995)
- In narrative discourse, clients with severe HIs differed from normal subjects on both language and information structures. Those with severe injuries evidenced disruption in understanding and relating story structure. This may account for the perception by others of disorganized discourse among these individuals. Reasons for the impairment in story structure may differ and may relate to severity of the initial injury, localization of the brain lesions, and age at time of injury. (Chapman, et al., 1992)
- When compared with a group of normal controls and with a group of children with dysarthria secondary to cerebral palsy, those with dysarthria secondary to TBI performed as well as the normal controls on measures of maximum sound prolongation and range of pitch. However, they produced very long responses on measures of maximum repetition rate (/pa/ /ta/ /ka/). Implications of the results are that children with TBI

have previously developed normal speech-motor patterns and can use the correct muscles if given adequate time. (Wit et al., 1994)

PROGNOSIS

Each year nearly 5 million children sustain an HI. Of these, 4,000 die as a result of the injury and 15,000 require prolonged hospitalization. Although there are individual variations, young children who sustain a serious HI generally have less favorable outcomes than adolescents or adults who sustain a similar injury. One reason for this is that the myelin sheath, which provides some protection, is not as fully developed in young children. Also, many HIs in very young children are a result of abuse, which frequently occurs on more than one occasion. (Iskowitz, 1996)

REFERENCES

Blosser JL, R DePompei. *Pediatric Traumatic Brain Injury: Proactive Intervention.* San Diego, Calif: Singular Publishing Group, Inc. 1994.

Campbell TF, CA Dollaghan. Speaking rate, articulatory speed, and linguistic processing in children and adolescents with severe traumatic brain injury. *Journal of Speech and Hearing Research.* 1995;38(4):864–75.

Chapman SB, KA Culhane, HS Levin, H Harward, D Mendelsohn, L Ewing-Cobbs, JM Fletcher, D Bruce. Narrative discourse after closed head injury in children and adolescents. *Brain & Language.* 1992;43(1):42–65.

Feldman H. Language development after early unilateral brain injury: a replication study. In: Tager-Flusberg H, ed. *Constraints on Language Acquisition: Studies of Atypical Children.* Hillsdale, NJ: Lawrence Erlbaum Associates, Publishers. 1994:75–90.

Iskowitz M. Unpredictable outcomes in pediatric TBI. *Advance for Speech-Language Pathologists & Audiologists.* 1996;6(40):3,9.

Iskowitz M. Overcoming obstacles of pediatric TBI. *Advance for Speech-Language Pathologists & Audiologists.* 1997;7(24):5.

Kerr T. Community re-entry program for teens with TBI. *Advance for Speech-Language Pathologists & Audiologists.* 1994;4(33):15.

Kriel RL, LE Krach, MG Luxenberg, C Chun. Recovery of language skills in children after prolonged unconsciousness. *Journal of Neurological Rehabilitation.* 1995;9(3):145–50.

Paul-Cohen R. The role of the speech-language pathologist in the treatment of mild brain injury: a community-based approach. In: Mandel S, RT Sataloff, SR Schapiro, eds. *Minor Head Trauma: Assessment, Management, and Rehabilitation.* New York: Springer-Verlag. 1993:261–71.

Shoemaker A. Managing narrative deficits in TBI. *Advance for Speech-Language Pathologists & Audiologists.* 1996;6(27):5,38.

Ylvisaker M. Communication outcome in children and adolescents with traumatic brain injury. *Neuropsychological Rehabilitation.* 1993;3(4):367–87.

Ylvisaker M, P Hartwick, B Ross, N Nussbaum. Cognitive assessment. In: Savage R, G Wolcott, eds. *Educational Dimensions of Acquired Brain Injury.* Austin, Tex: Pro-Ed. 1994:69–119.

Ylvisaker M, S Szekeres, J Haarbauer-Krupa, B Urbanczyk, T Feeney. Speech and language intervention. In: *Educational Dimensions of Acquired Brain Injury.* Savage R, G Wolcott, eds. Austin, Tex: Pro-Ed. 1994:185–235.

Ylvisaker M, S Szekeres, P Hartwick, P Tworek. Cognitive intervention. In: Savage R, G Wolcott, eds. *Educational Dimensions of Acquired Brain Injury.* Austin, Tex: Pro-Ed. 1994:121–84.

Wit J, B Maassen, FJM Gabreels, G Thoonen, et al. Traumatic versus perinatally acquired dysarthria: assessment by means of speech-like maximum performance tasks. *Developmental Medicine & Child Neurology.* 1994;36(3):221–29.

Zarella S. Strategies and modifications assist students with TBI. *Advance for Speech-Language Pathologists & Audiologists.* 1995;5(19):7.

Huntington's Disease (HD)

DESCRIPTION

Also known as Huntington's chorea, HD is an autosomal-dominant disorder usually beginning in middle age (35 to 50 years) but that may occur at any age. It is characterized by choreiform movements and progressive intellectual deterioration. Incidence is from 4 to 8 in 100,000; males and females are equally affected. Symptoms may include personality changes ranging from apathy or irritability to manic-depressive illness, as well as unsteady gait, involuntary movements, slurred speech, impaired judgment, and difficulty swallowing. Other motor manifestations include flicking movements of the extremities, facial grimacing, ataxia, and dystonia.

ETIOLOGY

HD is a result of atrophy of the caudate nucleus with degeneration of the small-cell population and decreases in levels of the neurotransmitters y-aminobutyric acid (GABA) and substance P. Each child of a parent with HD has a 50% chance of inheriting the HD gene. If both parents have the gene the risk to each child is 75%. Those who do inherit the gene will develop the disease. Those who have at least one parent with HD but who do not develop the disease do not pass it on to their children.

SPEECH AND LANGUAGE DIFFICULTIES

• Syllable repetitions and other perseverations.
• Increased voice-onset-time (VOT).
• Errors in place of articulation.
• Dysarthria may develop as the disease progresses.
• In later stages, clients may become mute.
• Impaired comprehension of affective and propositional prosody.

ASSOCIATED AND OTHER DIFFICULTIES

• Irregular and slowed motor execution.
• Involuntary movements.
• Loss of social inhibition.
• Low threshold for frustration.
• Cognitive decline.
• Dementia.
• Impaired memory for recent and remote events, although immediate memory may be relatively spared.
• Handwriting becomes large, slow, and accomplished with effort.
• Emotional impairment including depression, irritability, schizophrenia-like symptoms, obsessions, and abnormal sexual behavior.
• Constant involuntary movements cause significant number of calories to be burned, resulting in increased and often unsatisfied hunger.
• Weight loss.
• Dysphagia, characterized by neck and trunk hyperextension; involuntary movements of head, body, and oral motor structures; absent or inefficient mastication; irregular breathing patterns; pharyngeal dysmotility; and uncoordinated vocal cord adduction/abduction. (Cherney, 1994)
• Incontinence in later stages of the disease.

ASSESSMENT
- Administer *Boston Diagnostic Aphasia Examination (BDAE)*.
- Evaluate for dysphagia.
- Assess articulation and evaluate for dysarthria. (See Appendix A)

INTERVENTION TECHNIQUES
- Position for proper trunk and leg support.
- Work with other team members to prevent or minimize weight loss.
- For those with bradykinetic features, use iced-lemon stimuli to clear pharyngeal residue after each swallow. (Miller and Groher, 1992)
- When feeding, present spoon but wait for client to take the food from it; this may reduce frequency of tongue pushing bolus out of the oral cavity. (Miller and Groher, 1992)
- Provide cues when word-finding difficulties are evident.
- Providing multiple-choice answers may aid recall.

RESULTS OF RECENT STUDIES
- Dysarthria does not affect speech timing impairment. (Volkman, et al., 1992)
- Decrease in range of modulation of speech rate. (Volkman, et al., 1992)
- In those clients exhibiting Broca's aphasia, the aphasia may result from a loss of "the motor sequence programmer." (Volkman, et al., 1992)
- Confrontation naming is problematic for HD clients with even mild dementia. (Frank, et al., 1996)
- Similar to a group of normal subjects, clients with HD exhibited more difficulty with letter fluency tasks than with category fluency tasks. Clients with HD were, however, significantly impaired on both tasks. Their performance is indicative of initiation and retrieval problems secondary to disruption of frontostriatal circuits. (Rosser and Hodges, 1994)
- Compared with clients with Alzheimer's disease, clients with HD exhibit less memory impairment. Their difficulty appears to be in the operation of effective retrieval strategies to search for information stored in memory. (Rosser and Hodges, 1994)
- Compared with clients with Alzheimer's disease, clients with HD do less well on tasks of initiation. (Rosser and Hodges, 1994)

PROGNOSIS

The disease is progressive. Ultimately, clients lose both physical and mental ability for self-care. Common causes of death are dysphagia, either directly from suffocation or aspiration or indirectly from starvation, and cardiac failure. Death usually occurs within 10 to 20 years after the onset of symptoms.

REFERENCES

Brin MF, S Fahn, A Blitzer, LO Ramig, C Stewart. Movement disorders of the larynx. In: Blitzer A, ME Brin, CT Sasaki, S Fahn, KS Harris, eds. *Neurological Disorders of the Larynx*. New York: Thieme Medical Publishers, Inc. 1992:267–70.

Brookshire RH. *An Introduction to Neurogenic Communication Disorders,* 4th ed. St. Louis, Mo: Mosby Year Book. 1992:230.

Cherney LR. *Clinical Management of Dysphagia in Adults and Children,* 2nd ed. Gaithersburg, Md: Aspen Publishers, Inc. 1994:20–21.

Crawford H. A weighty issue: maintaining weight diminishes impact of Huntington's. *Advance for Speech-Language Pathologists & Audiologists.* 1998;8(17):4.

Frank EM, HL McDade, WK Scott. Naming in dementia secondary to Parkinson's, Huntington's and Alzheimer's Diseases. *Journal of Communication Disorders.* 1996;29:183–97.

Hertrich I, H Ackerman. Acoustic analysis of speech timing in Huntington's disease. *Brain & Language.* 1994;47(2):182–96.

Marmer L. Gambling against Huntington's. *Advance for Speech-Language Pathologists & Audiologists.* 1995;5(20):16–17.

Miller RM, ME Groher. General treatment of neurologic swallowing disorders. In: Groher ME, ed. *Dysphagia Diagnosis and Management,* 2nd ed. Boston: Butterworth-Heinemann. 1992:211–13.

Morris M. Dementia and cognitive changes in Huntington's disease. In: Weiner WJ, AE Lang, eds. *Behavioral Neurology of Movement Disorders*. New York: Raven Press. 1995:187–200.

Rosser A, JR Hodges. Initial letter and semantic category fluency in Alzheimer's disease, Huntington's disease, and progressive supranuclear palsy. *Journal of Neurology, Neurosurgery, and Psychiatry.* 1994;57(11):1389–94.

Volkman J, H Hefter, HW Lange, HJ Freund. Impairment of temporal organization of speech in basal ganglia diseases. *Brain & Language.* 1992;43(3):386–99.

Motor Neuron Disease (MND)

DESCRIPTION

MND refers to a progressive disorder of the nervous system, generally in the anterior horn cells of the spinal cord, the motor nuclei of the brainstem, and the corticospinal tracts. Several distinct disorders fall under the umbrella of MND:

1. Amyotrophic lateral sclerosis (ALS).
   (See also Amyotrophic Lateral Sclerosis.)
2. Primary lateral sclerosis (PLS) and progressive pseudobulbar palsy (PSB). Both are rare variants of MND characterized by gradually increasing signs of muscle stiffness.
3. Progressive muscular atrophy (PMA). A variation occurs in which anterior horn cell involvement is greater than corticospinal involvement. Muscle wasting and weakness begin in the hands and becomes more generalized over a period of time. Onset may begin at any age.
4. Progressive bulbar palsy (PBP). Predominantly involved are the muscles innervated by cranial nerves and corticobulbar tracts, leading to progressive difficulty with chewing, swallowing, and talking. Inappropriate emotional responses may also be seen.

ETIOLOGY

Specific etiologies of MND are not known. Lesions above the medulla produce contralateral weakness, while lesions below the medulla result in ipsilateral weakness. Lesions above the brainstem result in minimal weakness of jaw muscles and involvement of the lower half of facial muscles. Upper MND results in spasticity, which increases over time. Lower MND results in weakness and wasting of muscles.

SPEECH AND LANGUAGE DIFFICULTIES

• Dysarthria.
• Although rare, aphasia and dementia may occur.

ASSOCIATED AND OTHER DIFFICULTIES
- Dysphagia.
- Respiratory complications.

ASSESSMENT
- Assess for dysphagia.
- Assess for dysarthria. (See Appendix A.)

INTERVENTION TECHNIQUES
- Provide therapy for dysphagia.
- Provide therapy for dysarthria.
- As intelligibility decreases, consider use of augmentative and alternative communication (AAC) and work with the client and caregivers to provide an appropriate system.

RESULTS OF RECENT STUDIES
- Thirteen patients with MND underwent cricopharyngeal myotomy (CPM) with the following results: one died of cardiorespiratory arrest 48 hours after surgery; another developed a pharyngocutaneous fistula. Follow-up information, by questionnaires completed by clients or family members and, in some cases, by return visits to the clinic, was available for 11 of the 12 persons who survived the operation. Of these, 3 achieved excellent swallowing results and 6 achieved good swallowing results, which were maintained for 6 months after surgery; 2 people continued to have poor swallowing. One person had some improvement in voice that lasted less than 3 months; 2 experienced steady deterioration in voice over the 6 months following surgery; 2 initially reported no change in voice, followed by deterioration within 3 months after surgery; and 1 was aphonic both presurgery and postsurgery. Choking episodes were less frequent after surgery for 6 people, and for 3 of these the improvement was maintained for more than 6 months. Five of those who underwent and survived CPM died during periods from 9 to 18 months after surgery. In the same study, 7 people underwent pharyngostomy. Complications occurred in 6 of these cases; within 10 months of surgery, 5 persons had died. (Leighton, et al., 1994)

PROGNOSIS

ALS (See also Amyotrophic lateral sclerosis [ALS])

- For PBP, death generally occurs in 1 to 3 years, often as a result of the dysphagia and respiratory complications.
- For PMA, progression is gradual and survival of more than 25 years is possible.
- For PLS and PSB, deterioration is gradual; generally several years elapse before there is total disability.

REFERENCES

Caselli RJ, AJ Windebank, RC Petersen, T Komori, JE Parisi, H Okazaki, E Kokmen, R Iverson, RP Dinapoli, NR Graff-Radford, SD Smith. Rapidly progressive aphasic dementia and motor neuron disease. *Annals of Neurology.* 1993;33(2):200–7.

Hughes TAT, CM Wiles. Palatal and pharyngeal reflexes in health and in motor neuron disease. *Journal of Neurology, Neurosurgery, and Psychiatry.* 1996;61:96–98.

Kelley WN. *Textbook of Internal Medicine*, Vols. 1 and 2, 3rd ed. Philadelphia: Lippincott-Raven Publishers. 1997:361–7.

Leighton SEJ, MJ Burton, WS Lund, GM Cochrane. Swallowing in motor neurone disease. *Journal of the Royal Society of Medicine.* 1994;87:801–5.

Multi-Infarct Dementia (MID)

DESCRIPTION

MID, or arterioscleroric dementia, is the second most common type of dementia after Alzheimer's disease (AD); it is the cause of 20% of all cases of dementia. In another 15% of cases, it occurs concurrently with AD. It is more prevalent in men and generally occurs after age 70 years.

ETIOLOGY

MID is a progressive cerebrovascular disease secondary to multiple cerebral infarctions.

SPEECH AND LANGUAGE DIFFICULTIES

- Impairments in short- and long-term memory.
- Impairments in reasoning, abstract thinking, and judgment.

ASSOCIATED AND OTHER DIFFICULTIES

- Changes in personality.
- Difficulty with impulse control.
- Attention deficits.
- Difficulty with fine motor control.
- Depression is common.

ASSESSMENT

- Evaluation and assessment should be ongoing as status changes over time.
- Administer tests for aphasia.
- Evaluate pragmatic and discourse skills.
- Evaluate semantics. Administer *Boston Naming Test.*

INTERVENTION TECHNIQUES

- Keep in mind that the client's ability to generalize is severely limited; treatment goals must be functional and specific.

RESULTS OF RECENT STUDIES

- In a study comparing loss of prosody in clients with AD and in clients with multi-infarct dementia, prosodic loss was found to be more frequent and more severe in those with AD. Differences between the two groups were significant for emotional and intrinsic aprosody; differences were not significant for intellectual or inarticulate aprosody. (Pérez Trullen and Modrego Pardo, 1996)

PROGNOSIS

MID is a progressive condition.

REFERENCES

Grossman M, M D'Esposito, E Hughes, K Onishi, N Biassou, T White-Devine, KM Robinson. Language comprehension profiles in Alzheimer's disease, multi-infarct dementia, and frontotemporal degeneration. *Neurology.* 1996;47(1):183–9.

Pérez Trullen JM, PJ Modrego Pardo. Comparative study of aprosody in Alzheimer's disease and in multi-infarct dementia. *Dementia.* 1996;7:59–62.

Ramasubbu R, SH Kennedy. Factors complicating the diagnosis of depression in cerebrovascular disease, Part II—neurological deficits and various assessment methods. *Canadian Journal of Psychiatry.* 1994;39(10):601–7.

Ripich DN, TT Threats. Multi-infarct dementia and communication. *Topics in Stroke Rehabilitation.* 1994;1(2):87–99.

Multiple Sclerosis (MS)

DESCRIPTION

A slowly progressive disease of the central nervous system (CNS) resulting in multiple and varied neurologic symptoms, usually marked by periods of exacerbation and remission. The condition is more prevalent in temperate climates than in the tropics, and women are affected somewhat more often than men. Onset is generally between the ages of 20 and 40 years.

There are five classes of MS:

1. Relapsing and remitting (70% of young people with MS), characterized by virtually full recovery after each episode.
2. Chronic progressive, characterized by gradual worsening over time with no remissions.
3. Combined relapsing and remitting with chronic progression, characterized by a gradual deterioration over time with periods of relative remission.
4. Benign (20%), characterized by nearly normal function, a normal life span, and little progression of the disease.

5. Malignant (5% to 10%), characterized by rapid and extensive involvement leading to death within a short time.

ETIOLOGY

A specific cause is unknown although some immunologic abnormality is
suspected. Demyelination occurs in plaques or islands throughout the
CNS.

SPEECH AND LANGUAGE DIFFICULTIES

- Oral and facial apraxia.
- Aphasia may occur; typically nonfluent motor aphasia, with good recov-
ery.
- Paraphasic errors.
- Subtle difficulties with reading, word-finding, memory, attention, ab-
stract reasoning, and speed of information processing.
- Dysarthria, typically mixed spastic-ataxic, resulting in harsh voice qual-
ity, articulation deficits, and impaired ability to control volume.
- Speech is slow, often referred to as measured or scanned.
- Dysphonia, characterized by hypernasality, impaired pitch control, inap-
propriate habitual pitch, and breathiness.

ASSOCIATED AND OTHER DIFFICULTIES

- Dysphagia may be present, characterized by impaired ability to hold the
bolus anteriorly and laterally, delayed initiation of pharyngeal swallow,
reduced pharyngeal peristalsis, and, in later stages, laryngeal adduction.
(Cherney, 1994)
- Persons with severe MS may experience periods of hypoxemia during
oral intake.
- Peripheral hearing loss and/or central auditory deficits.
- Tinnitus.
- Facial numbness.
- Intention tremor.
- Nystagmus.
- Ataxia.
- Impaired attention, memory, and/or perception.
- Disorganized thinking.

- Inefficient processing of information.
- Difficulty processing abstract information.
- Difficulty learning new material.
- Difficulty with recent memory.
- Visual impairments.
- Inappropriate social behavior.
- Fatigue.
- Spasticity.
- Loss of normal bladder control.

ASSESSMENT

- Assess for dysphagia.
- Assess for dysarthria. (See Appendix A.)
- Administer *Arizona Battery for Communication Disorders of Dementia* (ABCD).
  (See Results of Recent Studies)
- Administer the *Test of Language Competence—Expanded* (TLC-E).
- Administer *The Word Test*.
- If evaluation for augmentative and alternative communication (AAC) is warranted, consider carefully visual deficits and deficits in motor skills. (Beukelman and Mirenda, 1992)

INTERVENTION TECHNIQUES

- Consider use of palatal lift to treat hypernasality. (Johnson, 1995)
- Provide strategies to improve intelligibility.
- Teach compensatory strategies before problems occur, i.e., organization of daily routines, lists, calendars. (Zarrella, 1995)
- Suggest more frequent, smaller meals to reduce fatigue. (Zarrella, 1995)
- To prevent or reduce hypoxemia during oral intake, use careful feeding techniques combined with a careful selection of food textures. (Rogers, et al., 1993)

RESULTS OF RECENT STUDIES

- In response to a questionnaire, 44% of clients with MS indicated that their speech and/or voice are impaired as a result of the disease, 18%

reported difficulty making themselves understood when speaking, and 33% indicated difficulty with mastication and swallowing. Yet, only 2% to 3% had seen a speech-language pathologist. (Hartelius and Svenson, 1994)

- On the *Arizona Battery of Communication Disorders* (ABCD), four clients with MS scored lower than a control group on the following subtests: Object Description, Generative Naming, Concept Definition, Generative Writing, and Picture Description. On other subtests of the ABCD, there were no significant differences between the two groups. Results indicate that the ABCD may be sensitive to some subtle linguistic impairments of MS, although not sensitive to cognitive impairments of this group. (Wallace and Holmes, 1993)
- Cases have been reported of resolution of dysarthria and other physical symptoms following application of electromagnetic fields. (Sandyk, 1995)

PROGNOSIS

The course of the disease is highly varied and unpredictable. Often initial remissions may last several years, but over time the periods between exacerbations grow shorter. On average, the illness lasts more than 25 years, but this is highly variable.

REFERENCES

Beukelman DR, P Mirenda. *Augmentative and Alternative Communication: Management of Severe Communication Disorders in Children and Adults.* Baltimore: Paul H. Brookes Publishing Co. 1992:317–19.

Cherney LR. *Clinical Management of Dysphagia in Adults and Children,* 2nd ed. Gaithersburg, Md: Aspen Publishers, Inc. 1994:19.

Hartelius L, P Svenson. Speech and swallowing symptoms associated with Parkinson's disease and multiple sclerosis: a survey. *Folia Phoniatrica & Logopedica.* 1994;46:9–17.

Johnson GR. Using a palatal lift to treat hypernasality in MS. *Advance for Speech-Language Pathologists & Audiologists.* 1995;5(36):17.

Kujala P, R Portin, J Ruutiainen. Language functions in incipient cognitive decline in multiple sclerosis. *Journal of the Neurological Sciences.* 1996;141(1–2):79–86.

Lethlean JB, BE Murdoch. Performance of subjects with multiple sclerosis on tests of high-level language. *Aphasiology.* 1997;11(1):39–57.

Rogers B, M Msall, D Shucard. Hypoxemia during oral feedings in adults with dysphagia and severe neurological conditions. *Dysphagia.* 1993;8(1):43–48.

Sandyk R. Resolution of dysarthria in multiple sclerosis by treatment with weak electromagnetic fields. *International Journal of Neuroscience.* 1995;83(1–2):81–92.

Sorensen P, S Brown, J Logemann, K Wilson, R Herndon. Communication disorders and dysphagia. *Journal of Neurologic Rehabilitation.* 1994;8(3):137–43.

Wallace G, S Holmes. Cognitive-linguistic assessment of individuals with multiple sclerosis. *Archives of Physical Medicine & Rehabilitation.* 1993;74(6):637–43.

Zarrella S, Managing MS. *Advance for Speech-Language Pathologists & Audiologists.* 1995;5(30):5.

Muscular Dystrophy (MD)

DESCRIPTION

There are several forms of MD:

1. Duchene dystrophy (DD) is the most common form of MD. It generally affects males, with symptoms first appearing between the ages of 3 and 7 years. The condition is marked by progressive muscle weakness, beginning in the pelvic girdle and affecting gait.

2. Becker muscular dystrophy (BMD) is a somewhat milder form of DD.

3. Oculopharyngeal muscular dystrophy (OPMD) is a rare, late-onset, progressive disease affecting the head, neck, and upper limbs. Most, although not all, cases occur among French Canadians.

4. Facioscapulohumeral muscular dystrophy (FSHD) (Landouzy-Dejerine) is characterized by weakness of the facial muscles and shoulder girdles. Onset is generally between the ages of 7 and 20 years, with early symptoms of difficulty with whistling, eye closure, and elevation of the arms.

5. Myotonic dystrophy (Steinert's disease) may occur at any age and with variable severity. Muscles of the hands are generally most affected. Other characteristics that may be present include premature balding, ptosis, and cataracts.

6. Limb-girdle dystrophy is characterized by weakness of pelvic and shoulder girdles.

ETIOLOGY

DD is an X-linked recessive disorder.

BMD is also an X-linked recessive disorder with genomic mutation at Xp21.

FSHD is an autosomal-dominant myopathy. The gene for FSHD has been located on the tip of the long arm of chromosome 4 in the band 4q35.

Steinert's disease is an autosomal-dominant disorder; the gene has been localized to 19q.

SPEECH AND LANGUAGE DIFFICULTIES

- Dysphonia.
- Hypernasality.
- Misarticulations, which may worsen as the disease progresses.

ASSOCIATED AND OTHER DIFFICULTIES

- Dysphagia—30% to 40% of those with OPMD experience dysphagia.
- High-frequency, sensorineural hearing loss associated with FSHD.
- May have dental abnormalities.
- Changes in craniofacial growth and development may result in excessive mandibular growth, emporomandibular joint dysfunction, and/or open bite.
- Average IQ of those with DD is 1 standard deviation (SD) below the norm.
- Mental retardation occurs frequently among those with Steinert's disease.
- Scoliosis.
- Lordosis.
- Flexion contractures.
- Foot drop may occur in FSHD.
- Retinal vascular disease is associated with FSHD.
- Ptosis is associated with OPMD and Steinert's disease.

ASSESSMENT

- Assess for dysphagia.

- Evaluate velopharyngeal competence. Work with a team of specialists including craniofacial specialists.
- Assess for dysarthria.

INTERVENTION TECHNIQUES

- Instruct family members and caregivers in signs and symptoms of dysphagia.
- Provide treatment for dysphagia.
- Provide articulation therapy.
- To treat flaccid dysarthria, work to improve support for speech breathing.
- Consider use of a prosthetic appliance to achieve velopharyngeal closure.
- Consider implementation of a system of augmentative and alternative communication (AAC) as intelligibility decreases.

(See also Hearing Loss—Children and Adolescents; Hearing Loss—Adults)

RESULTS OF RECENT STUDIES

No recent studies regarding communication skills were found in the literature.

PROGNOSIS

DD is progressive; most persons with the disorder are using a wheelchair between the ages 10 and 12 years. Death often occurs by 20 years. Most patients with BMD can still ambulate at age 16 years, and more than 90% live beyond age 20 years.

Life expectancy is normal in those with FSHD. In those with Steinert's disease, death occurs in the early 50s in severely affected individuals.

REFERENCES

Castell JA, DO Castell, A Duranceau, P Topart. Manometric characteristics of the pharynx, upper esophageal sphincter, esophagus, and lower esophageal sphincter in patients with oculopharyngeal muscular dystrophy. *Dysphagia.* 1995;10:22–26.

Duffy JR. *Motor Speech Disorders: Substrates, Differential Diagnosis, and Management.* St. Louis, Mo: Mosby. 1995:99–127.

Padberg GW, OF Brouwer, RJW de Keizer, G Dijkman, C Wijmenga, JJ Grote, RR Frants. On the significance of retinal vascular disease and hearing loss in facioscapulohumeral muscular dystrophy. *Muscle and Nerve.* 1995;Suppl 2:S73–S80.

Shoemaker A. Muscular dystrophy: specialized care needed for speech, swallowing. *Advance for Speech-Language Pathologists & Audiologists.* 1996;6(34):8,16.

Tiomny E, O Khilkevic, AD Korczyn, R Kimmel, A Hallak, J Baron, S Blumen, A Asherov, T Gikat. Esophageal smooth muscle dysfunction in oculopharyngeal muscular dystrophy. *Digestive Diseases and Sciences.* 1996;41(7):350–4.

Myasthenia Gravis (MG)

DESCRIPTION

An autoimmune disease characterized by muscle weakness, particularly muscles innervated by cranial nerves. Improvement is often seen with the use of cholinesterase-inhibiting drugs. Onset may occur at any age but generally occurs between the ages of 20 and 40 years. Females are affected more often than males. The most common symptoms are ptosis, diplopia, and muscle fatigue after exercise.

ETIOLOGY

Although the precipitating cause is unknown, MG is the result of an autoimmune attack on the acetylcholine receptor of the postsynaptic neuromuscular junction.

SPEECH AND LANGUAGE DIFFICULTIES

- Flaccid dysarthria characterized by hypernasality, imprecise articulation, and breathiness.
- Dysphonia.

ASSOCIATED AND OTHER DIFFICULTIES

- In infancy, poor suck and cry and feeding difficulties.
- Secondary respiratory infections.
- As the disease progresses, ocular muscles are affected in 85% of clients.
- Double vision.
- Fatigue.
- Proximal limb weakness.
- Dysphagia characterized by an overall reduction in the oral preparatory phase, reduced lingual motility, nasal regurgitation, reduced pharyngeal peristalsis, and slowed esophageal transit. (Cherney, 1994) Eating and swallowing deteriorate during the course of a meal due to fatigue. (Miller and Groher, 1992)

ASSESSMENT

- Assess for dysphagia.
- Assess for dysarthria.

INTERVENTION TECHNIQUES

- To improve eating and swallowing functions, limit energy output (including physical activity and excessive talking) just prior to meals. Provide foods that do not fall apart easily. (Miller and Groher, 1992)
- To treat dysarthria, teach conservation of strength by limiting duration of speaking. (Duffy, 1995)

RESULTS OF RECENT STUDIES

No recent studies regarding communication skills were found in the literature.

PROGNOSIS

Initially, death by apnea may occur. After age 10 years, exacerbations are less frequent.

REFERENCES

Cherney LR. *Clinical Management of Dysphagia in Adults and Children*, 2nd ed. Gaithersburg, Md: Aspen Publishers, Inc. 1994:21–22.

Duffy JR. *Motor Speech Disorders: Substrates, Differential Diagnosis, and Management.* St. Louis, Mo: Mosby. 1995:99–127.

Kelley WN. *Textbook of Internal Medicine*, Vols. 1 and 2, 3rd ed. Philadelphia: Lippincott-Raven Publishers. 1997:2457.

Kluin KJ, MB Bromberg, EL Feldman, Z Simmons. Dysphagia in elderly men with myasthenia gravis. *Journal of the Neurological Sciences.* 1996;138:49–52.

Magalini SI, SC Magalini. *Dictionary of Medical Syndromes,* 4th ed. Philadelphia: Lippincott-Raven Publishers. 1997:565.

Miller RM, ME Groher. General treatment of neurologic swallowing disorders. In: Groher, ME, ed. *Dysphagia Diagnosis and Management,* 2nd ed. Boston: Butterworth-Heinemann. 1992:208–9.

Neurofibromatosis Type 1 (NF1)

DESCRIPTION

Incidence of NF1, or von Recklinghausen disease, is 1 in 4,000 persons. Characteristics include café-au-lait spots, freckling, and peripheral neurofibromas. In a third of the cases, neurologic sequelae are present, generally appearing during puberty. In these cases, spinal cord compression may result. Tumors on cranial nerves may result in progressive blindness, dizziness, ataxia, or deafness. Learning disabilities occur among 30% to 45% of children with NF1; between 3% and 8% have some degree of intellectual impairment.

ETIOLOGY

An inherited autosomal-dominant disorder. The gene for NF1 is on chromosome number 17.

SPEECH AND LANGUAGE DIFFICULTIES

- Relatively high incidence of verbal and linguistic deficits, although these may be mild.

ASSOCIATED AND OTHER DIFFICULTIES

- Seizures occur in about 20% of cases.
- Gradual hearing loss may develop as a result of a tumor on the eighth cranial nerve.
- Neurofibroma on the optic nerve may develop and result in squinting or blurred or double vision.
- Intellectual impairment occurs in 2% to 5% of cases.
- Learning disabilities, hyperactivity, and or speech/language problems occur in 50% of cases.
- Headaches.
- Short stature.
- Scoliosis.
- Dermal neurofibromatosis—nonmalignant lesions that appear anywhere on the body—generally beginning to appear after puberty.
- Poor organizational skills.
- Attention deficits.
- Impulsivity.
- Decreased ability to perceive social cues.

ASSESSMENT

- Be aware that language deficits may be present although performance on various subtests may be less than 2 standard deviation (SD) below norms.
- Assess receptive, expressive, and pragmatic skills in depth.
- Conduct hearing screening and refer to audiologist as indicated.

INTERVENTION TECHNIQUES

- Provide structure in learning environments.

RESULTS OF RECENT STUDIES

No recent studies regarding communication skills were found in the literature.

PROGNOSIS

In most cases the disease is progressive.

REFERENCES

Gilbert P. *The A-Z Reference Book of Syndromes and Inherited Disorders: A Manual for Health, Social and Education Workers.* New York: Chapman & Hall. 1993:154–7.

Jones KL. *Smith's Recognizable Patterns of Human Malformation,* 5th ed. Philadelphia: W.B. Saunders Co. 1997:508–9.

North K, P Joy, D Yuille, N Cocks, P Hutchins. Cognitive function and academic performance in children with neurofibromatosis type 1. *Developmental Medicine and Child Neurology.* 1995;37:427–36.

Thoene JG, NP Coker, eds. *Physicians' Guide to Rare Diseases.* New York: Dowden Publishing Co. 1995:108.

Parkinson's Disease (PD)

DESCRIPTION

PD is an idiopathic, slowly progressive, degenerative central nervous system (CNS) disorder with four characteristic features: slowness and poverty of movement, muscular rigidity, resting tremors, and postural instability. Mean age of onset is 57 years, although juvenile parkinsonism, with onset in childhood or adolescence, does occur. Approximately 0.4% of the population under 40 years and 1% of the population over 65 years are affected. Males and females are affected about equally. Early symptoms, in 50% to 80% of clients, include a resting "pin-rolling" tremor of one hand. The tremor is greatest at rest and is enhanced by emotional tension or fatigue; it is diminished during movement and is absent during sleep. Tremor may become less pronounced as the disease progresses. Other early signs include frequent blinking, lack of facial expression, poverty of movement, and gait abnormality.

ETIOLOGY

Loss of the pigmented neurons of the substantia nigra, locus ceruleus, and other brainstem dopaminergic cell groups resulting in the depletion of the neurotransmitter dopamine in these areas. Secondary parkinsonism may occur as a result of neuroleptic drugs or, less commonly, as a result of carbon monoxide or manganese poisoning, hydrocephalus, or structural lesions such as tumors or infarcts involving the midbrain or basal ganglia.

SPEECH AND LANGUAGE DIFFICULTIES

- Dysarthria.
- Rapid or variable rate of speech.
- Decreased volume.
- Shallow respiration.
- Monotone.
- Decreased movement of articulators leading to decrease in precise production of speech.
- Difficulty initiating speech.
- Difficulty controlling breath support for proper phrasing.
- Inappropriate silences and pauses during conversation.
- Perseveration.
- Syntax deficits.
- Palilalia (repetition of an isolated word, phrase, or sentence with increasing rate and decreasing intelligibility) may be present but is rare.
- Hoarse voice with strained and breathy voice quality.
- Hypernasality may occur but is not common.
- Some medications may have a negative effect on speech production, making it more rapid and less distinct.

ASSOCIATED AND OTHER DIFFICULTIES

- Dysphagia, characterized by tongue tremor and reduced initiation of lingual movement, repetitive tongue-pumping action, delayed pharyngeal

swallow and reduced pharyngeal peristalsis, inadequate laryngeal elevation and/or closure, repetitive involuntary reflux, upper esophageal sphincter dysfunction, and reduced esophageal peristalsis. (Cherney, 1994)
- Progressive rigidity.
- Slowness and poverty of movement.
- Difficulty initiating movement.
- Burning or aching of feet or lower legs.
- Sleep disturbances.
- Resting tremor.
- Postural instability.
- Impaired visuospatial skills.
- Memory impairments.
- Increasing difficulty with decision-making.
- Loss of olfactory function.
- Masklike face with diminished blinking and decreasing ability to show emotions on the face.
- Stooped posture.
- Difficulty initiating walking, with shuffling gait and short steps.
- Increasing difficulty with activities of daily living (ADLs).
- Dementia is common in later stages of the disease and is more common in early stages among those whose symptoms of PD begin after age 70 years.
- Depression.

ASSESSMENT
- Perform a thorough oral-motor evaluation.
- Assess for dysarthria. (See Appendix A.)
- Assess respiration, phonation, and articulation.
- Assess language and cognitive status, including naming, verbal fluency, word retrieval, reading comprehension, auditory comprehension and written language. Consider use of portions of the *Western Aphasia Battery* (WAB) or the *Boston Diagnostic Aphasia Examination* (BDAE).
- Evaluate orientation, short-term memory and attention. Consider use of the *Mini-Mental State Examination* (MMSE). Deficits in these areas indicate a poor prognosis for benefit from therapy.

- Administer pure-tone audiological screening and refer to audiologist if a hearing loss is suspected.
- Assess home and work-related communication needs. Recommend communication aids as appropriate.
- To assess for augmentative and alternative communication (AAC) intervention, consider: cognitive/linguistic skills, motor skills, willingness to use AAC, and possible hearing impairments of listeners.
- Assess thoroughly for dysphagia. Be aware that patients with PD are often unaware of their swallowing difficulties.

INTERVENTION TECHNIQUES

- Before beginning a program of therapy, assess efficacy of such a program, taking into consideration factors such as the client's awareness of deficits and motivation to improve, cognitive abilities, and family support.
- Treat for dysphagia.
- Improve volume and maintenance of voicing by teaching phrasing.
- Use masking noise ('Lombard effect') to increase vocal intensity. (Adams and Lang, 1992)
- To improve intelligibility, teach overarticulation.
- Decrease rate through use of pacing technique. Also consider use of Delayed Auditory Feedback (DAF).
- Administer Lee Silverman Voice Treatment (LSVT) focusing on increasing loudness. (Trace, 1996) (See also Ramig, 1995)
- Have client point on alphabet board to first letter of each spoken word. This reduces rate of speaking while also giving listener additional information.
- In cases of severe difficulties with intelligibility, consider use of AAC.
- When using writing to aid communication, instruct client to write only one word at a time to compensate for microwriting, commonly seen in PD.
- Use portable amplification system to increase loudness.
- Consider use of artificial larynx to counteract severe voicing disorders, although motor difficulties and/or dysarthria may be contraindications.
- Instruct family members and others in techniques for optimal communication.

RESULTS OF RECENT STUDIES

- Decrease in range of modulation of speech rate. (Volkman, et al., 1992)
- Dysarthria does not affect speech timing impairment. (Volkman, et al., 1992)
- In those clients also exhibiting Broca's aphasia, the deficits may result from a loss of "the motor sequence programmer." (Volkman, et al., 1992)
- Clients with PD typically exhibit cognitive deficits only for complex situations. These deficits include impairments associated with cortical regions other than the frontal lobe. (Robbins, et al., 1994)
- A relationship has been demonstrated between performance on cognitive shifting tasks and severity of motor symptoms. (Van Spaendonck, et al., 1996)
- When comparing clients who are older at age of onset with those who are younger at age of onset, those who are older exhibit a more rapid progression of the disease and a higher incidence of cognitive impairment and dementia. (Levin and Katzen, 1995)
- Those whose motor signs first appear on the left side of the body consistently perform more poorly on cognitive tasks than do those whose motor symptoms first appeared on the right side of the body. (Levin and Katzen, 1995)
- Some clients are now undergoing pallidotomy—a procedure involving the cutting of a surgical lesion into a portion of the brain called the globus pallidum (GP). Patients frequently experience complete or nearly complete relief of symptoms of rigidity, slowness of movement, and tremor with improved walking and balance. (Kerr, 1996)
- In response to a questionnaire, 70% of clients with PD indicated that their speech and/or voice are impaired as a result of the disease, 42% reported difficulty making themselves understood when speaking, and 41% indicated difficulty with mastication and swallowing. Yet, only 2% to 3% had seen a speech-language pathologist. (Hartelius and Svenson, 1994)

PROGNOSIS

Although PD is a slowly progressive condition, life expectancy is near normal.

REFERENCES

Adams SG, AE Lang. Can the Lombard effect be used to improve low voice intensity in Parkinson's disease? *European Journal of Disorders of Communication.* 1992;27:121–7.

Beukelman DR, P Mirenda. *Augmentative and Alternative Communication: Management of Severe Communication Disorders in Children and Adults.* Baltimore: Paul H. Brookes Publishing Co. 1992:319–24.

Brin MF, S Fahn, A Blitzer, LO Ramig, C Stewart. Movement disorders of the larynx. In: Blitzer A, ME Brin, CT Sasaki, S Fahn, KS Harris, eds. *Neurological Disorders of the Larynx.* New York: Thieme Medical Publishers, Inc. 1992:249–51.

Brookshire RH. *An Introduction to Neurogenic Communication Disorders,* 4th ed. St Louis, Mo: Mosby Year Book. 1992:250.

Cherney LR. *Clinical Management of Dysphagia in Adults and Children,* 2nd ed. Gaithersburg, Md: Aspen Publishers, Inc. 1994:20.

DePippo KL. Management of communication dysfunction. In: Cohen AM, WJ Weiner, eds. *The Comprehensive Management of Parkinson's Disease.* New York: Demos Publications. 1994:75–88.

Hartelius L, P Svenson. Speech and swallowing symptoms associated with Parkinson's disease and multiple sclerosis: a survey. *Folia Phoniatrica & Logopedica.* 1994;46: 9–17.

Kelley WN. *Textbook of Internal Medicine,* Vols. 1 and 2, 3rd ed. Philadelphia: Lippincott-Raven Publishers. 1997:2388–9.

Kerr T. The promise of pallidotomy: patients with PD risk surgery for relief. *Advance for Speech-Language Pathologists & Audiologists.* 1996;6(8):5,38.

Leopold NA, MC Kagel. Prepharyngeal dysphagia in Parkinson's disease. *Dysphagia.* 1996;11:14–22.

Levin BE, HL Katzen. Early cognitive changes and nondementing behavioral abnormalities in Parkinson's Disease. In: Weiner WJ, AE Lang, eds. *Behavioral Neurology of Movement Disorders.* New York: Raven Press. 1995:85–95.

Lieberman P, E Kako, J Friedman, G Tajchman, LS Feldman, EB Jiminez. Speech production, syntax comprehension, and cognitive deficits in Parkinson's disease. *Brain and Language.* 1992;43:169–89.

Parris RK. Management of swallowing dysfunction. In: Cohen AM, WJ Weiner, eds. *The Comprehensive Management of Parkinson's Disease.* New York: Demos Publications. 1994:89–102.

Ramig LO. Speech therapy for patients with Parkinson's disease. In: Koller WC, G Paulson. *Therapy of Parkinson's Disease,* 2nd ed. New York: Marcel Dekker, Inc. 1995:539–550.

Reid WGJ, MA Hely, JGL Morris, GA Broe, M Adena, DJO Sullivan, PM Williamson. A longitudinal study of Parkinson's disease: clinical and neuropsychological correlates of dementia. *Journal of Clinical Neuroscience.* 1996;3(4):327–33.

Robbins TW, MJ Ames, AM Owen, KW Lange, AJ Lees, PN Leigh, CD Marsden, NP Quinn, BA Summers. Cognitive deficits in progressive supranuclear palsy, Parkinson's disease, and multiple system atrophy in tests sensitive to frontal lobe dysfunction. *Journal of Neurology, Neurosurgery, and Psychiatry.* 1994;57(1–4):79–88.

Trace R. Giving Parkinson's disease the LSVT treatment. *Advance for Speech-Language Pathologists & Audiologists.* 1996;6(8):6–7.

Van Spaendonck KPM, HJC Berger, MWIM Horstink, EL Buytenhuijs, AR Cools. Executive functions and disease characteristics in Parkinson's disease. *Neuropsychologia.* 1996;34(7):617–26.

Volkman J, H Hefter, HW Lange, HJ Freund. Impairment of temporal organization of speech in basal ganglia diseases. *Brain & Language.* 1992;43(3):386–99.

Pick's Disease

DESCRIPTION

A degenerative disease affecting neurons in the cerebral cortex.

ETIOLOGY

Etiology is unknown. Atrophy affects primarily the frontal and temporal lobes.

SPEECH AND LANGUAGE DIFFICULTIES

- Anomia.
- Circumlocutions.
- Echolalia.
- Deterioration of articulation skills.
- Receptive skills are often preserved.
- Repetition of stories or events.
- Decrease in comprehension of both spoken and written messages.
- Decline in confrontation naming skills.
- In final stages, may become mute.

ASSOCIATED AND OTHER DIFFICULTIES

- Changes in personality and emotional states are generally among the first symptoms of the disease.
- Apathy
- Disinhibition of behavior.
- Decrease in judgment and insight.
- Repetitive behavior patterns.

ASSESSMENT

- Assess overall receptive, expressive, and pragmatic skills.

INTERVENTION TECHNIQUES

- Work with the client as well as with caregivers to maximize effectiveness of communication.
- Encourage use of gestures and consider use of PACE therapy (promoting aphasics' communicative effectiveness). (Carlomango, 1994)

RESULTS OF RECENT STUDIES

- In a comparative study of language functioning of persons with Alzheimer's disease, multi-infarct dementia or frontotemporal degeneration (FD), those with FD demonstrated sentence comprehension difficulty due to impaired processing of grammatical phrase structures. (Grossman, et al., 1996).

PROGNOSIS

The condition is progressive, with progressive dementia. Death is often due to aspiration pneumonia or to infection.

REFERENCES

Bayles KA. Language in aging and dementia. In: Kirshner HS, ed. *Handbook of Neurological Speech and Language Disorders*. New York: Marcel Dekker, Inc. 1995:364–5.

Brookshire RH. *An Introduction to Neurogenic Communication Disorders,* 4th ed. St. Louis, Mo: Mosby Year Book. 1992:228.

Carlomango S. *Pragmatic Approaches to Aphasia Therapy*. San Diego, Calif: Singular Publishing Co, Inc. 1994.

Grossman M, M D'Esposito, E Hughes, K Onishi, N Biassou, T White-Devine, KM Robinson. Language comprehension profiles in Alzheimer's disease, multi-infarct dementia, and frontotemporal degeneration. *Neurology*. 1996;47(1):183–89.

Magalini SI, SC Magalini. *Dictionary of Medical Syndromes*, 4th ed. Philadelphia: Lippincott-Raven Publishers. 1997:33.

Pillon B, B Dubois, Y Agid. Cognitive deficits in non-Alzheimer's degenerative diseases. *Journal of Neural Transmission* Supplementum. 1996;47:61–71.

Postpolio (Poliomyelitis) Syndrome (PPS)

DESCRIPTION

Synonyms for PPS include postpolio muscular atrophy, late effects of polio, postpolio sequelae, and postpolio progressive muscular atrophy (PPMA). The condition could potentially affect half of the original 1.63 million polio survivors. PPS is a syndrome characterized by muscle fatigue, decreased endurance, weakness, and muscle atrophy, occurring several decades after an attack of paralytic poliomyelitis. Most likely to be affected are older persons and those whose initial episode of polio was more severe.

ETIOLOGY

The cause is thought to be associated with further loss of anterior horn cells, although this has not been proven. Another theory is that the observable symptoms are due to long-term overuse of healthy muscles as compensation for muscles weakened in the original episode of polio.

SPEECH AND LANGUAGE DIFFICULTIES

- Flaccid dysarthria.
- Changes in speech resonance and/or respiratory/phonatory changes may occur.

- May develop a hoarse voice.
- Oral motor weakness including weakness of the tongue, lips, and jaw.
- Hypernasality.
- Shallow or irregular breathing pattern due to weak muscles of the diaphragm, ribs, or abdomen.
- Decreased volume.
- Difficulty with phrasing.
- Unilateral weakness of tongue or palate.

ASSOCIATED AND OTHER DIFFICULTIES

- Dysphagia characterized by excessive tongue movements, difficulty with bolus control, delayed pharyngeal swallow, reduced pharyngeal peristalsis, upper esophageal sphincter dysfunction, and gastroesophageal reflux. (Cherney, 1994)
- Muscle weakness, which may be progressive.
- Fatigue.
- Varying degrees of pain.
- Changes in gait pattern.
- Decreased ability for weight bearing.
- New or increased difficulty with activities of daily living (ADL).

ASSESSMENT

- Evaluate for dysphagia, including oral sensorimotor examination.
- Evaluate strength of cough and ability to clear the throat. Inability to cough or clear the throat signals increased potential for aspiration.
- Obtain videofluoroscopic studies.
- Evaluate current speech skills, including intelligibility, oral-motor skills, and breath support.
- Polio survivors should be assessed and monitored periodically over the long term for evidence of decreasing function.

INTERVENTION TECHNIQUES

- Treat for dysphagia.
- To treat flaccid dysarthria, work to increase support for speech breathing.

RESULTS OF RECENT STUDIES

• New swallowing difficulties are reported by about 20% of all polio survivors and are most common among those with bulbar involvement at the time of their acute poliomyelitis. (Ivanyi, et al., 1994)

PROGNOSIS

Symptoms are variable among polio survivors.

REFERENCES

Cherney LR. *Clinical Management of Dysphagia in Adults and Children,* 2nd ed. Gaithersburg, Md: Aspen Publishers, Inc. 1994:22.

Duffy JR. *Motor Speech Disorders: Substrates, Differential Diagnosis, and Management.* St. Louis, Mo: Mosby. 1995:99–127.

Ivanyi B, SSKS Phoa, M de Visser. Dysphagia in postpolio patients: a videofluorographic follow-up study. *Dysphagia.* 1994;9:96–98.

Sonies BC. Long-term effects of post-polio on oral-motor and swallowing function. In: Halstead LS, G Grimby, eds. *Post-Polio Syndrome.* St. Louis, Mo: Mosby. 1995:125–37.

Windebank AJ. Differential diagnosis and prognosis. In: Halstead LS, G Grimby, eds. *Post-Polio Syndrome.* St. Louis, Mo: Mosby. 1995:69–88.

Primary Progressive Aphasia (PPA)

DESCRIPTION

Gradual deterioration of speech, comprehension, reading, and writing skills with preservation of nonverbal cognitive skills for several years. Cases that begin after the age of 65 years may have a more rapid progression. Age of onset is generally between 40 and 75 years. Ratio of males to females is 2 to 1.

ETIOLOGY

Asymmetrical atrophy in the left temporal and central parietal areas is often evident on neuroimaging.

SPEECH AND LANGUAGE DIFFICULTIES

- Verbal apraxia, with severity increasing as the disease progresses.
- Anomia.
- Mild agrammatism.
- Dysfluencies.
- Language production may be fluent or nonfluent. Fluent production often contains phonological, morphological, and semantic paraphasias and circumlocutions.
- Dysarthria may develop in later stages.
- May develop mutism.

ASSOCIATED AND OTHER DIFFICULTIES

- Limb apraxia.
- Apathy.
- Irritability.
- Lack of insight.
- Dysphagia may develop in later stages.

ASSESSMENT

- Administer *Western Aphasia Battery (WAB)*. Re-administer over time to document changes.
- Assess oral-motor skills.
- Assess for dysphagia. Re-assess periodically with the passage of time or when symptoms are reported.

INTERVENTION TECHNIQUES

- Extensive therapy is generally not indicated. Teach compensatory strategies, such as the use of writing, and help the client and family members to understand the nature of the illness. (Kertesz and Munoz, 1997)
- Early in the course of the disease, work with the client to establish a system of gestures.
- Work on pairing verbal and gestural responses. (Schneider, et al., 1996)
- Work on functional tasks specific to each client.
- Treat for dysphagia as indicated.

RESULTS OF RECENT STUDIES

No recent studies regarding communication skills were found in the literature.

PROGNOSIS

The course of the disease is variable and is frequently of long duration. Several cases have been reported of persons functioning well for 5 to 12 years despite their inability to speak.

REFERENCES

Gibson E. Progressive aphasia: three explanations. *Australian Journal of Human Communication Disorders*. 1995;23(1):24–34.

Iskowitz M. Primary progressive aphasia: behavioral treatment yields mixed outcomes. *Advance for Speech-Language Pathologists & Audiologists*. 1997;7(10):8–9,18.

Karbe H, A Kertesz, M Polk. Profiles of language impairment in Primary Progressive Aphasia. *Archives of Neurology*. 1993;50:193–201.

Kertesz A, D Munoz. Clinical and pathological characteristics of primary progressive aphasia and frontal dementia. *Journal of Neural Transmission* (Supplementum). 1996; 47:133–41.

Kertesz A, DG Munoz. Primary progressive aphasia. *Clinical Neuroscience*. 1997;4:95–102.

Schneider SL, CK Thompson, B Luring. Effects of verbal plus gestural matrix training on sentence production in a patient with primary progressive aphasia. *Aphasiology*. 1996;10(3):297–317.

Progressive Supranuclear Palsy (PSP)

DESCRIPTION

Onset of PSP, also known as Steele-Richardson-Olszewski syndrome, occurs in late middle age and is manifested by loss of voluntary eye movements, bradykinesia, muscular rigidity with progressive axial dystonia, pseudobulbar palsy (spastic weakness of the pharyngeal musculature causing dysphagia and dysarthria with emotional lability), and dementia.

ETIOLOGY

Etiology is unknown. Degeneration of neurons in the basal ganglia and the brainstem is noted while the cortex remains intact.

SPEECH AND LANGUAGE DIFFICULTIES

• Dysarthria is often an early symptom.
• Acquired stuttering.
• Echolalia.
• Decreased initiation of conversational speech.
• Palilalia.
• Memory impairments, including rapid forgetting, increased sensitivity to interference, and difficulty employing memory search strategies.

ASSOCIATED AND OTHER DIFFICULTIES

• Dysphagia, characterized by hyperextended neck posture, excessive lingual and velar movements, impaired oral bolus transport, and delayed initiation of pharyngeal swallow. (Cherney, 1994)
• Drooling.
• Dementia.
• Emotional lability.
• Forgetfulness.
• Slowness of thought.
• Changes in personality with apathy, depression, and irritability.
• Motor impersistence.
• Limb and trunk bradykinesia.
• Rigidity.
• Spasticity.
• Ataxia.
• Ocular and visual disturbances.

ASSESSMENT

- Administer *Boston Naming Test (BNT)*.
- Assess for dysphagia.
- Assess for dysarthria. (See Appendix A.)

INTERVENTION TECHNIQUES

- To modify rate, consider use of pacing board and use of delayed auditory feedback. (Duffy, 1995)
- Treat for dysphagia when present.
- Assist caregivers in employing strategies to facilitate conversation.

RESULTS OF RECENT STUDIES

- Difficulties noted (forgetfulness, slowness of thought, changes in personality with apathy and depression, impaired ability to manipulate acquired language, enhanced grasp reflexes, and motor impersistence) are indications of frontal lobe involvement. (Robbins, et al., 1994)
- Although language impairment is not generally associated with PSP, three clients demonstrated verbal adynamia or dynamic aphasia, characterized by unimpaired performance on tasks of naming from pictures, naming from verbal descriptions, and intact word and sentence comprehension, accompanied by considerable impairment on tasks requiring active initiation and search strategies (letter and category fluency, and sentence completion), and on tasks of narrative language production. Perseveration was noted as the disease progressed, and over time the clients became mute. (Esmonde, et al., 1996)
- Similar to a group of control subjects, clients with PSP had more difficulty with letter fluency tasks than with category fluency tasks. Clients with PSP were significantly impaired on both tasks. Difficulties appear to relate to difficulty with initiation and retrieval, secondary to disruption of frontostriatal circuits. (Rosser and Hodges, 1995)
- Compared to those with Alzheimer's disease, clients with PSP do less well on tests of initiation. (Rosser and Hodges, 1995)
- While semantic memory is impaired in those with Alzheimer's as well as those with PSP, episodic memory is relatively spared in those with PSP. (van der Kurk and Hodges, 1995)

- In a group of 44 clients with PSP all had mixed dysarthria. The dysarthria differed from that of clients with Parkinson's disease because of the presence of spastic and occasionally ataxic components, and differed from that of clients with pseudobulbar palsy because of the presence of hypokinetic and ataxic components. (Kluin, et al., 1993)
- In a group of 44 clients with PSP, more than half exhibited dysphagia. The presence or degree of dysphagia was not related to the severity of dysarthria. (Kluin, et al., 1993)

PROGNOSIS

Death generally occurs 5 to 7 years after onset.

REFERENCES

Brookshire RH. *An Introduction to Neurogenic Communication Disorders,* 4th ed. St. Louis, Mo: Mosby Year Book. 1992:230.

Cherney LR. *Clinical Management of Dysphagia in Adults and Children,* 2nd ed. Gaithersburg, Md: Aspen Publishers, Inc. 1994:20.

Cohen S, M Freedman. Cognitive and behavioral changes in the Parkinson-plus syndromes. In: Weiner WJ, AE Lang, eds. *Behavioral Neurology of Movement Disorders.* New York: Raven Press. 1995:139–42.

Duffy JR. *Motor Speech Disorders: Substrates, Differential Diagnosis, and Management.* St. Louis, Mo: Mosby. 1995:128–44.

Esmonde T, E Giles, J Xuereb, J Hodges. Progressive supranuclear palsy presenting with dynamic aphasia. *Journal of Neurology, Neurosurgery, and Psychiatry.* 1996;60(4): 403–10.

Kluin KJ, NL Foster, S Berent, S Gilman. Perceptual analysis of speech disorders in progressive supranuclear palsy. *Neurology.* 1993;3(1):563–6.

Robbins TW, MJ Ames, AM Owen, KW Lange, AJ Lees, PN Leigh, CD Marsden, NP Quinn, BA Summers. Cognitive deficits in progressive supranuclear palsy, parkinson's disease, and multiple system atrophy in tests sensitive to frontal lobe dysfunction. *Journal of Neurology, Neurosurgery, and Psychiatry.* 1994;57(1–4):79–88.

Rosser A, JR Hodges. Initial letter and semantic category fluency in Alzheimer's disease, Huntington's disease, and progressive supranuclear palsy. *Journal of Neurology, Neurosurgery, and Psychiatry.* 1995;57(11):1389–94.

van der Kurk PR, JR Hodges. Episodic and semantic memory in Alzheimer's disease and progressive supranuclear palsy: a comparative study. *Journal of Clinical and Experimental Neuropsychology.* 1995;17(3):459–71.

Pseudobulbar Palsy (PBP)

DESCRIPTION

A motor neuron disease of unknown origin characterized by progressive degeneration of corticospinal tracts and/or anterior horn cells and/or bulbar motor nuclei. It is one of a group of lower and upper motor neuron diseases. Median age of onset is 55 years. Incidence is greater in males.

ETIOLOGY

Muscles affected are those innervated by cranial nerves and corticobulbar tracts. Etiology varies and may include multiple strokes, head injuries, multiple sclerosis, or brain tumors.

SPEECH AND LANGUAGE DIFFICULTIES

- Slow and labored speech with imprecise articulation.
- Low pitch.
- Monopitch.
- Pitch breaks.
- Distorted vowels.
- Harsh/strained vocal quality.
- Slow rate.
- Hypernasality.
- Hyperactive jaw reflex.
- Positive sucking reflex.

ASSOCIATED AND OTHER DIFFICULTIES

- Bilateral facial paralysis.
- Dysphagia.
- Difficulty swallowing; danger of aspiration.
- Drooling.
- Hemiparesis.
- Bradykinesia.
- Incontinence.
- Labile and inappropriate emotional responses.

ASSESSMENT

- Administer *Frenchay Dysarthria Assessment.*
- Assess for dysphagia.

INTERVENTION TECHNIQUES

- Goal of therapy is to maximize intelligibility. Teach pragmatic strategies such as modifying length of utterances, employing repair strategies, self-monitoring, and orientation to topic.
- Work on improved breath support and control.
- Address phonation and voice quality through relaxation techniques.
- Emphasize gentle, easy articulation, rather than preciseness.
- To treat dysphagia, position the client in an upright position with the neck flexed and provide foods that maintain a cohesive bolus. Ensure adequate hydration. Avoid foods that are sticky, dry, hard to chew, or crumble easily. As necessary, provide verbal cues before and during the eating process and provide an environment free of distractions. (Miller, et al., 1993)

RESULTS OF RECENT STUDIES

No recent studies regarding communication skills were found in the literature.

PROGNOSIS

Prognosis is poor. Death often occurs in 1 to 3 years, often from respiratory complications.

REFERENCES

Miller RM, ME Groher, KM Yorkston, TS Rees. Speech, language, swallowing, and auditory rehabilitation. In: DeLisa JA, BM Gans, eds. *Rehabilitation Medicine: Principles and Practice,* 2nd ed. Philadelphia: J.B. Lippincott Co. 1993:201–26.

Murdoch BE, EC Thompson, DG Theodoros. Spastic dysarthria. In: McNeil MR, ed. *Clinical Management of Sensorimotor Speech Disorders.* New York: Thieme. 1997:287–310.

Shy-Drager Syndrome

DESCRIPTION

A rare, progressive, autonomic failure of the nervous system. Intellectual and sensory systems generally remain intact. The disease is more common in men. Symptoms generally first appear between the ages of 40 and 75 years.

ETIOLOGY

A multiple systems degeneration in which signs of more widespread neurologic damage occur, including autonomic dysfunction with cerebellar ataxia, Parkinsonism, corticospinal, and corticobulbar tract dysfunction and amyotrophy.

SPEECH AND LANGUAGE DIFFICULTIES

- Vocal fold paresis. Tracheostomy may be necessary, and, in some cases as a last resort, total laryngectomy.
- Hoarseness and vocal stridor.
- Intermittent glottal fry.
- Hypernasality may occur.
- Monotony of voice.
- Dysarthria.
- Slow, deliberate speaking rate.

ASSOCIATED AND OTHER DIFFICULTIES

- Urinary and rectal incontinence.
- Iris atrophy.
- External ocular palsies.
- Atrophy of distal muscles.
- Rigidity.
- Tremor.
- Generalized weakness.
- Impaired handwriting.
- Dysphagia may develop later.

ASSESSMENT
- Assess for dysphagia.
- Assess for dysarthria. (See Appendix A.)
- Assess voice quality and vocal hygiene.

INTERVENTION TECHNIQUES
- Work on modifying rate and prosody to improve intelligibility. (Duffy, 1995)
- To modify rate, consider use of pacing board and use of delayed auditory feedback.
- Treat for dysphagia as indicated.

RESULTS OF RECENT STUDIES
No recent studies regarding communication skills were found in the literature.

PROGNOSIS
Bulbar dysfunction may result in death. Average duration of survival following onset of orthostatic hypotension is 7 to 8 years; average duration of survival following onset of neurologic symptoms is 4 years. Death generally occurs by aspiration, sleep apnea, or cardiac arrhythmia.

REFERENCES

Bawa R, HH Ramadan, SJ Wetmore. Bilateral vocal cord paralysis with Shy-Drager syndrome. *Otolaryngology—Head and Neck Surgery.* 1993;109:911–4.

Duffy JR. *Motor Speech Disorders: Substrates, Differential Diagnosis, and Management.* St. Louis, Mo: Mosby. 1995:166–88.

Love RJ, WG Webb. *Neurology for the Speech-Language Pathologist*, 3rd ed. Boston: Butterworth-Heinemann. 1996:189–90.

Thoene JG, NP Coker, eds. *Physicians' Guide to Rare Diseases.* New York: Dowden Publishing Co. 1995:374.

Chapter 4

Psychosocial and Psychiatric Disorders

- Asperger's syndrome (AS)
- Autism
- Childhood disintegrative disorder (CDD)
- Fluency disorders—adolescents and adults
- Fluency disorders—children
- Pervasive Developmental Disorder—Not Otherwise Specified (PDD-NOS)
- Schizophrenia

Asperger's Syndrome (AS)

DESCRIPTION

AS falls within the spectrum of autism-like disorders. Those with the disorder are generally among the more able of those with autism. Males are more frequently affected by a ratio of 7 to 1.

ETIOLOGY

Cause is unclear. Cerebral damage has been postulated, as has organic deficiency of brain function.

SPEECH AND LANGUAGE DIFFICULTIES

- Attainment of early speech and language milestones is normal, but deficits emerge in the areas of syntax and semantics.
- Vocabulary irregularities. May use obscure words while vocabulary of more common words is deficient.
- Memorization skills may mask difficulty in processing information and context.
- Difficulty with speech prosody, facial expression, gaze, and gesture.
- Severe deficits in pragmatic skills.
- Difficulty understanding jokes, metaphors, etc.
- Difficulty referring to self with pronouns.
- Deficit in understanding listener's needs in communicating in a social context. (Fine, et al., 1994)
- Speech delivery may be flat and monotonous.

ASSOCIATED AND OTHER DIFFICULTIES

- Seizure disorder.
- Severe impairment in social interactions.
- Restricted and repetitive patterns of behavior, interests, and activities.
- Prefer strict adherence to routines and schedules.
- May experience motor delays or clumsiness in preschool years.

Diagnostic Criteria for Asperger's Disorder

A. Qualitative impairment in social interaction, as manifested by at least two of the following:
   (1) marked impairment in the use of multiple nonverbal behaviors such as eye-to-eye gaze, facial expression, body postures, and gestures to regulate social interaction
   (2) failure to develop peer relationships appropriate to developmental level
   (3) a lack of spontaneous seeking to share enjoyment, interests, or achievements with other people (e.g., by a lack of showing, bringing, or pointing out objects of interest to other people)
   (4) lack of social or emotional reciprocity
B. Restricted repetitive and stereotyped patterns of behavior, interests, and activities, as manifested by at least two of the following:
   (1) encompassing preoccupation with one or more stereotyped and restricted patterns of interest that is abnormal either in intensity or focus
   (2) apparently inflexible adherence to specific, nonfunctional routines or rituals
   (3) stereotyped and repetitive motor mannerisms (e.g., hand or finger flapping or twisting, or complex whole-body movements)
   (4) persistent preoccupation with parts of objects
C. The disturbance causes clinically significant impairment in social, occupational, or other important areas of functioning.
D. There is no clinically significant general delay in language (e.g., single words used by age 2 years, communicative phrases used by age 3 years).
E. There is no clinically significant delay in cognitive development or in the development of age-appropriate self-help skills, adaptive behavior (other than in social interaction), and curiosity about the environment in childhood.
F. Criteria are not met for another specific pervasive developmental disorder or schizophrenia.

Source: Reprinted with permission from the *Diagnostic and Statistical Manual of Mental Disorders,* Fourth Edition. Copyright 1994 American Psychiatric Association.

ASSESSMENT

- Assess receptive language, expressive language, and pragmatic skills and pinpoint areas of weakness.

INTERVENTION TECHNIQUES

- Address pragmatic skills.
- Teach scripts for successful social interactions.
- Work with potential employers and co-workers to foster an understanding of the condition and the strengths of the client, as well as eccentricities inherent in the disorder.

RESULTS OF RECENT STUDIES

- In one study comparing boys with AS; those with autism; those with deficits in attention, motor control, and perception (DAMP); and those with receptive developmental speech disorder, the following findings were reported: AS is associated with higher full-scale and verbal IQ than autism; AS is not associated with better pragmatic skills than autism. (Ramberg, et al., 1996)
- In a study comparing gaze of an adult with AS, an adult with a schizoid personality disorder, and a normal control during short, unstructured interactions with a volunteer, it was found that the person with AS looked at the volunteer significantly less often during times when the volunteer was speaking. However, there were not significant differences in eye gaze when the volunteer was listening. (Tantam, et al., 1993)

PROGNOSIS

Improvement is often seen over time, especially after adolescence. Some type of employment is possible for many with the disorder, particularly in jobs involving a regular routine.

REFERENCES

Berthier ML, A Bayes, ES Tolosa. Magnetic resonance imaging in patients with concurrent Tourette's disorder and Asperger's syndrome. *Journal of the American Academy of Child & Adolescent Psychiatry.* 1993;32(3):633–9.

Fine J, G Bartolucci, P Szatmari, G Ginsberg. Cohesive discourse in pervasive developmental disorders. *Journal of Autism and Developmental Disorders.* 1994;24(3):315–29.

Ghaziuddin M, L Gerstein. Pedantic speaking style differentiates Asperger syndrome from high-functioning autism. *Journal of Autism and Developmental Disorders.* 1996; 26(6):585–95.

Gilbert P. *The A-Z Reference Book of Syndromes and Inherited Disorders: A Manual for Health, Social and Education Workers.* New York: Chapman & Hall. 1993:31–33.

Ramberg C, S Ehlers, A Nydén, M Johansson, C Gillberg. Language and pragmatic functions in school-age children on the autism spectrum. *European Journal of Disorders of Communication.* 1996;31:387–414.

Smith MD, JS Damico. *Childhood Language Disorders.* New York: Thieme Medical Publishers, Inc. 1996:160–3.

Tantam D, D Holmes, C Cordess. Nonverbal expression in autism of Asperger type. *Journal of Autism and Developmental Disorders.* 1993;23(1):111–33.

Thoene JG, NP Coker, eds. *Physicians' Guide to Rare Diseases.* New York: Dowden Publishing Co. 1995:269–70.

Autism

DESCRIPTION

A syndrome beginning in early childhood characterized by:
- Abnormal social relationships.
- Language disorder with impaired understanding, echolalia, and pronominal reversal (using "you" instead of "I" or "me").
- Rituals and compulsive behaviors.
- Uneven intellectual development.

Autism occurs more frequently in males by a ratio of 3 to 1. Symptoms usually appear in the first year of life. Incidence is approximately 15 in every 10,000 births. A third of those with autism also have epilepsy. Hallmarks of the disorder are difficulties in the areas of socialization, communication, and imagination. Among those with autism, 3% to 9% demonstrate normal intellectual functioning, 10% to 20% are mildly involved, and 70% to 80% are severely involved. (Stahl, 1995)

ETIOLOGY

Although specific etiology is unknown, autism is now believed to be a disorder of brain development. There is strong evidence of a genetic factor. Disorders in which autism is present with a higher than chance occurrence rate include Fragile X syndrome, Cornelia de Lang syndrome, and tuberous sclerosis. (See accompanying chapters in this book)

SPEECH AND LANGUAGE DIFFICULTIES

- May develop language skills normally until about 15 months, then regresses and loses acquired skills.
- Impairment in verbal and nonverbal communication.
- Impairment or absence of nonverbal communication such as pointing, gesturing, head shakes, and nods.
- Good articulation skills but poor intonation and/or prosody.
- Frequent dysfluencies.
- Likely to provide too much or too little information when speaking.
- Difficulty using pronouns.
- Difficulty with abstract language.
- Echolalia.
- Perseverative and/or irrelevant language.
- May read at above-average level but lack comprehension of what has been read.
- Poor pragmatic skills.
- Failure to understand intentionality in others' behavior.
- Deficit in understanding listener's needs in communicating in a social context. (Fine, et al., 1994)
- In discourse, difficulties include lack of communicative intent, noncommunicative use of language, difficulty with turn-taking, and difficulty switching listener-speaker roles.
- Failure to develop a theory of mind—an understanding of make-believe, deception, or inferential communication.

ASSOCIATED AND OTHER DIFFICULTIES

- Extreme aloneness and, in very young children, failure to cuddle.
- Avoidance of eye contact.

- Self-injurious behaviors.
- Insistence on sameness; resistance to change.
- Self-stimulation.
- Rituals.
- Morbid attachment to familiar objects.
- Hyperacusis, or consistently inappropriate responses to sounds or complaints of uncomfortable levels of sounds in response to sounds that are not perceived as uncomfortably loud to average persons.
- Repetitive acts.
- Limited repertoire and range of interests.
- Lack of symbolic play.
- Avoidance of social initiations of others.
- Impairment in reciprocal social interactions.
- Irregular sleep pattern.
- Sensory processing deficits resulting in abnormal responses to sensory input.

ASSESSMENT

- With preschool-aged and other young children, assess caregiver/child interactions.
- With preschool children, evaluate and assess skills on several different occasions and in different settings. Children may demonstrate different communicative skills in different environments.
- Assess, in the client's natural settings, the communication repertoires currently being used. Assessment should include evaluations of behaviors used to express intentions, systems of gestural and vocal communication, ability to repair conversation breakdowns, topic maintenance, and turn-taking skills. (Wetherby and Prizant, 1992)
- Assess communication style of those interacting with the client, i.e., facilitative versus directive.
- Administer the *Pre-Linguistic Autism Diagnostic Observation Schedule* (PL-ADOS) to aid in differentiation between young children with autism and children with other developmental delays. (DiLavore, et al., 1995)
- Administer the *Autism Diagnostic Observation Schedule* (ADOS).
- Evaluate appropriateness of implementing augmentative communication.

Diagnostic Criteria for Autistic Disorder

A. A total of six (or more) from (1), (2), and (3), with at least two from (1) and one each from (2) and (3):

(1) qualitative impairment in social interaction, as manifested by at least two of the following:

    (a) marked impairment in the use of multiple nonverbal behaviors such as eye-to-eye gaze, facial expression, body postures, and gestures to regulate social interaction

    (b) failure to develop peer relationships appropriate to developmental level

    (c) a lack of spontaneous seeking to share enjoyment, interests, or achievement with other people (e.g., by a lack of showing, bringing, or pointing out objects of interest)

    (d) lack of social or emotional reciprocity

(2) qualitative impairments in communication as manifested by at least one of the following:

    (a) delay in, or total lack of, the development of spoken language (not accompanied by an attempt to compensate through alternative modes of communication such as gestures or mime)

    (b) in individuals with adequate speech, marked impairment in the ability to initiate or sustain a conversation with others

    (c) stereotyped and repetitive use of language or idiosyncratic language

    (d) lack of varied, spontaneous make-believe play or social imitative play appropriate to developmental level

(3) restricted repetitive and stereotyped patterns of behavior, interests, and activities, as manifested by at least one of the following:

    (a) encompassing preoccupation with one or more stereotyped and restricted patterns of interest that is abnormal either in intensity or focus

    (b) apparently inflexible adherence to specific, nonfunctional routines or rituals

continues

(c) stereotyped and repetitive motor mannerisms (e.g., hand or finger flapping or twisting, or complex whole-body movements)

(d) persistent preoccupation with parts of objects

B. Delays or abnormal functioning in at least one of the following areas, with onset prior to 3 years of age: (1) social interaction, (2) language as used in social communication, or (3) symbolic or imaginative play.

C. The disturbance is not better accounted for by Rett syndrome or childhood disintegrative disorder.

Source: Reprinted with permission from *Diagnostic and Statistical Manual of Mental Disorders,* Fourth Edition. Copyright 1994 American Psychiatric Association.

INTERVENTION TECHNIQUES

(NOTE: The use of facilitated communication to enhance the communication skills of persons with autism has been reported in the literature. The reader should be aware that use of this technique is controversial. References on the use of facilitated communication may be found in Appendix D.)

- Work with audiologist to rule hearing loss in or out.
- Base communication goals on developmental and functional criteria.
- Involve the entire family in intervention with young children. Facilitate interactions that nurture and encourage communication development.
- Help caregivers and others to establish consistency, predictability, and structure for the child.
- Encourage caregivers and others to communicate with the child at his/ her language age rather than chronological age and to use natural gestures.
- Use imitation of a young child's movements to facilitate attention to people, social contingency, and turn-taking. (Klinger and Dawson, 1992)
- Expand the child's ability to indicate requests and to label.
- Work on developing a socially acceptable way to express protest and rejection.

- Facilitate language development through inclusion in an integrated preschool program.
- Encourage turn-taking skills and conversational repair strategies.
- Encourage symbolic play using one object to symbolize another, e.g., using a block as a telephone or a finger as a baby's bottle.
- Understand that behavioral deficits in autism are generally the result of a combination of excessive sensory stimulation and an internal chemical trigger. Techniques include providing a safer, less disruptive source for stimulation (such as a providing a koosh ball), providing sustained physical exercise, and providing sensory integration training. (Fox, 1994)
- Structure the environment to reduce an overload of sensory stimulation while providing sensory input. For example, keep work and play areas free of clutter, provide vestibular and proprioceptive input such as a rocking chair or a bean bag chair. Provide visual supports such as schedules and calendars, labels and signs, and color coding of materials. (Mora and Kashman, 1997)
- Language may be perceived as just noise. Present language on tapes, CDs, etc., allowing the client to focus on just the words without any visual distractions. (Fox, 1994)
- Beginning in preschool years, use the Picture Exchange Communication System (PECS). Teach child to place picture in hand of adult in exchange for desired object. (Trace, 1994)
- When echolalia is present, receptive understanding of what is expressed cannot be assumed. Provide the client with a strong receptive foundation of knowledge, beginning with actual objects and moving on to pictures and photographs. (Fox, 1994)
- Conveying information visually is often more successful than repeatedly conveying the same message auditorily. (Fox, 1994)
- With young children, implement language intervention within a whole language curriculum environment. (Trace, 1993)
- Use Pivotal Response Training (PRT) to teach children to engage in symbolic play. Principles of PRT include turn-taking, reinforcing attempts at appropriate responses, frequent task variation, allowing child's choice of activities, interspersing maintenance tasks, and using natural consequences. (Stahmer, 1995)
- Consider use of auditory integration training (AIT). (See Results of Recent Studies)

- Provide order and routine in scheduling. (Fox, 1994)
- Provide visual cues to help with sequencing of activities.
- Emphasize learning of functional skills, i.e., making change, buying and ordering food, etc.
- Address pragmatic skills, including eye contact, turn-taking, following commands, and topic maintenance.
- Consider use of some form of augmentative communication. Few persons with autism reach intellectual, language, and social levels necessitating complex, expensive devices. Consider various forms of picture boards and notebooks. (Siegel, 1996)
- Assist parents as they select an educational program for their child. Factors to be considered include the ability to individualize programming to meet each child's needs, a family component, opportunities for integration with nondisabled peers, and a strong social communication emphasis. Other factors to be considered include the training of the staff, opportunities for regular in-service training for staff, the length of the program day and week, and staff-to-student ratio. (Iskowitz, 1998b)
- Work to gradually introduce clients to a wider variety of foods.

RESULTS OF RECENT STUDIES

Four subtypes of autism have been identified:

1. typically autistic with abnormal verbal and nonverbal communication, aloofness, impaired social skills, and sensory disturbances.
2. similarly autistic but with a moderate to severe mental disability.
3. high-functioning, overactive, and aggressive.
4. a group with impairments in social and language skills, restricted interests, and a family history of learning problems. (Eaves, et al., 1994)

- One young child (nearly 3 years old) diagnosed with autism was given 10 treatments of hyperbaric oxygen therapy (HBOT). Improvements in mood, a sense of humor, and increased social contact were noted, raising the possibility that an intrauterine stroke or stroke at birth had occurred. It is recommended that young children diagnosed with autism have a complete neurological evaluation to determine if there is any brain injury. A finding of brain injury may prompt consideration of HBOT. (Iskowitz, 1998a)

- Children with autism enrolled in one of several intensive early intervention (EI) programs serving children with autism all had the following characteristics in common: significant acceleration of developmental rates and significant gains in IQ; significant language gains; improved social behavior and decreased symptoms of autism. By age 5 years, 75% of autistic children who attended these EI programs had some useful speech. (Rogers, 1996)
- In children with autism, more echolalia is present when adults use high linguistic constraint utterances (direct questions, directives) than when low constraint utterances (commenting, reflective questioning) are used. Immediate echoes are more likely to follow high constraint adult utterances, while delayed echoes are more likely to follow low constraint utterances. Delayed echoes show more evidence of comprehension than do immediate echoes. (Rydell and Mirenda, 1994)
- Deficits in speech and gestural communication skills in children with autism may be due in part to apraxia. Presence of apraxia must be evaluated when considering augmentative and alternative communication (AAC) options. (Prizant, 1996)
- In one study of the effects of auditory integration therapy (AIT), both the experimental and the control group had decreased levels of inappropriate behavior. In other studies, parents and teachers have noted positive effects of AIT, including children becoming calmer and less disturbed by changes in their environment. (Gelman, 1996)
- As described by their parents, autistic girls with mild or no mental handicaps were judged as less severely handicapped in communication and social skills at young ages than were a matched group of autistic boys. But among the same groups as adults, the females were judged as more socially impaired than were the males. A possible explanation is that as adults males may participate in more nonverbal activities with peers, i.e., sports. (McLennan, et al., 1993)
- Preverbal children between the ages of 3 and 5 years were matched with a similar group of children diagnosed with developmental language disorder (DLD). Those with autism were less likely to engage in joint attention. Adults used more literal and fewer conventional bids for joint attention with autistic children while using fewer literal and more conventional bids with children with DLD. (Mcarthur and Adamson, 1996)

- Following specific training in sociodramatic play, children with autism exhibited an increase in the ability to role play, increases in make-believe, and the ability to play with ambiguous and nonexistent objects and an increase in persistence in play. (Thorp, et al., 1995)
- Children with autism did significantly better recalling words used in subject-performed tasks than they did with words on straight word lists. A group of controls performed about equally well on both tasks. (Summers and Craik, 1994)
- In a study comparing adults with autism with a group of adults who had a childhood diagnosis of receptive language delay (RLD), the adults with autism were significantly more impaired on all measures (total inappropriacy rate, positive inappropriacy rate, empty turn rate, and initiation rate). Pragmatic impairments may be due either to a failure of intention or a failure of execution. Inappropriacy due to impairment of intention was much more common among those with autism than among those with RLD. (Eales, 1993)
- In conversation, when compared with a group of subjects with Asperger's disorder, those with higher-functioning autism referred more often to the physical world and less often to previous conversational text, making sustained conversation difficult. (Fine, et al., 1994)
- Individual adults with autism were paired with examiners under the following conditions:
  1. both the participant and the examiner spoke.
  2. the participant spoke and the examiner typed.
  3. the participant typed and the examiner spoke.
  4. both the participant and the examiner typed.
  Mean length of response was significantly lower under the first condition, possibly indicating visual strengths and auditory weakness. (Forsey, et al., 1996)
- High-functioning adults with autism show several language and pragmatic deficits similar to those of adults with right hemisphere damage. (Ozonoff and Miller, 1996)

PROGNOSIS

Autism is a life-long condition.

REFERENCES

Baltaxe CA, N D'Angiola. Cohesion in the disclosure interaction of autistic, specifically language-impaired, and normal children. *Journal of Autism & Developmental Disorders.* 1992;22(1):1–21.

Bettison S. The long-term effects of auditory training on children with autism. *Journal of Autism and Developmental Disorders.* 1996;26(3):361–74.

Brown J, PA Prelock. Brief report: the impact of regression on language development in autism. *Journal of Autism & Developmental Disorders.* 1995;25(3):305–9.

DiLavore PC, C Lord, M Rutter. The pre-linguistic autism diagnostic observation schedule. *Journal of Autism & Developmental Disorders.* 1995;25(4):355–79.

Eales MJ. Pragmatic impairments in adults with childhood diagnoses of autism or developmental receptive language disorder. *Journal of Autism & Developmental Disorders.* 1993;23(4):593–617.

Eaves LC, HH Ho, DM Eaves. Subtypes of autism by cluster analysis. *Journal of Autism & Developmental Disorders.* 1994;24(1):3–22.

Fine J, G Bartolucci, P Szatmari, G Ginsberg. Cohesive discourse in pervasive developmental disorders. *Journal of Autism and Developmental Disorders.* 1994;24(3):315–329.

Forsey J, EKR Bird, J Bedrosian. Brief report—the effects of typed and spoken modality combinations on the language performance of adults with autism. *Journal of Autism & Developmental Disorders.* 1996;26(6):643–9.

Fox S. Educational strategies address pragmatic and behavioral deficits in autism. *Advance for Speech-Language Pathologists & Audiologists.* 1994;4(6):12–13.

Frith U. Social communication and its disorder in autism and Asperger syndrome. *Journal of Psychopharmacology.* 1996;10(1):48–53.

Gelman J. Reining in AIT: clinicians call for stricter guidelines, more research. *Advance for Speech-Language Pathologists & Audiologists.* 1996;6(1):4,11.

Iskowitz M. Making a case for HBOT. *Advance for Speech-Language Pathologists & Audiologists.* 1998a;8(1):6–9.

Iskowitz M. Selecting an education program. *Advance for Speech-Language Pathologists & Audiologists.* 1998b;8(1):11–13.

Klinger LG, G Dawson. Facilitating early social and communicative development in children with autism. In: Warren SF, J Reichle, eds. *Causes and Effects in Communication and Language Intervention.* Baltimore: Paul H. Brookes Publishing Co. 1992:157–86.

Mcarthur D, LB Adamson. Joint attention in preverbal children—autism and developmental language disorders. *Journal of Autism & Developmental Disorders.* 1996;26(5):481–96.

McLennan JD, C Lord, E Schopler. Sex differences in higher functioning people with autism. *Journal of Autism & Developmental Disorders.* 1993;23(2):217–27.

Mora J, N Kashman. Strategies for sensory integration. *Advance for Speech-Language Pathologists & Audiologists.* 1997;7(50):20–22.

Ozonoff S, JN Miller. An exploration of right-hemisphere contributions to the pragmatic impairments of autism. *Brain and Language.* 1996;52:411–34.

Parker R. Incorporating speech-language therapy into an applied behavior analysis program. In: Maurice C, ed. *Behavioral Intervention for Young Children with Autism: A Manual for Parents and Professionals.* Austin, Tex: Pro-Ed. 1996:297–306.

Prizant BM. Brief report: communication, language, social, and emotional development. *Journal of Autism & Developmental Disorders.* 1996;26(2):173–8.

Prizant BM, AM Wetherby. Communication in preschool autistic children. In: Schopler E, ME Van Bourgondien, MM Bristol, eds. *Preschool Issues in Autism.* New York: Plenum Press. 1993:95–128.

Rogers SJ. Brief report: early intervention in autism. [Review, 10 refs] *Journal of Autism & Developmental Disorders.* 1996;26(2):243–6.

Rydell PJ, P Mirenda. Effects of high and low constraint utterances on the production of immediate and delayed echolalia in young children with autism. *Journal of Autism & Developmental Disorders.* 1994;24(6):719–35.

Shoemaker A. Preparing children for life: addressing speech and language issues in autism. *Advance for Speech-Language Pathologists & Audiologists.* 1997;7(1):7,16.

Siegel B. *The World of the Autistic Child: Understanding and Treating Autistic Spectrum Disorders.* New York: Oxford University Press. 1996:253–73.

Stahl C. Treating autism through the lifespan. *Advance for Speech-Language Pathologists & Audiologist.* 1995;5(14):16.

Stahmer AC. Teaching symbolic play skills to children with autism using pivotal response training. *Journal of Autism & Developmental Disorders.* 1995;25(2):123–43.

Summers JA, FI Craik. The effects of subject-performed tasks on the memory performance of verbal autistic children. *Journal of Autism & Developmental Disorders.* 1994; 24(6):773–83.

Tager-Flushberg H. Brief report: current theory and research on language and communication in autism. *Journal of Autism & Developmental Disorders.* 1996;26(2):169–72.

Thorp DM, AC Stahmer, L Schreibman. Effects of sociodramatic play training on children with autism. *Journal of Autism & Developmental Disorders.* 1995;25(3):265–82.

Towbin KE. Pervasive developmental disorder. In: Cohen DJ, FR Volkmar, eds. *Handbook of Autism and Pervasive Developmental Disorders,* 2nd ed. New York: John Wiley & Sons. 1997:123–47.

Trace R. Integrated preschools offer benefits to children with autism. *Advance for Speech-Language Pathologists & Audiologists.* 1993;3(7):8.

Trace R. Using picture exchange to teach functional communication skills to children with autism. *Advance for Speech-Language Pathologists & Audiologists.* 1994;4(17):6.

Wetherby AW, BM Prizant. Facilitating language and communication development in autism: assessment and intervention guidelines. In: Berkell DE, ed. *Autism: Identification, Education, and Treatment.* Hillsdale, NJ: Lawrence Erlbaum Associates. 1992:107–34.

Childhood Disintegrative Disorder (CDD)

DESCRIPTION

The American Psychiatric Association's *Diagnostic and Statistical Manual of Mental Disorders*, 4th ed. (DSM-IV), lists the following criteria for the diagnosis of CDD: normal development for at least 2 years; a significant loss of previously acquired skills in the areas of language, social skills, toileting skills, and play or motor abilities before age 10 years; a concomitant development of abnormal functioning in at least two of the following three areas: social interaction, communication, or repetitive patterns of behavior or activities. The disorder, also known as Heller's syndrome, is not better accounted for by another childhood-onset pervasive developmental disorder (PDD) or by schizophrenia. (See accompanying Table.)

Males are affected in greater numbers than females, in ratios ranging from 4 to 1 to 8 to 1. Onset is later than 3 years and may be sudden or develop over time. In some cases there seems to be a precipitating event such as the birth of a sibling, accidental injury, or hospital admission for elective surgery.

ETIOLOGY

Etiology is unknown but neurobiological factors are suspected. Electroencephalographic (EEG) abnormalities are generally present.

SPEECH AND LANGUAGE DIFFICULTIES

• Loss or marked regression in communication skills, both receptive and expressive.

ASSOCIATED AND OTHER DIFFICULTIES

• Difficulty with social interactions.
• Resistance to change.
• Overactivity.

Diagnostic Criteria for Childhood Disintegrative Disorder

A. Apparently normal development for at least the first 2 years after birth as manifested by the presence of age-appropriate verbal and nonverbal communication, social relationships, play, and adaptive behavior.

B. Clinically significant loss of previously acquired skills (before age 10 years) in at least two of the following areas:
   (1) expressive or receptive language
   (2) social skills or adaptive behavior
   (3) bowel or bladder control
   (4) play
   (5) motor skills

C. Abnormalities of functioning in at least two of the following areas:
   (1) qualitative impairment in social interaction (e.g., impairment in nonverbal behaviors, failure to develop peer relationships, lack of social or emotional reciprocity)
   (2) qualitative impairments in communication (e.g., delay or lack of spoken language, inability to initiate or sustain a conversation, stereotyped and repetitive use of language, lack of varied make-believe play)
   (3) restricted, repetitive, and stereotyped patterns of behavior, interests, and activities, including motor stereotypes and mannerisms.

D. The disturbance is not better accounted for by another specific pervasive developmental disorder or by schizophrenia.

Source: Reprinted with permission from the *Diagnostic and Statistical Manual of Mental Disorders,* Fourth Edition. Copyright 1994 American Psychiatric Association.

- Excessive fearfulness and anxiety.
- Deterioration in self-help skills (particularly bowel and bladder control).
- Deterioration in intellectual functioning.
- Seizure disorder.

ASSESSMENT

- Assess all areas of communication skills—receptive language, expressive language, and pragmatic skills.

INTERVENTION TECHNIQUES

- Encourage participation in early intervention program and provide language development activities within the program.
- Provide language development and communication interaction modeling for parents and caregivers.

RESULTS OF RECENT STUDIES

No recent studies were found in the literature.

PROGNOSIS

Static as well as progressive forms of the disorder have been noted. Prognosis seems to be somewhat worse than for those with autism. (Volkmar and Rutter, 1995) Most clients function in the moderate to severe range of mental retardation.

REFERENCES

American Psychiatric Association, *Diagnostic and Statistical Manual of Mental Disorders,* Fourth Edition. Washington, DC: American Psychiatric Association. 1994.

Volkmar FR. Childhood disintegrative disorder: issues for DSM-IV. *Journal of Autism and Developmental Disorders.* 1992;22(4):625–42.

Volkmar FR, M Rutter. Childhood disintegrative disorder: results of the *DSM-IV* field test. *Journal of the American Academy of Child and Adolescent Psychiatry.* 1995;34(8): 1092–5.

Volkmar FR, A Klin, W Marans, DJ Cohen. Childhood disintegrative disorder. In: Cohen, DJ, FR Volkmar, eds. *Handbook of Autism and Pervasive Developmental Disorders,* 2nd ed. New York: John Wiley & Sons. 1997:47–59.

Fluency Disorders—
Adolescents and Adults

DESCRIPTION
(See also Fluency Disorders—Children)

ETIOLOGY
There are cases of adult-onset neurogenic stuttering, in some instances secondary to vascular brain damage.

(See also Fluency Disorders—Children)

SPEECH AND LANGUAGE DIFFICULTIES
- Repetition of sounds, syllables, and/or single-syllable words.
- Prolongation of voiced or voiceless sounds.
- Blocks such as stoppage of the flow of air or voice.
- Secondary behaviors in the form of escape behaviors (i.e., eye blinks, head nods, insertion of "uh") and avoidance behaviors (i.e., changing words, avoiding situations).

ASSOCIATED AND OTHER DIFFICULTIES
- Development of negative feelings about oneself and the ability to speak.
- Most antidepressant medications increase stuttering.

ASSESSMENT
- Administer *Self-Efficacy Scale for Adolescents* or *Self-Efficacy Scale of Adult Stutterers* (SESAS).
- Administer pretreatment and posttreatment assessment of the clients' perception of their speech performance through use of the *Speech Performance Questionnaire.*
- Obtain and analyze a speech sample.
- Differentiate stuttering from cluttering.
- Engage in trial therapy, using a variety of techniques during the evaluation, and assess the client's responses.

INTERVENTION TECHNIQUES

- As a clinician, be familiar with the tenets of stuttering modification therapy and fluency shaping therapy. Based on each client's needs, decide on a course of therapy that utilizes one of these approaches or a combination of the two. (Guitar, 1998)
- As one component of therapy, consider use of delayed auditory feedback (DAF) and/or a computer-aided device that teaches proper breathing and voice onset. (Guteri, 1995)
- Have adolescents, as well as adults, set their own goals for therapy.
- Address age-appropriate issues during therapy sessions.
- When working with adolescents, address social and pragmatic skills as well as speech skills. (Iskowitz, 1997a)
- Provide counseling relative to the emotional aspects of stuttering.
- As a clinician, be willing to demonstrate dysfluent speech in real-life situations.
- As one part of therapy, consider use of visualization and guided imagery techniques. (Scott, 1998b)
- Consider client enrollment in an intensive, residential treatment program.
- Help clients come to terms with their moments of stuttering; help them to recognize avoidances, substitutions, etc.
- Provide instruction in fluency skills of prolongation, easy onset, soft contacts, and appropriate phrasing.
- Provide for some supervised maintenance following completion of treatment.

RESULTS OF RECENT STUDIES

- There are those who recover from periods of stuttering without the assistance of treatment. In a study designed to determine if the speech of such persons is perceptually different from those who have never stuttered, a group of judges analyzed videotaped speech samples of the two groups. Results showed that there were differences; the speech of those who had at one time stuttered was judged to have a higher frequency of part-word repetitions and to sound less natural. (Finn, 1997)
- In a study of the effects of altered auditory feedback (AAF) on scripted telephone conversations of nine adults who stutter, significant results were noted. Stuttering frequency was reduced 55% under the condition of

frequency altered feedback (FAF) and 60% under the condition of DAF. (Zimmerman, et al., 1997)

PROGNOSIS

Emphasis is on improved ease of communication, with resulting improvement in the quality of life.

REFERENCES

Boberg E, D Kully. Long-term results of an intensive treatment program for adults and adolescents who stutter. *Journal of Speech and Hearing Research*. 1994;37:1050–9.

Bojleveld H, Y Lebrun, H van Dongen. A case of acquired stuttering. *Folia Phoniatrica & Logopedica*. 1994;46:250–3.

Finn P. Adults recovered from stuttering without formal treatment: perceptual assessment of speech normalcy. *Journal of Speech, Language, and Hearing Research*. 1997; 40(4):821–31.

Guitar B. *Stuttering: An Integrated Approach to Its Nature and Treatment,* 2nd ed. Baltimore: Williams & Wilkins. 1998.

Guteri GO. Clinicians discuss role of fluency devices in stuttering therapy. *Advance for Speech-Language Pathologists & Audiologists*. 1995;5(18):6–7,15.

Iskowitz M. Communication skills approach to stuttering. *Advance for Speech-Language Pathologists & Audiologists*. 1997a;7(37):6.

Iskowitz M. Supervised maintenance essential after stuttering treatment. *Advance for Speech-Language Pathologists & Audiologists*. 1997b;7(19):10.

Scott, A. Coming to terms with stuttering. *Advance for Speech-Language Pathologists & Audiologists*. 1998a;8(19):12,24.

Scott A. Visualizing fluency. *Advance for Speech-Language Pathologists & Audiologists*. 1998b;8(5):10–11.

Trace R. When the fluency disorder is 'cluttering.' *Advance for Speech-Language Pathologists & Audiologists*. 1993;3(10):11.

Trace R. Counseling addresses life issues of people who stutter. *Advance for Speech-Language Pathologists & Audiologists*. 1996;6(19):6–7,16.

Wedmore S. Early childhood stuttering: SEA workshop participants share ideas. *Advance for Speech-Language Pathologists & Audiologists*. 1997;7(35):4.

Zarella S. Therapy program bolsters self-esteem of students. *Advance for Speech-Language Pathologists & Audiologists*. 1995;5(18):8.

Zimmerman S, J Kalinowski, A Stuart, M Rastatter. Effect of altered auditory feedback on people who stutter during scripted telephone conversations. *Journal of Speech, Language, and Hearing Research*. 1997;40(5):1130–4.

Fluency Disorders—Children

DESCRIPTION

"Stuttering is characterized by an abnormally high frequency or duration of stoppages in the forward flow of speech. These stoppages usually take the form of: (a) repetitions of sounds, syllables, or one-syllable words; (b) prolongations of sounds; or (c) 'blocks' of airflow or voicing in speech." (Guitar, 1998)

Prevalence is estimated to be about 1% during the school years. Although very young males and females are affected about equally, the ratio of males to females steadily increases from 3 to 1 in first grade to 5 to 1 in third grade.

ETIOLOGY

An exact cause and a single cause of dysfluent speech have not been discovered. Numerous theories have been proposed. One of these theories is that there is some genetic basis to stuttering. It has also been shown that those who stutter exhibit higher levels of muscle activity during speech production. (Wedmore, 1997) Other theories are directed toward sensory-motor coordination, central auditory processing differences, and differences in cerebral dominance for language.

SPEECH AND LANGUAGE DIFFICULTIES

- Repetition of sounds, syllables, and/or single-syllable words.
- Prolongation of voiced or voiceless sounds.
- Blocks such as stoppage of the flow of air or voice.
- Secondary behaviors in the form of escape behaviors (i.e., eye blinks, head nods, insertion of "uh") and avoidance behaviors (i.e., changing words, avoiding situations).
- A higher percentage of children who stutter have articulation and language problems than do fluent speakers.
- Poor performance in processing speech in the right ear.

Developmental Levels of Dysfluency

Normal
Dysfluency

All of the following criteria must be met:
(a) No more than 10 dysfluencies per 100 words
(b) Most dysfluencies are multisyllable word and phrase repetitions
(c) Repetitions consist of two or fewer units per repetition
(d) Repetitions are slow and regular in tempo
(e) All dysfluencies are produced in a relaxed manner
(f) The child seems hardly aware of the dysfluencies

Borderline
Stuttering

(a) More than 10 dysfluencies per 100 words
(b) Dysfluencies may consist of part-word repetitions, single-syllable word repetitions, and prolongations
(c) Repetitions may be more than two per unit
(d) Dysfluencies are loose and relaxed

Beginning
Stuttering

(a) Dysfluencies are tense and hurried
(b) Dysfluencies may consist of rapid repetitions; pitch rises during repetitions and prolongations; difficulty beginning airflow or phonation; signs of facial tension
(c) The stutterer shows awareness of his or her dysfluencies
(d) Escape behaviors to terminate blocks may be used

Intermediate
Stuttering

(a) Blocks are tense, shutting off sound or voice
(b) Repetitions and prolongations may also be present
(c) Escape behaviors are used to terminate blocks

continues

	(d) Blocks are often anticipated and avoidance behaviors are used prior to feared words
	(e) Difficult situations are anticipated and may be avoided
	(f) Fear, embarrassment, and shame are present
Advanced Stuttering	(a) Blocks are often long, tense; tremors of the lips, tongue, and/or jaw may often be present
	(b) Repetitions and prolongations are generally present
	(c) Complex patterns of escape and avoidance behaviors are present
	(d) Emotions of fear, embarrassment, and shame are strongly present

Source: Adapted with permission from B. Guitar, *Stuttering: An Integrated Approach to Its Nature and Treatment,* 2nd Ed., © 1998, Williams & Wilkins.

ASSOCIATED AND OTHER DIFFICULTIES

- Development of negative feelings and attitudes about oneself and the ability to speak.
- Cognitive stress increases dysfluencies.
- Ritalin may increase stuttering.

ASSESSMENT

- Prior to seeing a preschool-aged child, ask the parents to furnish an audiotape of the child speaking in a typical home situation.
- Observe one or both parents, and other family members if possible, interacting with the child.
- In young children, assess the interrelatedness of the complexity of speech, the length of utterance, and rate. (Trace, 1992)
- Administer *Stuttering Prediction Instrument for Young Children* (SPI).
- Administer *Stuttering Severity Instrument,* 3rd ed. (SSI-3).

- In addition to assessing fluency, evaluate receptive and expressive language skills, articulation skills, cognitive development, and social-emotional development.
- Following the assessment, determine if the child is experiencing normal dysfluency, borderline stuttering, beginning stuttering, or intermediate stuttering and discuss this information and its implications with the parents. (See accompanying Table.)

INTERVENTION TECHNIQUES

- Encourage use of fluency-enhancing techniques among those interacting with the child. These include using a slowed rate of speech, eliminating demands for complex responses, and acknowledgment of the child's feelings. (Wedmore, 1997)
- Use words young child can understand, i.e., "hard" and "soft" rather than "tense" and "relaxed."
- Involve children in both group and individual therapy.
- Teach the child to recognize muscle tension and how to use this knowledge to pull out of a dysfluency. (Wedmore, 1997)
- Instruct in the use of proper diaphragmatic breathing. (Wagaman, et al., 1993)
- Provide consultation to teachers on techniques to enhance fluency in the classroom.
- Consider group therapy or camp settings to bring together children who stutter.

RESULTS OF RECENT STUDIES

- Several studies have sought to differentiate early childhood stuttering from normal developmental dysfluencies. Results indicate that regarding frequency, children who stutter are dysfluent at least twice as often as children who don't stutter; those who stutter produce more within-word dysfluencies; and associated, nonspeech behaviors are present even in very young children who stutter. (Zebrowski, 1995)

PROGNOSIS

Although different studies yield differing figures regarding the percentage of children who fully recover from stuttering, it can be said generally that between 50% and 85% of children who stutter recover with or without professional help. (Guitar, 1998)

REFERENCES

Guitar B. *Stuttering: An Integrated Approach to Its Nature and Treatment,* 2nd ed. Baltimore: Williams & Wilkins. 1998.

Maske-Cash WS, RE Curlee. Effect of utterance length and meaningfulness on the speech initiation times of children who stutter and children who do not stutter. *Journal of Speech and Hearing Research.* 1995;38:18–25.

Shoemaker A. Empowering children who stutter. *Advance for Speech-Language Pathologists & Audiologists.* 1997a;7(19):9.

Shoemaker A. Providing fluency services in the schools. *Advance for Speech-Language Pathologists & Audiologists.* 1997b;7(19):8,16.

Trace R. Stuttering: early intervention is the key to successful treatment. *Advance for Speech-Language Pathologists & Audiologists.* 1992;2(25):9,14.

Wagaman JT, RG Miltenberger, RE Arndorfer. Analysis of a simplified treatment for stuttering in children. *Journal of Applied Behavior Analysis.* 1993;26(1):53–61.

Wedmore S. Early childhood stuttering: SEA workshop participants share ideas. *Advance for Speech-Language Pathologists & Audiologists.* 1997;7(35):4.

Zarella, S. Fluency program bolsters self-esteem of students. *Advance for Speech-Language Pathologists & Audiologists.* 1995;5(18):8.

Zebrowski PM. The topography of beginning stuttering. *Journal of Communication Disorders.* 1995;28:75–91.

Pervasive Developmental Disorder— Not Otherwise Specified (PDD-NOS)

(See also Autism)

DESCRIPTION

A syndrome similar to autism but with a later age of onset: 30 months to 12 years. Sometimes referred to as atypical autism or subthreshold.

ETIOLOGY

No single cause of PDD has been identified. Etiology is likely a combination of genetic, congenital, and life events factors.

SPEECH AND LANGUAGE DIFFICULTIES

- Visual skills are generally superior to verbal skills.
- Echolalia.
- Severe articulation deficits.
- Socially awkward communication skills.
- Difficulty understanding prepositions, pronouns, and "wh" questions.
- Difficulty with turn-taking.
- Deficit in understanding listener's needs in communicating in a social context. (Fine, et al., 1994)

ASSOCIATED AND OTHER DIFFICULTIES

- May have visual/spatial processing deficits.
- Aloofness.
- Inappropriate affect.
- Intense need for schedules and routines.
- Delays in social development.
- May have delays in motor development.
- Risk avoidance and purposeful failure.
- Learned helplessness.

ASSESSMENT

- Assess receptive and expressive language skills.
- Observe behavior and note strengths and weaknesses.
- Administer *The MacArthur Communicative Development Inventories* (CDI).
- Administer *Communication and Symbolic Behavior Scales* (CSBS).

INTERVENTION TECHNIQUES

- Early intervention is essential.

- Encourage caregivers and others to communicate with the child at his or her language age rather than chronological age and to use natural gestures.
- In preschool settings, work with other disciplines to provide integrated therapy within the classroom. (Scott, 1998b)
- Intervention should be interactive; approaches that use immediate tangible rewards, as well as approaches that teach isolated skills, should be avoided.
- Capitalize on visual strengths by using pictures and other visual aids to teach language skills.
- Consider use of cued speech. (Beck, 1998)
- Capitalize on desire for patterns by using many examples to teach a specific language skill.
- Provide many successes to counteract fear of failure.
- Capitalize on interest in a specific subject to teach language skills as they relate to that subject.
- Provide therapy in small groups to address social skills.
- Consider use of some form of augmentative communication. Few persons with autism or PDD reach intellectual, language, and social levels necessitating complex, expensive devices. Consider various forms of picture boards and notebooks. (Siegel, 1996)
- Consider that early use of augmentative and alternative communication (AAC) may facilitate development of natural speech. (Scott, 1998c)
- Be aware of the effects on development of poor or inadequate diet. Provide assistance in this area by systematically introducing clients to a variety of foods. (Scott, 1998a)

RESULTS OF RECENT STUDIES

No recent studies regarding communication skills were found in the literature.

PROGNOSIS

Few longitudinal studies have been completed. Outcome is thought to be somewhat better than expectations for autism and somewhat less favorable than expectations for Asperger's syndrome. (Towbin, 1997) (See also Autism; Asperger's syndrome.)

REFERENCES

Beck PH. Sound approach. *Advance for Speech-Language Pathologists & Audiologists.* 1998;8(27):30–31.

Fine J, G Bartolucci, P Szatmari, G Ginsberg. Cohesive discourse in pervasive developmental disorders. *Journal of Autism and Developmental Disorders.* 1994;24(3):315–29.

Iskowitz M. Targeting strengths to teach language: strategies for higher functioning children with PDD. *Advance for Speech-Language Pathologists & Audiologists.* 1997;7(37):9,16.

Kirchner DM. Atypical cognitive, linguistic, and social development in children with pervasive developmental disorders of childhood. In: Smith MD, JS Damico, eds. *Childhood Language Disorders.* New York: Thieme Medical Publishers. 1996;157–97.

Scott A. Diet and development. *Advance for Speech-Language Pathologists & Audiologists.* 1998a;8(10):16–17.

Scott A. Improving natural speech. *Advance for Speech-Language Pathologists & Audiologists.* 1998b;8(7):9.

Scott A. Integrated therapy: an effective classroom approach for children with severe or multiple disabilities. *Advance for Speech-Language Pathologists & Audiologists.* 1998c;8(10):6–9.

Siegel B. *The World of the Autistic Child: Understanding and Treating Autistic Spectrum Disorders.* New York: Oxford University Press. 1996:253–73.

Smith J, H Diller. Ensuring success for late-talking children. *Advance for Speech-Language Pathologists & Audiologists.* 1997;7(48):29–31.

Smith MD, JS Damico. *Childhood Language Disorders.* New York: Thieme Medical Publishers. 1996;161–2.

Towbin KE. Pervasive developmental disorder. In: Cohen DJ, FR Volkmar, eds. *Handbook of Autism and Pervasive Developmental Disorders,* 2nd ed. New York: John Wiley & Sons. 1997:123–47.

Schizophrenia

DESCRIPTION

Schizophrenia is a generally chronic mental disorder characterized by symptoms involving disturbances of thought, perception, feeling, and behavior. Six specific criteria for the diagnosis include:

- Delusions, hallucinations, formal thought disorder.
- Deterioration from a previous level of functioning.
- Duration of the illness for at least 6 months.
- Generally, onset before age 45 years.
- Symptoms not due to mood disorders.
- Symptoms not due to organic disorder or mental retardation.

Onset of schizophrenia in childhood or adolescents occurs in approximately 3 in 10,000 youngsters.

ETIOLOGY

Etiology is uncertain and likely involves a complex interaction between inherited and environmental factors.

Documented anatomical and physiological irregularities include reduced metabolic and blood-flow functioning in frontal areas, enlarged lateral ventricles, and temporal lobe asymmetries.

SPEECH AND LANGUAGE DIFFICULTIES

- Poverty of speech.
- Mutism may develop.
- Abrupt changes in subject during conversation.
- In children, language may be vague, overelaborate, circumstantial, and/or impoverished in content.
- Difficulty with speaker-listener roles.
- Deficits in pragmatic skills.
- Auditory processing deficits.
- Memory deficits.
- Word-finding difficulties.
- Echolalia.
- Perseveration.
- Semantic paraphasias.
- Loose associations.
- Use of unclear and ambiguous references.
- Use of fewer parts of speech and fewer different words.

- Decreased or absent use of gestures.
- Long pauses between clauses and increased use of hesitation phrases ("ah" or "uh").
- Decreased use of cohesive ties such as "and," "but," and "so."
- Substitutions of words with similar meanings, leading to confusion on the part of the listener.
- Dysarthria, which may be a result of antipsychotic drugs.
- Inappropriate stress patterns.
- Rapid changes in melody and pitch.
- Seemingly meaningless repetition of words and phrases.
- Tendency to pun or rhyme words may be present.
- May exhibit dysfluencies.

ASSOCIATED AND OTHER DIFFICULTIES
- High incidence of learning disabilities.
- Increasing difficulty with clear, goal-directed thinking.
- Blunting and incongruity of affect.
- Depression.
- Elation.
- Excitement.
- Hallucinations. While auditory hallucinations are most common, hallucinations involving sight, smell, taste, and touch may also occur.
- Delusions involving persecution, jealousy, grandeur, hypochondria, religious ideas, and sexual identity.
- Posturing.
- Disturbances in movement ranging from overactivity to decreased movement and stupor.
- Exaggerated mannerisms.
- Withdrawal from external reality.

ASSESSMENT
- Assess short-term memory skills. Deficits in this area may contribute to disorganization of narratives.
- Assess ability to name words in a category.
- Administer the *Porch Index of Communicative Abilities* (PICA).
- Administer the *Scale for Assessment of Thought, Language and Communication Disorders* (TLC).

INTERVENTION TECHNIQUES

- For those clients with persistent 'voices,' improve ability to organize thoughts into narrative and discourse. (Hoffman and Satel, 1993)
- Provide group intervention, focusing on nonverbal communication, social language, listening and attending skills, cognitive language skills, specific functional communication, and humor. (Scott, 1998)

RESULTS OF RECENT STUDIES

- In a study of 42 children and adolescents diagnosed with schizophrenia, 83% exhibited difficulty with pragmatics, 81% had difficulty with prosody, 72% had auditory processing deficits, 64% showed deficits in abstract language, 62% had deficits in both receptive and expressive vocabulary, 53% had fluency disorders, 51% had deficits in receptive and expressive syntax, 38% had articulation deficits, and 26% had voice disorders. (Baltaxe and Simmons, 1995)
- On selected measures of language functioning, such as the repetition of words subtest of the *Boston Diagnostic Aphasia Examination*, the *Boston Naming Test*, the *Token Test*, the spontaneous speech subtest of the *Western Aphasia Battery* and *Raven's Coloured Progressive Matrices*, the performance of clients with speech disordered schizophrenia did not differ from that of clients with fluent aphasia. (Landre, et al., 1992)
- The speech of clients with schizophrenia shows longer switching pauses, increased frequency of long within-clause pauses, and increased frequency of false starts and repetitions following within-clause pauses, suggesting difficulty in formulating thoughts and finding words to express thoughts. (Alpert, et al., 1994)
- In one study, the *PICA* scores of clients with thought-disorder schizophrenia were significantly lower than the scores of clients with schizophrenia without thought disorders. (Landre and Taylor, 1995)
- Preliminary investigations indicate that the signing of deaf persons with schizophrenia shows many of the same types of disorders as does the verbal language of hearing persons with schizophrenia. (Thacker, 1994)

PROGNOSIS

About 30% of affected persons recover completely. Most others show some improvement. Relapse is common without adequate follow-up services and maintenance of medication.

REFERENCES

Alpert M, A Clark, ER Pouget. The syntactic role of pauses in the speech of schizophrenic patients with alogia. *Journal of Abnormal Psychology*. 1994;103(4):750–7.

Baltaxe CAM, JQ Simmons III. Speech and language disorders in children and adolescents with schizophrenia. *Schizophrenia Bulletin*. 1995;21(4):677–91.

Caplan R. Communication deficits in childhood schizophrenia spectrum disorders. *Schizophrenia Bulletin*. 1994;20(4):671–83.

Caplan R, D Guthrie, JG Foy. Communication deficits and formal thought disorder in schizophrenic children. *Journal of the American Academy of Child & Adolescent Psychiatry*. 1992;31(1):151–9.

Duffy JR. *Motor Speech Disorders: Substrates, Differential Diagnosis, and Management*. St. Louis, Mo: Mosby. 1995.

Hoffman RE, SL Satel. Language therapy for schizophrenic patients with persistent 'voices.' *British Journal of Psychiatry*. 1993;162:755–8.

Landre NA, MA Taylor. Formal thought disorder in schizophrenia linguistic, attentional, and intellectual correlates. *The Journal of Nervous and Mental Disease*. 1995; 183(11):673–80.

Landre NA, MA Taylor, KP Kearns. Language functioning in schizophrenic and aphasic patients. *Neuropsychiatry, Neuropsychology, and Behavioral Neurology*. 1992;5(1):7–14.

Scott A. Speech and psychosis. *Advance for Speech-Language Pathologists & Audiologists*. 1998;8(13):13–15.

Steffy RA. Cognitive deficits in schizophrenia. In: Dobson KS, PC Kendall, eds. *Psychopathology and Cognition*. San Diego, Calif: Academic Press, Inc. 1993:429–72.

Thacker AJ. Formal communication disorder: sign language in deaf people with schizophrenia. *British Journal of Psychiatry*. 1994;165:818–23.

Vita A, M Dieci, GM Giobbio, A Caputo, L Ghiringhelli, M Comazzi, M Garbarini, AP Mendini, C Morganti, F Tenconi, B Cesana, G Invernizzi. Language and thought disorder in schizophrenia: brain morphological correlates. *Schizophrenia Research*. 1995;15:243–51.

Chapter 5

Metabolic and Endocrine Disorders

- Hypothyroidism
- Pendred syndrome
- Prader-Willi syndrome (PWS)
- Williams syndrome (WS)
- Wilson's disease (WD)

Hypothyroidism

DESCRIPTION

Neonatal hypothyroidism (cretinism) is characterized by respiratory distress, cyanosis, jaundice, poor feeding, a hoarse cry, and retardation of bone growth. Childhood (juvenile) hypothyroidism is characterized by growth retardation, delayed dentition, and mental impairment. Treatment within the first month of life is essential for preventing severe developmental problems. Adults may also develop hypothyroidism, often as a result of treatment for hyperthyroidism.

ETIOLOGY

A deficiency in thyroid activity, probably the result of an autoimmune disease.

SPEECH AND LANGUAGE DIFFICULTIES

- Articulation deficits.
- Hoarse voice quality.
- Slow rate of speaking.

ASSOCIATED AND OTHER DIFFICULTIES

- Early delays in motor skills, which may later resolve.
- May be of short stature.
- Dull facial expression.
- Memory deficits.
- Psychosis may develop.

ASSESSMENT

- In very young children, assess feeding skills.
- Evaluate articulation skills.
- Assess receptive and expressive language skills.

INTERVENTION TECHNIQUES

- Assist parents in providing optimal conditions for feeding.
- Provide therapy to foster development of receptive and expressive language skills.
- Provide therapy for articulation deficits as indicated.

RESULTS OF RECENT STUDIES

No recent studies regarding communication skills were found in the literature.

PROGNOSIS

Hypothyroidism is treated with replacement therapy. With this treatment, prognosis is very good.

REFERENCE

Gottschalk B, RA Richman, L Lewandowski. Subtle speech and motor deficits of children with congenital hypothyroid treated early. *Developmental Medicine and Child Neurology*. 1994;36:216–20.

Pendred Syndrome

DESCRIPTION

A disorder of the thyroid gland resulting in congenital deafness. Goiter may be present. Between 7.5% and 10% of congenital deafness may be attributed to this disorder. Males and females are equally affected. Malformation of the cochlea is one characteristic of the syndrome.

ETIOLOGY

Mapping of the disorder is to chromosome 7q31, with autosomal-recessive inheritance.

SPEECH AND LANGUAGE DIFFICULTIES

(See Hearing Loss—Children and Adolescents; Hearing Loss—Adults)

ASSOCIATED AND OTHER DIFFICULTIES

• Moderate to severe sensorineural hearing loss that is greater in higher frequencies. In some cases the loss is progressive.

(See also Hearing Loss—Children and Adolescents; Hearing Loss—Adults)

ASSESSMENT

(See Hearing Loss—Children and Adolescents; Hearing Loss —Adults)

INTERVENTION TECHNIQUES

(See Hearing Loss—Children and Adolescents; Hearing Loss—Adults)

RESULTS OF RECENT STUDIES

No recent studies regarding communication skills were found in the literature.

PROGNOSIS

A normal life span should be expected. Intelligence is generally within the normal range.

REFERENCES

Fritsch MH, A Sommer. *Handbook of Congenital and Early Onset Hearing Loss*. New York: Igaku-Shoin Medical Publishers, Inc. 1991:103–5.

Reardon W, RC Trembath. Pendred Syndrome. *Journal of Medical Genetics.* 1996; 33:1037–40.

Prader-Willi Syndrome (PWS)

DESCRIPTION

A multisystem disorder affecting males more often than females. Incidence figures range from 1 in 15,000 to 1 in 30,000. Primary characteristics include infantile hypotonia, failure to thrive, short stature, and impaired intellectual and behavioral functioning. In early childhood, hyperphagia leads to obesity that can result in life-threatening heart and lung complications if not controlled. Sexual development stops before puberty.

ETIOLOGY

A disorder of chromosome deletion; generally a deletion affecting the long arm of chromosome number 15.

SPEECH AND LANGUAGE DIFFICULTIES

- Articulation errors.
- Flaccid dysarthria.
- Hypernasal speech.
- Repetitive speech, such as persistent questioning.
- May perseverate on favorite topics.
- Deficits in processing information.
- Deficits in expressive language skills including grammatical errors and incomplete sentence structure.
- Deficits in pragmatic skills including difficulty in the areas of turn-taking, topic maintenance, and proximity.

ASSOCIATED AND OTHER DIFFICULTIES

- Intellectual impairment. Severity varies.
- Food-related behavior problems including excessive appetite, absent sense of satiation, and obsession with eating.
- May develop insulin-dependent diabetes.
- Scoliosis.
- Osteoporosis.

- High threshold for pain.
- May have poor fine and gross motor coordination.
- Hypotonia.
- Self-injurious behaviors.
- Lability of mood.
- Impulsiveness.

ASSESSMENT

- Assess language skills, in both familiar and unfamiliar settings on an annual basis.
- Assess pragmatic skills.
- Assess articulation skills.

INTERVENTION TECHNIQUES

- Consider some form of nonverbal communication during preschool years.
- Begin early to work on decision-making skills.
- Address pragmatic skills.

RESULTS OF RECENT STUDIES

No recent studies regarding communication skills were found in the literature.

PROGNOSIS

Reduced life expectancy is related to morbid obesity. Some increase in maladaptive behaviors during adolescence and early adult life may be seen.

REFERENCES

Clarke DJ, H Boer, MC Chung, P Sturmey, T Webb. Maladaptive behavior in Prader-Willi syndrome in adult life. *Journal of Intellectual Disability Research*. 1996;40(Pt 2):159–65.

Downey DA, CL Knutson. Speech and language issues. In: Greenswag LR, RC Alexander, eds. *Management of Prader-Willi Syndrome,* 2nd ed. New York: Springer-Verlag. 1995: 142–55.

Gilbert P. *The A-Z Reference Book of Syndromes and Inherited Disorders: A Manual for Health, Social and Education Workers*. New York: Chapman & Hall. 1993:168–71.

Jones KL. *Smith's Recognizable Patterns of Human Malformation,* 5th ed. Philadelphia: W.B. Saunders Co. 1997:202–3.

Thoene JG, NP Coker, eds. *Physicians' Guide to Rare Diseases*. New York: Dowden Publishing Co. 1995:125.

Williams Syndrome (WS)

DESCRIPTION

Typical characteristics of the syndrome are elfin-like facial features, supravalvular aortic stenosis, and mental retardation. The syndrome occurs in 1 in 25,000 births, with both sexes being equally affected.

ETIOLOGY

A genetic defect involving the vascular, connective tissue, and central nervous systems. Several genes are generally missing. Many cases are also caused by an unidentified defect in the ability to metabolize vitamin D.

SPEECH AND LANGUAGE DIFFICULTIES

- Comprehension is more limited than expressive skills would indicate.
- Expressive language is characterized by inappropriate use of clichés and stereotyped phrases. Higher-level grammar and semantics may be impaired.
- Hoarse voice.

ASSOCIATED AND OTHER DIFFICULTIES

- Difficulties in feeding as an infant, due partially to profuse vomiting and irritability.
- Constipation; poor weight gain.

- May have severe learning disabilities.
- Attention deficits, including distractibility and impulsiveness.
- Marked deficits in spatial skills in contrast to relatively preserved language skills.
- Wide mouth with dental abnormalities including microdontia, missing teeth, and enamel hypoplasia.
- Approximately 61% of children have otitis media.
- Growth retardation and short stature.
- Microcephaly.
- Mild hypotonia in childhood progressing to increased tone with advancing age.
- Delayed motor development may occur.
- Renal and cardiovascular abnormalities.
- Joint contractures.
- Early puberty is common.
- High rates of emotional and behavioral disturbance, characterized by poor concentration and attention-seeking behaviors.
- Excessive anxiety.
- Hypersensitivity to sounds.
- Eating and sleeping difficulties.
- Poor peer relationships.
- Outgoing and excessively affectionate toward adults.
- Deficits in visuospatial abilities.

ASSESSMENT
- Fully assess receptive and expressive language skills. Reassess periodically over time to monitor development in these areas.
- Assess pragmatic skills.

INTERVENTION TECHNIQUES
- Provide early intervention services.
- Provide functional therapy for language and pragmatic deficits.

RESULTS OF RECENT STUDIES
No recent studies regarding communication skills were found in the literature.

PROGNOSIS

Most adults are not able to live independently. Some experience premature death.

REFERENCES

Chapman CA, A du Plessis, BR Pober. Neurologic findings in children and adults with Williams syndrome. *Journal of Child Neurology*. 1995;11(1):63–65.

Jones KL. *Smith's Recognizable Patterns of Human Malformation,* 5th ed. Philadelphia: W.B. Saunders Co. 1997:118–9.

Marmer L. Rare genetic disorder: treatment for Williams syndrome focuses on function. *Advance for Speech-Language Pathologists & Audiologists*. 1996;6(48):15.

Messer DJ. *The Development of Communication: From Social Interaction to Language.* New York: John Wiley & Sons. 1994:273–5.

Scott GS, TL Layton. Epidemiologic principles in studies of infectious disease outcomes: pediatric HIV as a model. *Journal of Communication Disorders*. 1997;30:303–24.

Thoene JG, NP Coker, eds. *Physicians' Guide to Rare Diseases*. New York: Dowden Publishing Co. 1995:162.

Udwin O, M Davies, P Howlin. A longitudinal study of cognitive abilities and educational attainment in Williams syndrome. *Developmental Medicine & Child Neurology*. 1996; 38(11):1020–9.

Vicari S, D Brizzolara, GA Carlesimi, G Pezzini, V Volterra. Memory abilities in children with Williams syndrome. *Cortex*. 1996;32:503–14.

Wilson's Disease (WD)

DESCRIPTION

WD is caused by a disturbance in copper (Cu) metabolism. Incidence figures range from 1 in 30,000 to 1 in 100,000 across all ethnic and geographic populations. First symptoms generally appear in adolescence although they may appear at any age between 5 and 50 years. In 40% to 50% of cases the initial illness may be an episode of acute hepatitis that is often misdiagnosed as infectious mononucleosis. In 40% to 50% of cases, the first signs are disturbances of the central nervous system characterized by any of the following: tremors, dystonia, dysarthria, dysphagia, drooling, open-mouthedness, or incoordination. Sensory disturbances are not present, except for headache. In 5% to 10% of clients, the disease is first noted in Kayser-Fleischer rings during a refractive eye examination, in repeated miscarriages, renal Cu deposits, or abnormally high urinary excretion of amino acids, uric acids, phosphate, calcium, or glucose.

ETIOLOGY

WD is transmitted in an autosomal-recessive fashion and is a fatal disturbance in Cu metabolism. About 1.1% of the world's population—50 million individuals—are heterozygous carriers of one WD gene. The gene has recently been mapped to chromosome number 13.

SPEECH AND LANGUAGE DIFFICULTIES

- Decrease in range of modulation.
- Decrease in variability of speech rate.
- Dysarthria.

ASSOCIATED AND OTHER DIFFICULTIES

- Jaundice and vomiting, which are symptoms of liver disease.
- Kayser-Fleischer rings (green-yellow pigmented rings encircling the cornea).
- Drooling.
- Dysphagia.
- Tremor.
- Spasticity.
- Muscle rigidity.
- Double vision.
- Loss of dexterity over time.
- Predisposition to gallstones.
- Osteoporosis.
- Cardiac arrhythmia.

ASSESSMENT

- Assess for dysphagia.

- Assess for general speech intelligibility and for dysarthria. (See Appendix A)

INTERVENTION TECHNIQUES

- To modify rate, consider use of pacing board and use of delayed auditory feedback. (Duffy, 1995)
- Treat for dysphagia.

RESULTS OF RECENT STUDIES

Dysarthria does not affect speech timing impairment. (Volkman, et al., 1992)

PROGNOSIS

The disease is always fatal, usually before the age of 30 years.

REFERENCES

Duffy JR. *Motor Speech Disorders: Substrates, Differential Diagnosis, and Management.* St. Louis, Mo: Mosby. 1995:166–88.

Thoene, JG, NP Coker, eds. *Physicians' Guide to Rare Diseases.* New York: Dowden Publishing Co. 1995:247–8.

Volkman J, H Hefter, HW Lange, HJ Freund. Impairment of temporal organization of speech in basal ganglia diseases. *Brain & Language.* 1992;43(3):386–99.

Yarze JC, P Martin, SJ Muñoz, LS Friedman. Wilson's disease: current status. *The American Journal of Medicine.* 1992;92:643–54.

Chapter 6

Musculoskeletal and Connective Tissue Disorders

- Polymyositis/dermatomyositis
- Progressive systemic sclerosis (scleroderma) (PSS) (SSc)
- Sjögren's syndrome (SS)
- Systemic lupus erythematosus (SLE)

Polymyositis/Dermatomyositis

DESCRIPTION

Polymyositis is a systemic connective tissue disease characterized by inflammatory and degenerative changes in the muscles. Similar involvement of the skin, which occurs frequently, is referred to as dermatomyositis.

The disease may appear at any age. In children the characteristic time of appearance is between the ages of 5 and 10 years, and in adults between the ages of 40 and 60 years. Females are twice as likely as males to be affected. Incidence in the general population is 0.5 to 10 per 1 million, with a somewhat higher incidence among Black Americans.

ETIOLOGY

Etiology is unknown.

SPEECH AND LANGUAGE DIFFICULTIES

• Dysphonia.

ASSOCIATED AND OTHER DIFFICULTIES

• Muscle weakness. Muscles of the hands, feet, and face are not involved.
• Limb contractures may develop.
• Dysphagia.
• Weight loss.

ASSESSMENT

• Assess for dysphagia.
• Assess voice quality.
• Assess adequacy of respiratory function.
• Assess oral-motor function.

INTERVENTION TECHNIQUES

• Provide therapy for dysphagia.

- Suggest smaller, more frequent meals to reduce fatigue.
- To treat flaccid dysarthria, work to improve support for speech breathing.
- Provide therapy for voice disorders as they occur.

(See also Voice Disorders)

RESULTS OF RECENT STUDIES

No recent studies regarding communication skills were found in the literature.

PROGNOSIS

Remissions may occur, particularly in children.

Death is often the result of dysphagia, malnutrition, aspiration pneumonia, or respiratory failure.

REFERENCES

Duffy JR. *Motor Speech Disorders: Substrates, Differential Diagnosis, and Management.* St. Louis, Mo: Mosby. 1995:99–127.

Iskowitz M. Managing polymyositis. *Advance for Speech-Language Pathologists & Audiologists.* 1998;8(8):13–15.

Progressive Systemic Sclerosis (Scleroderma) (PSS) (SSc)

DESCRIPTION

Characteristics include diffuse fibrosis, degenerative changes, and vascular abnormalities in the skin, articular structures, and intestinal organs. The disease is about four times more common in women than in men. Severity and manifestation are variable, but all organs may be affected, with the exceptions of the brain and the liver.

ETIOLOGY

A rare autoimmune disease of unknown cause. Hardening of tissue is caused by overproduction of the protein collagen.

SPEECH AND LANGUAGE DIFFICULTIES

- Difficulty with vocalization due to shrinking tissues around the mouth.
- When the vocal folds are involved, hoarseness may result. Or, muscles that control the vocal cords or larynx may become weak.
- Sjögren's syndrome (a scarring of the salivary glands inside the mouth, resulting in dry mouth and multiple speech and dental problems) may develop.
- Gastroesophageal reflux may cause hoarseness, laryngitis, and hearing problems.
- Oral or laryngeal cancers may develop as a complication of reflux.
- Development of "seal bark" (a burplike sound probably as a result of gas originating in the abdomen).

ASSOCIATED AND OTHER DIFFICULTIES

- Esophageal dysfunction.
- Dysphagia.
- Gastroesophageal reflux disease (GERD).
- Hearing loss.
- Vestibular disturbances.

ASSESSMENT

- Perform hearing screening and refer to audiologist as indicated.
- Evaluate for dysphagia.
- Evaluate voice production.

INTERVENTION TECHNIQUES

- Treat for dysphagia as indicated.
- Assist the client in adjustment to loss of hearing. (See also Hearing Loss—Adults)
- Instruct the client in principles of good vocal hygiene and provide voice therapy as indicated.

RESULTS OF RECENT STUDIES

No recent studies regarding communication skills were found in the literature.

PROGNOSIS

Progression is varied and unpredictable. The disease may remain unprogressive for long periods of time. Prognosis is poor if cardiac, pulmonary, or renal manifestations appear early.

REFERENCES

Berrettini S, C Ferri, N Pitaro, P Bruschini, A Latorraca, S Sellari-Franceschini, G Segnini. Audiovestibular involvement in systemic sclerosis. *Otolaryngology—Head and Neck Surgery.* 1994;56:195–8.

Iskowitz M. Scleroderma: not one of the usual suspects. *Advance for Speech-Language Pathologists & Audiologists.* 1997;7(1):11,42.

Sjögren's Syndrome (SS)

DESCRIPTION

A chronic, systemic inflammatory disorder characterized by dryness of the mouth, eyes, and other mucous membranes. Onset occurs in middle age; 80% to 90% of cases are female.

ETIOLOGY

Etiology is unknown. SS is an autoimmune disease involving the endocrine glands, especially the lacrimal and salivary glands. Possible contributing factors may be infectious, allergic, autoimmune, congenital, or familial.

SPEECH AND LANGUAGE DIFFICULTIES

• Decreased diadochokinetic rates.

ASSOCIATED AND OTHER DIFFICULTIES

- Dryness of eyes and mouth.
- Joint inflammation.
- Dysphagia.
- Excessive dental cavities.

ASSESSMENT

- Evaluate for dysphagia.
- Evaluate for adequacy of diet and nutritional intake.
- Evaluate adequacy of speech production.

INTERVENTION TECHNIQUES

Treat for dysphagia.

RESULTS OF RECENT STUDIES

No recent studies regarding communication skills were found in the literature.

PROGNOSIS

SS is a chronic disease. Its course is generally mild for several years, after which lymphoma or reticular cell sarcoma may develop.

REFERENCES

Magalini SI, SC Magalini. *Dictionary of Medical Syndromes,* 4th ed. Philadelphia: Lippincott-Raven Publishers. 1997:745.

Rhodus NL, K Moller, S Colby, J Bereuter. Articulatory speech performance in patients with salivary gland dysfunction: a pilot study. *Quintessence International.* 1995;26(11): 805–10.

Rhodus NL, K Moller, S Colby, J Bereuter. Dysphagia in patients with three different etiologies of salivary gland dysfunction. *ENT Journal.* 1995;74(1):39–48.

Systemic Lupus Erythematosus (SLE)

DESCRIPTION

An inflammatory connective tissue disorder, SLE generally affects young women, although children may also be affected. Incidence is higher among Asians.

ETIOLOGY

An autoimmune disease of unknown etiology.

SPEECH AND LANGUAGE DIFFICULTIES

• Hoarseness.

ASSOCIATED AND OTHER DIFFICULTIES

• Oral mucosal lesions.
• Dry mouth.
• Salivary gland dysfunction.
• Dysphagia.
• Temporomandibular joint arthritis.
• Laryngeal involvement; laryngeal edema.
• Vocal cord paralysis.
• Headaches.
• Personality changes.
• Renal involvement—may be benign and asymptomatic or progressive and fatal.

ASSESSMENT

• Evaluate for dysphagia.
• Evaluate for nutrition and adequacy of diet.
• Evaluate voice quality.

INTERVENTION TECHNIQUES

• Treat for dysphagia.

(See also Voice Disorders)

RESULTS OF RECENT STUDIES

No recent studies regarding communication skills were found in the literature.

PROGNOSIS

SLE is a chronic and relapsing condition with periods (sometimes years) of remission. The 10-year survival rate in most developed countries is greater than 95%.

REFERENCES

Rhodus NL, K Moller, S Colby, J Bereuter. Dysphagia in patients with three different etiologies of salivary gland dysfunction. *ENT Journal*. 1995;74(1):39–48.

Woo P, J Menelsohn, D Humphrey. Rheumatoid nodules of the larynx. *Otolaryngology—Head and Neck Surgery*. 1995;113:147–50.

Chapter 7

Sensory Disorders

- Dual-sensory impairment
- Hearing loss—adults
- Hearing loss—children and adolescents

Dual-Sensory Impairment

DESCRIPTION

The Helen Keller National Center (HKNC) defines a person who is deaf-blind as someone "(1) with central visual acuity of 20/200 or worse in the better eye with corrective lenses and/or a visual field size of 20 degrees or less in the better eye (180 degrees being the maximum possible), or with a progressive visual loss whose prognosis is seen as leading to one or both of these conditions; (2) who has either a chronic hearing impairment so severe that most speech cannot be understood with optimum amplification or a progressive hearing loss whose prognosis is seen as leading to this condition; and (3) for whom the combination of impairments described in clauses 1 and 2 causes extreme difficulty in attaining independence in daily life activities, achieving psychological adjustment, or obtaining a vocation." (Helen Keller National Center Act, 29 U.S.C., Chapter 206, Section 1901) (Everson, 1995) Usher syndrome is the leading cause of deaf-blindness in early adulthood. (See also Usher syndrome)

ETIOLOGY

There are four categories of deaf-blindness:

- Congenital deaf-blindness occurs among those who are born with dual sensory losses or who experience these losses early in the developmental period. Causes include congenital rubella syndrome, CHARGE association (See also CHARGE association), prematurity, and prenatal or perinatal trauma.
- Adventitious deaf-blindness occurs among those who acquire sensory losses later in life, after language has developed. Causes include diseases resulting in high fever, diabetes, encephalitis, trauma, and accumulation of toxins in the body.
- Congenital deafness and adventitious blindness occurs among those who are born deaf or hearing impaired and experience visual loss later in life. The most common etiology is Usher syndrome.
- Congenital blindness and adventitious deafness occurs among those who are born with visual impairments and acquire a hearing loss later in life.

SPEECH AND LANGUAGE DIFFICULTIES
- Receptive language deficits due to inability or diminished ability to receive input either visually or auditorially.
- Expressive language deficits.

ASSOCIATED AND OTHER DIFFICULTIES
- Those with acquired visual and/or hearing loss must adjust to a new self-concept.
- May have limited life experiences.

ASSESSMENT
- Assess formal and idiosyncratic methods of communication currently being used as well as communicative intent of maladaptive behaviors.
- Assess current and future communicative needs of the client.

INTERVENTION TECHNIQUES
- Instruct in Tadoma method—having client place a hand over the face and neck of the person speaking to monitor facial actions associated with speaking.
- Instruct in tactual reception of fingerspelling into the palm.
- Instruct in tactual reception of signing.
- Assist the client in making adjustments to new means of communicating as visual and/or hearing skills deteriorate.
- If necessary, use the skills of an interpreter when working with clients whose primary means of communication is through American Sign Language (ASL), Signed English, or fingerspelling.
- Work with the client and other team members to design systems of communication.
- Assist the client in using communication strategies in functional settings.

RESULTS OF RECENT STUDIES
No recent studies regarding communication skills were found in the literature.

PROGNOSIS

Potential for independent living is highly variable.

REFERENCES

Everson JM, ed. *Supporting Young Adults Who Are Deaf-Blind in Their Communities: A Transition Planning Guide for Service Providers, Families, and Friends.* Baltimore: Paul H. Brookes Publishing Co. 1995.

Reed CM, LA Delhorne, NI Durlach, SD Fischer. A study of the tactual reception of sign language. *Journal of Speech and Hearing Research.* 1995;38:477–89.

Hearing Loss—Adults

DESCRIPTION

The American College of Occupational Medicine (ACOM) defines occupational noise-induced hearing loss as a slowly developing hearing loss over a long period (several years) as a result of exposure to continuous or intermittent loud noise. (Sataloff and Sataloff, 1993). Occupational noise-induced hearing loss is always sensorineural and is almost always bilateral. Other causes of adult-onset hearing loss include severe head trauma, viral infections, hereditary hearing loss, ototoxicity, and acoustic neuromas. While instances of traumatic hearing loss are rare, they do occur. In at least one case, sensorineural hearing loss occurred subsequent to air bag inflation. (Iskowitz, 1997c)

ETIOLOGY

A conductive hearing loss is caused by a lesion in the external auditory canal or the middle ear, while a sensorineural loss is caused by a lesion in the inner ear or eighth cranial nerve. Characteristics of sensory hearing loss include a mild to moderate loss of speech discrimination, improved discrimination with increasing intensity, presence of recruitment, and high sensitivity for small increments in intensity. Sensorneural hearing losses are characterized by severe loss of speech discrimination skills, absence of recruitment, and poor sensitivity for small increments in intensity.

SPEECH AND LANGUAGE DIFFICULTIES
- Difficulty understanding the speech of others. In cases of profound loss, deterioration of the client's speech clarity may occur.
- Speech volume may increase.
- Monotone may develop.

ASSOCIATED AND OTHER DIFFICULTIES
- Attempts to minimize, deny, or disguise the loss.
- Difficulty hearing and/or localizing warning signals.
- Depression.
- Decrease in self-confidence.
- Social isolation.
- Embarrassment.
- Fatigue.
- Anger.

ASSESSMENT
- Assess current speech skills.

INTERVENTION TECHNIQUES
- Give the client a clear understanding of the hearing loss and its effects.
- Provide the client with some information regarding the articulation of specific sounds. Such knowledge can be useful when one is no longer able to auditorially monitor his/her own speech production.
- Instruct the client to use a combination of speech reading techniques (including interpretation of facial expressions, body movements, and gestures) and auditory training techniques. (Miller, et al., 1993)
- Assist clients in learning to maximize their visual skills.
- Offer group sessions for elderly clients with recent onset of hearing loss. Sessions can offer information on topics such as conversation strategies and assistive technology, and, more importantly, allow group members to share experiences and brainstorm solutions. (Iskowitz, 1997b)
- Provide information regarding closed captioning.

RESULTS OF RECENT STUDIES

No recent studies regarding communication skills were found in the literature.

PROGNOSIS

No statements regarding prognosis or outcome were found in the literature.

REFERENCES

Iskowitz M. Brain injury and hearing loss may result in greater overall deficit. *Advance for Speech-Language Pathologists & Audiologists.* 1997a;7(35):7,19.

Iskowitz M. Collaborative problem-solving for elderly patients. *Advance for Speech-Language Pathologists & Audiologists.* 1997b:7(50):10–11.

Iskowitz M. Traumatic hearing loss following air bag inflation. *Advance for Speech-Language Pathologists & Audiologists.* 1997c;7(44):5.

Miller RM, ME Groher, KM Yorkston, TS Rees. Speech, language, swallowing, and auditory rehabilitation. In: DeLisa JA, BM Gans. *Rehabilitation Medicine: Principles and Practice,* 2nd ed. Philadelphia: J.B. Lippincott Co. 1993:217–26.

Sataloff RT, J Sataloff. Occupational hearing loss. In: Sataloff RT, J Sataloff, eds. *Hearing Loss,* 3rd ed. New York: Marcel Dekker, Inc. 1993:371–402.

Sataloff RT, J Sataloff, C Copeland, DS Hirshout. Hearing loss: handicap and rehabilitation. In: Sataloff RT, J Sataloff, eds. *Hearing Loss,* 3rd ed. New York: Marcel Dekker, Inc. 1993:417–32.

Hearing Loss—
Children and Adolescents

DESCRIPTION

About 1 in 600 neonates has a congenital hearing loss, and many more acquire hearing loss during the neonatal period and beyond. Approximately 1.8% of youth younger than 18 years have some hearing impairment. Incidence of severe, inherited childhood deafness is about 1 in 2,000 births. Hearing loss may be conductive, involving a defect in the transmission of sound energy through the outer and middle ear; sensorineural, involving inability of the cochlea to convert mechanical energy into electrical impulses or inability of the auditory nervous system to recognize these impulses; or mixed.

ETIOLOGY

Risk factors include history of early hearing loss in a parent or close relative; congenital infections such as toxoplasmosis, syphilis, rubella or cytomegalovirus (CMV); craniofacial abnormalities, especially of the pinna and ear canal; birth weight less than 1,500 gm; high levels of hyperbilirubinemia; high levels of toxic drugs; bacterial meningitis; prolonged mechanical ventilation; Apgar scores of less than 4 at 5 minutes; lack of spontaneous respiration by 10 minutes or persistent hypotonia up to 2 hours after birth; or findings associated with syndromes that include sensorineural hearing loss. Otitis media (OM) may also lead to transient or permanent hearing loss. Another risk factor for hearing loss is congenital hypothyroidism (CH). Up to 20% of children with CH experience mild hearing loss. The loss may be conductive and/or sensorineural and is generally in the high frequency range. In some instances use of an antibiotic may induce hearing loss. The most common form of inherited hearing loss is autosomal recessive. Losses in this category are generally prelingual and profound. Several congenital malformations of the inner ear are known to cause sensorineural loss in children. These include large endolymphatic duct and sac syndrome (LEDSS), cochlear dysplasia, labyrinthine ossifications, and absent cochlear nerve.

SPEECH AND LANGUAGE DIFFICULTIES

- Delays in receptive language, expressive language, and speech development.
- Delays and deficits in the areas of syntax, morphology, semantics, pragmatics, and phonology.
- May exhibit difficulty controlling respiration for speech.
- Breathy, hoarse, or strained vocal quality.
- Pitch may be higher than normal.
- Monopitch or excessive pitch fluctuations.
- Difficulty controlling vocal intensity.

- Hypernasality or hyponasality.
- Multiple misarticulations, including omission, substitution, and distortion of consonants; voiced/voiceless errors; and substitution, neutralization, prolongation, and nasalization of vowels.

ASSOCIATED AND OTHER DIFFICULTIES

- Headaches, dizziness, or tinnitus may occur following recent cochlear implant.
- Tinnitus may be present in nearly half of those with hearing loss, whether or not they have received a cochlear implant.

ASSESSMENT

- Methods of testing hearing in high-risk infants include auditory brainstem response (ABR) testing and otoacoustic emissions (OAE) testing.
- Assess for canonical babbling by 11 months. This is absent in deaf infants; present in all others. (Eilers and Berlin, 1995)
- The National Institutes of Health (NIH) recommends hearing screening for all newborns by way of OAE testing prior to discharge from the hospital. Infants who fail the OAE testing should have additional ABR testing, and those who fail the ABR should receive a comprehensive hearing evaluation by no later than 3 months of age. (Trace, 1993b)
- Assess receptive, expressive, and pragmatic language skills.
- Administer *Test of Language Development* (TOLD).
- Assess articulation skills. Administer *Fisher-Logemann Test of Articulation Competence.*

INTERVENTION TECHNIQUES

- With very young children, provide therapy in home setting; work with the child as well as providing information, guidance, and empowerment to parents.
- Involve children in cooperative learning activities within the classroom: small group play or problem-solving activities requiring the active participation of all group members. (Trace, 1995a)
- Arrange for preferential seating in the classroom.
- For children with mild losses, consider assistive listening devices.

- Counsel parents to get child's attention before speaking and to reduce or eliminate distracting, competing sounds.
- Provide classroom activities for hearing and hearing impaired students explaining mechanics of hearing, hearing loss, amplification, etc. (Scott, 1998b)
- Help teach temporal concepts by identifying "first," "last," "then," "next," and "after" within sequences of activities. (Greenfield, 1998)
- Avoid oversimplification of language. Use complete, syntactically correct sentences and discourse.
- Expectations for students who use American Sign Language (ASL) should be the same as expectations for hearing students. Work with adolescents on developing functional communication skills in a variety of settings. (Shoemaker, 1997)
- To facilitate the development of writing skills, consider use of computers to make the actual task of writing less laborious. (Mander, et al., 1995)
- Help prepare children for implant surgery with explanations and role-playing.
- Understand that children with implants are able to hear the full range of sounds, and expect a higher level of performance from those who have implants.
- Provide intense auditory training as soon as possible following cochlear implant.
- Consider use of cued speech.
- Work with caregivers and with teachers to develop skills in interacting with children to foster conversational skills and social competence, i.e., guiding caregivers and teachers in asking "wh"questions.
- Work with teachers in the use of role-playing to teach and reinforce skills such as requests for clarification and topic maintenance.
- Encourage interactions between children, with less mediation from adults.
- Work with audiologist to present hearing conservation presentations to high school industrial arts classes. (Crawford, 1998)
- Provide information to caregivers regarding closed captioning.

RESULTS OF RECENT STUDIES

- Children between the ages of 5 and 9 years with mild to moderate hearing loss were matched with a group of normal hearing children with comparable receptive vocabulary knowledge. Children were presented with a novel word-learning task consisting of an acquisition phase and a retention phase. While half of the hearing-impaired students performed as well as the controls, the others performed more poorly than the higher-functioning hearing-impaired group and all of the controls on most measures of language, phonological processing, and novel word learning. Thus, the population of children with mild to moderate hearing loss may contain two distinct groups—normally developing children who have a hearing loss and children with language impairment who have a hearing loss. (Gilberston and Kamhi, 1995)

• Speech production skills and expressive language skills of children with mild hearing losses were compared along a continuum with the skills of normally developing children, and those with severe to profound hearing loss. In the areas of both speech production and expressive language the skills and performance of children with a mild loss were closer to the skills and performance of normally developing children than they were to the skills and performance of those with severe to profound losses. (Elfenbein, et al., 1994)

PROGNOSIS

Due to wide variations in a host of factors, such as degree and type of hearing loss, age of onset, presence of other disabling conditions and level of familial and educational supports, outcomes as to speech development, literacy, overall communication skills, educational outcome, and vocational options are highly variable. (Steinberg and Knightly, 1997)

REFERENCES

Anita SD, KH Kreimeyer. Social competence intervention for young children with hearing impairments. In: Odom SL, SR McConnell, MA McEvoy, eds. *Social Competence of Young Children with Disabilities*. Baltimore: Paul H. Brookes Publishing Co. 1992:135–64.

Crawford H. Talking shop: prevention program promotes hearing conservation at school and home. *Advance for Speech-Language Pathologists & Audiologists*. 1998;8(21):12.

Eilers RE, C Berlin. Advances in early detection in infants. *Current Problems in Pediatrics*. 1995;25(2):60–66.

Elfenbein JL, MA Hardin-Jones, JM Davis. Oral communication skills of children who are hard of hearing. *Journal of Speech and Hearing Research*. 1994;37(1):216–25.

Gilberston M, AG Kamhi. Novel word learning in children with hearing impairment. *Journal of Speech and Hearing Research*. 1995;38(3):630–42.

Greenfield M. Storytelling skills: exploring narrative production with children who are deaf. *Advance for Speech-Language Pathologists & Audiologists*. 1998;8(26):32–33.

Guilford P, S Ben Arab, S Blanchard, J Levilliers, J Weissenbach, A Belkahia, C Petit. A non-syndromic form of neurosensory, recessive deafness maps to the pericentromeric region of chromosome 13q. *Nature Genetics. 1994;*6:24–28.

Guteri GO. Teratogenic agents may cause hearing loss. *Advance for Speech-Language Pathologists & Audiologists*. 1994;5(28):8.

Iskowitz M. DNA mutations and deafness. *Advance for Speech-Language Pathologists & Audiologists*. 1998a;8(7):7–8.

Iskowitz M. High resolution: identifying lesions that cause sensorineural hearing loss in pediatrics. *Advance for Speech-Language Pathologists & Audiologists*. 1998b;8(25):10–11.

Iskowitz M. Tinnitus in children. *Advance for Speech-Language Pathologists & Audiologists*. 1998c;8(18):12–14.

Mander R, KM Wilson, MAR Townsend, P Thomson. Personal computers and process writing: a written language intervention for deaf children. *British Journal of Educational Psychology*. 1995;65:441–53.

Pratt S R, N Tye-Murray. Speech impairment secondary to hearing loss. In: McNeil MR, ed. *Clinical Management of Sensorimotor Speech Disorders*. New York: Thieme. 1997:345–87.

Rovet J, W Walker, B Bliss, L Buchanan, R Ehrlich. Long-term sequelae of hearing impairment in congenital hypothyroidism. *The Journal of Pediatrics*. 1996;128(6):776–83.

Scott A. Cochlear implants in the classroom: specialized training helps clinicians and educators accommodate students. *Advance for Speech-Language Pathologists & Audiologists*. 1998a;8(16):4–5.

Scott A. Education and acceptance. *Advance for Speech-Language Pathologists & Audiologists*. 1998b;8(11):10–12.

Scott A. High expectations: speech-language pathologists should expect better speech perception, speech production and language performance in children with implants. *Advance for Speech-Language Pathologists & Audiologists*. 1998c;8(16):10–11.

Shoemaker A. Home-based program teaches children, empowers parents. *Advance for Speech-Language Pathologists & Audiologists*. 1996a;6(38):8.

Shoemaker A. Progressive hearing loss: newborn screening reveals increased incidence. *Advance for Speech-Language Pathologists & Audiologists*. 1996b;6(34):5,7.

Shoemaker A. Great expectations: helping student ASL users develop functional communication skills. *Advance for Speech-Language Pathologists & Audiologists*. 1997;7(37):8,11.

Steinberg AG, CA Knightly. Hearing: sounds and silences. In: Batshaw ML, ed. *Children with Disabilities*, 4th ed. Baltimore: Paul H. Brookes Publishing Co. 1997:241–74.

Trace R. Cued speech facilitates learning and communication. *Advance for Speech-Language Pathologists & Audiologists*. 1993a;3(5):8.

Trace R. NIH Joint Commission advocate universal infant hearing screening in all states. *Advance for Speech-Language Pathologists & Audiologists*. 1993b;3(19):10–11.

Trace R. Cooperative learning benefits children with hearing loss. *Advance for Speech-Language Pathologists & Audiologists*. 1995a;5(41):9.

Trace R. 'Reading to speak' for children with hearing loss. *Advance for Speech-Language Pathologists & Audiologists*. 1995b;5(8):8.

Chapter 8

Otolaryngology and Head and Neck Cancers

- Cancer of the larynx (laryngectomy)
- Head and neck cancers
- Otitis media (OM) and otitis media with effusion (OME)
- Voice disorders

Cancer of the Larynx
(Laryngectomy)

DESCRIPTION

Approximately 12,000 Americans are diagnosed with laryngeal cancer each year. The majority are males. Treatment of the cancer may involve chemotherapy, irradiation, surgery, or any combination of these modalities. Surgery may be supraglottic laryngectomy, hemilaryngectomy, subtotal laryngectomy, or total laryngectomy.

ETIOLOGY

Most often laryngectomy is necessary to eradicate squamous cell carcinoma. The carcinoma is generally the result of excessive use of tobacco and alcohol.

SPEECH AND LANGUAGE DIFFICULTIES

- Aphonia due to surgical removal of the larynx, its intrinsic muscles, and the hyoid bone.

ASSOCIATED AND OTHER DIFFICULTIES

- Effects of radiation therapy may include loss of taste or smell and/or tongue sensitivity.
- Loss of appetite.
- Decrease in taste.
- Decrease in enjoyment of social aspects of meals.
- Dysphagia as a result of narrowing of the new pharyngeal lumen and resistance to the passage of a bolus.
- Increased risk of aspiration.
- Depression may develop.

ASSESSMENT

- Assess for dysphagia.
- Assess for potential to develop esophageal speech.

• In assessing for alaryngeal means of communication, consider intelligence, memory and mental function, manual dexterity, and eyesight. Assess the feasibility of a relative or caregiver managing the prothesis if it appears the client will be unable to do so.

INTERVENTION TECHNIQUES

• Meet with the client before surgery to discuss options for production of speech, to answer questions, and to establish a relationship with the client.
• When possible, begin speech therapy before the client leaves the hospital.
• Encourage presurgical and postsurgical visits by other laryngectomees; encourage and assist with laryngectomee support groups.
• Prior to surgery, whether a total or near-total laryngectomy will be required cannot be ascertained with certainty. Discuss with the client and family members communication options under both conditions.
• Immediately following near-total laryngectomy, instruct in the use of an artificial larynx, which the client will use until the voice shunt is operating well; 7 to 12 days after surgery, begin voice instruction.
• Consider an external prosthetic device such as an electrolarynx or a pneumatic reed.
• Consider a tracheal-esophageal puncture (TEP) with insertion of a small one-way valved prosthesis.
• Clients who are unable to manage the care of a standard prothesis may be candidates for an indwelling prothesis, which can be inserted by a speech-language pathologist or by an ear, nose, and throat specialist. Two criteria for its use are the size and shape of the stoma and the ability to pass air through the cricopharyngus.
• Consider esophageal speech.
• Consider injections of botulinum toxin to improve speech and swallowing functions. (Crary and Glowasky, 1996)
• Help the client to realize that others may initially feel uncomfortable, and teach strategies for assertiveness in initiating contacts.
• Encourage good habits from the beginning, i.e., encourage effortless air intake and discourage "double pumping" and facial grimacing. Discourage excessive digital pressure on the pharyngoesophageal (P-E) juncture and/or on a trachesophageal (T-E) puncture. Work to prevent stoma blast noise from the beginning. Teach consistency of tone and air intake time

before working on loudness and pitch variations. (McFarlane and Watterson, 1995)

- Provide a program of therapy to address dysphagia. Understand, through videofluorographic studies, exactly why the dysphagia is occurring.
- To reduce the risk of aspiration following supraglottic laryngectomy, instruct clients to hold their breath before and during the swallow (to close the true vocal folds) and to cough to clear any residue from the top of the airway before inhaling after the swallow. (Logemann, et al., 1994)
- Total laryngectomy in young children is quite rare. In addition to teaching sound production, therapists should realize that articulation and language expression skills may not have been learned prior to the surgery. (Heeneman, et al., 1996)

RESULTS OF RECENT STUDIES

- Trends in manner of speaking following laryngectomy are changing. In a recent study, 83% of those who had surgery prior to 1980 used esophageal speech compared to 39% of those who had surgery from 1980 through 1989. Use of an artificial larynx increased from 11% of those who had surgery before 1980 to 40% of those who had surgery between 1980 and 1989 and 38% of those who had surgery from 1985 to 1993. Ten percent of those who had surgery between 1980 and 1989 and 23% of those who had surgery between 1990 and 1993 used prosthetic-assisted speech. (Gelman, 1995b)
- Following pharyngoesophageal reconstruction with the radial forearm free flap, 88% of clients had no evidence of dysphagia and were on a regular diet. Following tracheoesophageal puncture (TEP) and prothesis, speech was judged superior to either esophageal speech or an electrolarynx. (Anthony, et al., 1994)
- In a study of clients who had undergone near-total laryngectomy, 76% achieved good speech. Twenty-one percent experienced severe aspiration, and in 10% reversal of the shunt was necessary. Severe aspiration and poor voice outcome were associated with development of a postoperative pharyngocutaneous fistula. (Suits, et al., 1996)
- A narrow esophageal lumen in combination with a hypertonic P-E segment may cause obstruction of a voice prothesis. The "Allan Johnson" modification of the Bivoma voice prothesis uses a stainless steel slide and has been used to remedy this situation. (Spraggs, et al., 1994)

Solutions to Speech Problems after Near-Total Laryngectomy

Problem	Causes	Solutions
Aphonia immediately after surgery	Edematous shunt; insufficiently healed voice shunt	Do not initiate efforts to inflate the voice shunt until some healing and reduction of edema have occurred, approximately 10 to 14 days after surgery when the nasogastric tube has been removed or as advised by the surgeon. Sutures and staples should be removed.
Aphonia 10 to 14 days after surgery	1. Edematous shunt; insufficiently healed shunt 2. Patient appears to be exhaling but is actually holding his or her breath	1. Continue shunt inflation procedure two or three times each day when the tracheostomy tube is removed for cleaning. 2. Use tissue or mirror to show that the patient is not exhaling; the tissue should move or the mirror should steam up.
Aphonia, dysphonia, or intermittent phonation 1 to 3 months after surgery	1. Insufficient exhalatory effort 2. Shunt may remain tight	1. Use tissue or mirror as above. 2. Continue shunt inflation procedure two or three times each day when the tracheostomy tube is removed for cleaning.

continues

Problem	Causes	Solutions
	3. Digital pressure at the stoma is too great, impeding vibration of the shunt	3. Apply lighter digital pressure at the stoma.
	4. Exhalation is too forceful, which causes the shunt to tighten and remain closed	4a. Exhale with less effort. 4b. Try different head positions.
	5. Excessive tension in the head and neck area and possibly through-out the body	5a. Perform relaxation procedures. 5b. Try different head positions.
	6. Angle of the thumb or finger at the stoma prevents the shunt from vibrating	6a. Reposition the thumb or finger; use a different digit or one on the other hand. 6b. Try covering the stoma with the same digit, but applying it in an upward, downward, or side-to-side movement. 6c. If the configuration of the stoma allows and air pressure at the stoma is not excessive, try a tracheostoma valve.

continues

Problem	Causes	Solutions
Aphonia or excessively "tight" sounding voice 4 to 6 months after surgery	1. Tight shunt 2. Tight shunt	1. Practice shunt inflation more often each day. 2. Surgeon considers revision or dilation of the shunt, but these procedures are usually deferred until 6 months after near-total laryngectomy. (After shunt dilation or revision, voice might not be produced for 7-10 days due to edema.)
Difficulty getting the voice "started" in the morning or after a period of not speaking	1. Shunt tightens slightly after a period of inactivity	1a. Continue talking to loosen the shunt and make voice production less effortful; the shunt will not close permanently even if it is used infrequently. 1b. Prolong a soft "ah" and produce seriatim speech such as counting. 1c. Try different head positions.
"Gurgly" voice quality	1. Accumulation of saliva in the pharynx at the superior end of the voice shunt	1a. Swallow more frequently; suck on sugarless candy to increase swallowing. 1b. Talk more; overall voice quality tends to improve with increased use of the voice. 1c. Sip warm liquid with no dairy products or sugar. 1d. Reduce consumption of dairy products. 1e. Gargle with warm water.

continues

Problem	Causes	Solutions
Distracting stomal noises at the end of exhalation while speaking	1. Poor valving of the stoma	1. Hold breath slightly at the end of the exhalation before removing thumb or finger to inhale.
Coughing when the stoma is occluded to produce voice	1. Excessive digital pressure at the stoma	1. Apply lighter digital pressure at the stoma.
	2. Sensitive stoma	2a. Wear a stoma button, which may help desensitize the stoma.
		2b. Gently touch and massage around the stoma to desensitize it.
	3. Poorly fitting stoma button	3. Check the fit of the stoma button and use a different size or style as needed.
Air leakage at the stoma around the thumb or finger when speaking	1. Inadequate occlusion of the stoma	1a. Try a different finger or the thumb for complete occlusion of the stoma.
		1b. Occlude the stoma over a cloth stoma cover or a foam stoma cover.
		1c. Wear a rubber "sticky finger" turned inside out to enlarge the thumb or finger.
		1d. Try wearing a stoma button.
		1e. Consider wearing a tracheostoma valve.

continues

Problem	Causes	Solutions
Liquid and/or bits of food appear at the stoma after swallowing	1. Shunt is too loose, leading to aspiration	1a. Swallow food and liquid together. 1b. Try thickened fluids. 1c. Change head positioning when swallowing. 1d. Apply digital pressure at neck. 1e. Undergo surgery to tighten or close the shunt permanently.

Source: Reprinted from R. Smee, *Laryngeal Cancer: Proceedings of the 2nd World Congress on Laryngeal Cancer,* Sydney 2–24 February, 1994, pp. 678–679, with permission from Elsevier Science.

PROGNOSIS

Secondary tumors occur at the rate of 3% to 5% per year. Abstinence or curtailed use of alcohol and tobacco is essential for a favorable prognosis.

REFERENCES

Advance Staff. Giving laryngectomee voice through artificial larynx, esophageal speech, TEP. *Advance for Speech-Language Pathologists & Audiologists.* 1993;3(20):6–7,18.

Anthony JP, MI Singer, DG Deschler, ET Dougherty, CG Reed, MJ Kaplan. Long-term functional results after pharyngoesophageal reconstruction with the radial forearm free flap. *American Journal of Surgery.* 1994;168(5):441–5.

Crary MA, AL Glowasky. Using botulinum toxin A to improve speech and swallowing function following total laryngectomy. *Archives of Otolaryngology—Head and Neck Surgery.* 1996;122:760–3.

Gelman J. Restoring communication to laryngectomee facilitates adjustment process. *Advance for Speech-Language Pathologists & Audiologists.* 1995a;5(46):8–9.

Gelman, J. Trends in alaryngeal speech: use of artificial larynx, prosthetic-assisted speech on the rise. *Advance for Speech-Language Pathologists & Audiologists.* 1995b; 5(46):5,15.

Heeneman H, DL MacRae, IR Nicholson. Laryngectomy in children: a psychological and speech-language pathology 20-year follow-up report. *The Journal of Otolaryngology.* 1996;25(5):342–5.

Iskowitz M. Indwelling prothesis: a new option for laryngectomees. *Advance for Speech-Language Pathologists & Audiologists.* 1997;7(8):10.

Kelley WN. *Textbook of Internal Medicine,* Vol. 1 and 2, 3rd ed. Philadelphia: Lippincott-Raven Publishers. 1997:1363–7.

Kerr AIG, S Denholm, RJ Sanderson, SJ Anderson. Blom-Singer prothesis—an 11 year experience of primary and secondary procedures. *Clinical Otolaryngology.* 1993; 18:184–7.

Kronenberger MB, AD Meyers. Dysphagia following head and neck cancer surgery [Review article, 52 refs]. *Dysphagia.* 1994;9(4):36–44.

Logemann JA, P Gibbons, AW Rademaker, BR Pauloski, PJ Kahrilas, M Bacon, J Bowman, E McCracken. Mechanisms of recovery of swallow after supraglottic laryngectomy. *Journal of Speech and Hearing Research.* 1994;37:965–74.

McFarlane SC, TL Watterson. General principles of working to develop alaryngeal speech. *Seminars in Speech and Language.* 1995;16(3):175–8.

Mendelsohn M. Dysphagia after treatment for laryngeal cancer. In: Smee R, GP Bridger, eds. *Laryngeal Cancer: Proceedings of the 2nd World Congress on Laryngeal Cancer, Sydney, 20-24 February 1994.* New York: Elsevier. 1994:705–8.

Miller RM, ME Groher, KM Yorkston, TS Rees. Speech, language, swallowing, and auditory rehabilitation. In: DeLisa JA, BM Gans, eds. *Rehabilitation Medicine: Principles and Practice,* 2nd ed. Philadelphia: J.B. Lippincott Co. 1993:205–6.

O'Leary IK, JM Heaton, RT Clegg , AJ Parker. Acceptability and intelligibility of tracheoesophageal speech using the Groningen valve. *Folia Phoniatrica & Logopedica.* 1994;46:180–7.

Spraggs PD, A Perry, AD Cheesman. The 'Allan Johnson' voice prothesis: a modification of the Bivona voice prothesis for immediate post-fitting aphonia after secondary tracheo-oesophageal puncture. *Journal of Laryngology & Otology.* 1994;108(7):579–81.

Suits GW, JI Cohen, EC Everts. Near-total laryngectomy: patient selection and technical considerations. *Archives of Otolaryngology—Head & Neck Surgery.* 1996;122(5): 473–5.

Thomas JE, RL Keith. The speech pathologist's role in speech rehabilitation after near-total laryngectomy. In: Smee R, GP Bridger, eds. *Laryngeal Cancer: Proceedings of the 2nd World Congress on Laryngeal Cancer, Sydney, 20–24 February 1994.* New York: Elsevier. 1994:676–80.

Trace R. Shared experiences and professional expertise benefit laryngectomee. *Advance for Speech-Language Pathologists & Audiologists.* 1994;4(15):12–13.

Head and Neck Cancers

DESCRIPTION

Oral cancers account for 5% of all cancers in men and 2% of cancers in women. Approximately 30,000 new cases occur in the United States each year. Patients with an oral squamous cancer have a 33% chance of developing at least one additional cancer in the mouth, pharynx, larynx, esophagus, or lung. Head and neck cancers are classified by size and by extent of involvement. A Stage I neoplasm is less than 2 cm or is localized to one anatomic site. A Stage II neoplasm measures between 2 cm and 4 cm or involves two areas within a site but without regional or distant metastasis. Stage III neoplasms are greater than 4 cm or involve three adjacent areas of the head and neck. Stage IV neoplasms are massive cancers that involve bone and cartilage and/or those that extend outside the site of origin.

ETIOLOGY

Sites of oral cancer are generally the floor of the mouth, the ventrolateral aspect of the tongue, and the soft palate.

SPEECH AND LANGUAGE DIFFICULTIES

- Muscle tension dysphonia may result from attempts to overcompensate for vocal problems.
- Vocal fold paralysis generally results in breathiness, hoarseness, high pitch, limited range, decreased intensity, and the need for frequent breath replenishment.
- Dysarthria.

ASSOCIATED AND OTHER DIFFICULTIES

- Salivary gland dysfunction.
- Dry mouth.
- Cranial radiation in children may produce progressive sensorineural hearing loss.
- Children who survive acute lymphoblastic leukemia (ALL) show a decline in intelligence.
- Radiation may produce decreased salivary flow, leading to increased dental caries, inflammation in the mucous lining, formation of necrotic ulcers, trismus (inability to open the jaw), and/or loss of taste and appetite.
- Radiation may destroy healthy tissue around the face and jaw.
- Radiation may increase the likelihood of atherosclerotic plaques in the cervical carotid arteries, which in turn increases the risk of stroke. (Ginsberg, 1998)
- Swallowing function may be impaired due to reduced range and coordination of tongue movements, delayed triggering of pharyngeal swallow, reduced tongue base retraction, and reduced efficiency of swallow. (Lazarus, et al., 1993a)
- Dysphagia and aspiration are common: Following glossectomy an intraoral skin graft best preserves tongue mobility. Next best is a myocutaneous flap. Following mandibulectomy, drooling is nearly always present if the anterior mandibular arch is removed, but is less common following removal of more lateral portions. Following hard palate

surgery, material enters the nose through the oronasal fistula. A prosthetic device generally corrects the problem. Following soft palate surgery, there is often a problem due to insufficient length for effective closure of the nasopharynx. Over time, the soft palate may adapt to this change. (Kronenberger and Meyers, 1994)

ASSESSMENT

- For clients presenting with glottic cancer, use videolaryngostroboscopy to view vibratory motion of vocal folds.
- Assess articulation skills postoperatively, in single words, in selected sentences, and in conversational speech.
- Assess swallowing function using videofluoroscopic studies.
- Assess for dysphagia.

INTERVENTION TECHNIQUES

- Counsel clients prior to surgery about potential speech and swallowing difficulties.
- Meet with clients prior to radiation therapy and provide exercises to prevent trismus. (Scott, 1998)
- Provide voice therapy postoperatively.
- Discourage clients from trying to force or strain their voice in attempts to improve vocal quality.
- To treat flaccid dysarthria, work to improve support for speech breathing.
- Provide therapy to develop modified swallowing techniques and counsel re: dietary requirements as necessary.
- Consider use of supraglottic, super-supraglottic, and Mendelsohn maneuvers to improve efficiency of swallow. (Lazarus, et al., 1993b)
- Change of posture may alleviate dysphagia. (Logemann, et al., 1994.)
- To provide therapy for dysphagia following surgery, learn exactly what was done in surgery and specifically what effects the procedures have on the swallowing function. (Crane, 1997)
- Following surgery such as thyroplasty for vocal fold medialization, patients should be provided therapy for breath control, relaxation techniques, and laryngeal function exercises. (Iskowitz, 1997b)
- Encourage participation in support groups. (Tilke, 1992)

RESULTS OF RECENT STUDIES

- Dysphagia following tongue resection is often transitory; some clients compensate with increased use of buccal musculature. Those who have a glossectomy involving the base of the tongue often have more persistent dysphagia. (Groher and Gonzalez, 1992)
- In a study of 30 clients, oral pharyngeal swallow efficiency (OPSE) was evaluated as a function of surgical variables including, volume resected; flap volume; ratio of flap volume to volume resected; percentage of oral tongue, tongue base; and anterior and lateral floor of mouth resected; and preservation of mandible. No significant differences were found based on volume of the surgical resection, volume of flap reconstruction, or the ratio between flap volume and volume resected. There was a negative correlation between OPSE and percentages of oral tongue and tongue base resected. (McConnel, et al., 1994)
- Swallowing problems in patients treated with external-beam radiation and adjuvant chemotherapy for newly diagnosed tumors included delayed triggering of pharyngeal swallow, reduced posterior motion of the tongue to the posterior pharyngeal wall, reduced laryngeal elevation, and reduced laryngeal closure during swallow. (Lazarus, et al., 1996)
- In a study of speech and swallowing function of surgically treated oral and oropharyngeal cancer clients, the level of functioning at 12 months after surgery was generally not significantly different from the level of functioning at 3 months postoperatively. Those who underwent postsurgery radiation showed some reversal of swallowing function at 6 months, with some improvement at 12 months postsurgery. (Pauloski, et al., 1994)
- Dysphagia and dysphonia often result from skull base surgery. To alleviate hypernasality and nasal reflux, unilateral adhesion of the palate to the posterior wall of the nasopharynx has achieved positive results. (Netterville and Vrabec, 1994)
- Following resection of the anterior tongue and floor of mouth distal flap reconstruction with maintenance of the mandibular arch, 16 clients showed significant functional impairment in speech and swallowing with generally no improvement by 3 months posthealing. Generally, clients achieved speech intelligibility scores of 50%, oral residues in excess of 50%, and oropharyngeal swallow efficiencies of less than 30. (Pauloski et al., 1993)

- In a study of child survivors of ALL and their siblings, memory deficits in the ALL group were found to be at the level of "central executive." Differences between the two groups were not found in spatial memory, list learning, visuospatial learning, pattern discrimination, or retention. Results showed that children in the ALL group did not use a cumulative rehearsal strategy for transfer of items from a memory buffer into short term memory. (Rodgers, et al., 1992)
- In a study of quality of life satisfaction among persons who had undergone successful treatment for head and neck cancer, pain, dysphagia, and difficulty with speech were the main determinants of satisfaction. (Morton, 1995)

PROGNOSIS

With proper treatment, survival rates for Stage I are about 90%, while survival rates are 75% for Stage II, 45% to 75% for Stage III, and less than 35% for Stage IV. Overall 5-year survival rates for Stages I and II are 65%. Patients over 70 years of age have better survival rates than younger patients.

REFERENCES

Crane R. Dysphagia and cancer: do your clinical homework. *Advance for Speech-Language Pathologists & Audiologists.* 1997;7(8):5,50.

Duffy JR. *Motor Speech Disorders: Substrates, Differential Diagnosis, and Management.* St. Louis, Mo: Mosby. 1995.

Fenton JE, H Brake, A Shirazi, MS Mendelsohn, MD Atlas, PA Fagan. The management of dysphagia in jugular foramen surgery. *The Journal of Laryngology and Otology.* 1996;110:144–7.

Ginsberg M. Complications of oral cancer treatment. *Advance for Speech-Language Pathologists & Audiologists.* 1998;8(21):28.

Groher ME, EE Gonzalez. Mechanical disorders of swallowing. In: Groher ME, ed. *Dysphagia Diagnosis and Management,* 2nd ed. Boston: Butterworth-Heinemann. 1992: 53–84.

Iskowitz M. Improving voice after cancer treatment. *Advance for Speech-Language Pathologists & Audiologists.* 1997a;7(8):8.

Iskowitz M. Managing unilateral vocal fold paralysis : the speech-language pathologist's role. *Advance for Speech-Language Pathologists & Audiologists.* 1997b;7(32):6.

Kronenberger MB, AD Meyers. Dysphagia following head and neck cancer surgery [Review, 52 refs]. *Dysphagia*. 1994;9(4):236–44.

Lazarus CL. Effects of radiation therapy and voluntary maneuvers on swallow functioning in head and neck cancer patients. *Clinics in Communication Disorders*. 1993a;3(4): 11–20.

Lazarus CL, JA Logemann, P Gibbons. Effects of maneuvers on swallowing function in a dysphagic oral cancer patient. *Head & Neck*. 1993b;15:419–24.

Lazarus CL, JA Logemann, BR Pauloski, LA Colangelo, PJ Kahrilas, BB Mittal, M Pierce. Swallowing disorders in head and neck cancer patients treated with radiotherapy and adjuvant chemotherapy. *Laryngoscope*. 1996;106(9 Pt 1):157–66.

Logemann JA, AW Rademaker, BR Pauloski, PJ Kahrilas. Effects of postural change on aspiration in head and neck surgical patients. *Otolaryngology—Head and Neck Surgery*. 1994;110:222–7.

McConnel FM, JA Logemann, AW Rademaker, BR Pauloski, SR Baker, J Lewin, D Shedd, MA Heiser, S Cardinale, S Collins, D Graner, BS Cook, F Milianti, T Baker. Surgical variables affecting postoperative swallowing efficiency in oral cancer patients: a pilot study. *Laryngoscope*. 1994;104(1 Pt 1):87–90.

Morton RP. Life-satisfaction in patients with head and neck cancer. *Clinical Otolaryngology*. 1995;20:499–503.

Netterville JL, JT Vrabec. Unilateral palatal adhesion for paralysis after high vagal injury. *Archives of Otolaryngology— Head & Neck Surgery*. 1994;120(2):218–21.

Pauloski BA, JA Logemann, AW Rademaker, FMS McConnel, MA Heiser, S Cardinale, D Shedd, J Lewin, SR Baker, D Graner, B Cook, F Millanti, S Collins, T Baker. Speech and swallowing function after anterior tongue and floor of mouth resection with distal flap reconstruction. *Journal of Speech and Hearing Research*. 1993;36:267–76.

Pauloski BR, JA Logemann, AW Rademaker, FMS McConnel, D Stein, Q Beery, J Johnson, MA Heiser, S Cardinale, D Shedd, D Graner, B Cook, F Millanti, S Collins, T Baker. Speech and swallowing function after oral and oropharyngeal resections: one-year follow-up. *Head & Neck*. 1994;16:313–22.

Rhodus NL, K Moller, S Colby , J Bereuter. Dysphagia in patients with three different etiologies of salivary gland dysfunction. *ENT Journal*. 1995;74(1):39–48.

Rodgers J, PG Britton, RG Morris, J Kernahan, AW Craft. Memory after treatment for acute lymphoblastic leukaemia. *Archives of Disease in Childhood*. 1992;67:266–8.

Scott A. Treating trismus. *Advance for Speech-Language Pathologists & Audiologists*. 1998;8(30):22–23.

Sessions RB, GF Martin, SD Miller, BI Solomon. Videolaryngostroboscopy for evaluation of laryngeal disorders. In: Blitzer A, MF Brin, S Fahn, CT Sasaki, KS Harris, eds. *Neurologic Disorders of the Larynx*. New York: Thieme Medical Publishers, Inc. 1992:140–46.

Shoemaker A. Progressive hearing loss: newborn screening reveals increased incidence. *Advance for Speech-Language Pathologists & Audiologists*. 1996;6(34):5,7.

Tilke B. Support groups: sometimes what patients need most is each other. *Advance for Speech-Language Pathologists & Audiologists*. 1992;2(21):19.

Trace R. Rehabilitation of cancer patients benefits from organ preservation protocols. *Advance for Speech-Language Pathologists & Audiologists.* 1993;3(20):10–11,13.

Otitis Media (OM) and Otitis Media with Effusion (OME)

DESCRIPTION

Otitis media (OM) can occur at any age but is most common in children between the ages of 3 months and 3 years. The condition is most common among Hispanic children, followed by Caucasian and then African-American children. Symptoms include persistent, severe earache, fever, nausea, vomiting, and diarrhea. Hearing loss may occur. Serious complications include acute mastoiditis, petrositis, labyrinthitis, facial paralysis, conductive and sensorineural hearing loss, epidural abscess, meningitis, brain abscess, lateral sinus thrombosis, subdural empyema, and otitic hydrocephalus. Symptoms of these impending complications include headache, sudden profound hearing loss, vertigo, and chills and fever. Those at some increased risk of developing OM include males, Caucasians, and Native Americans; those with a family history of OM; those in child care settings; and those exposed to second-hand smoke.

ETIOLOGY

OM is a bacterial or viral infection in the middle ear, usually secondary to an upper respiratory infection. Some studies have indicated that allergic reactions to some foods may cause excess mucous production and swelling of the eustachian tube. (Layton, 1996)

SPEECH AND LANGUAGE DIFFICULTIES

- Babbling in infancy may be delayed.
- Deficits in auditory sequential memory, auditory discrimination, and sound recognition.

- Difficulty discriminating voiced/voiceless pairs.
- Misarticulations.

ASSOCIATED AND OTHER DIFFICULTIES

- Mild to moderate conductive hearing impairment while the effusion is present.
- Sensorineural hearing loss affecting high frequencies may develop; sensorineural hearing loss is more frequent in adults with chronic OM.
- Easily distracted.
- Deficits in gross motor skills. Deficits generally resolve following myringotomy and placement of tympanostomy tubes.

ASSESSMENT

- Screen hearing and refer to audiologist as appropriate.
- Assess phonology.
- Assess receptive and expressive language skills.
- Administer *Sequenced Inventory of Communication Development, Revised* (SICD-R).

INTERVENTION TECHNIQUES

- To decrease incidence of OM, instruct caregivers not to feed infants who are in a supine position.
- Provide optimum listening environments.
- Provide and instruct others in the provision of language-rich environments.
- Use visual supports to aid in understanding what is being heard.
- Eliminate or reduce distracting, competing noise.
- Employ verbal redirection as needed to sustain attention.
- Consider use of low-gain hearing aids or FM system in classroom and/or therapy sessions.

RESULTS OF RECENT STUDIES

- Two-year-old children with early OM were followed from birth and compared with children without OM. The two groups did not differ on measures of receptive language but differed significantly on measures of expressive language and articulation. All members of the otitis-positive group showed delays in expressive language. On measures of articulation, this group had developed significantly fewer initial consonants and produced them less accurately. (Abraham, et al., 1996)

- Frequent episodes of OME in early childhood may affect the establishment of responsive interaction styles between mother and child. The child may appear unresponsive. Not receiving needed cues from the child, the mother may alter, and possibly decrease, her interactions with the child. (Robert, et al., 1995)
- Children with persistent hearing impairment due to OME were managed in the following ways: one group received an adenoidectomy and insertion of a tympanostomy tube, a second group underwent insertion of a tube without adenoidectomy, and a third group was treated nonsurgically. Both types of surgery had some positive effect on hearing and on the presence of OM at 6 months postoperatively, but the results at 12 months were no different than those obtained through natural resolution. (Dempster, et al., 1993)
- In one study, 125 children received a conventional pressure equalizing (PE) tube in one ear and a PE tube treated with silver oxide salt and silicon in the other ear. After 1 year there was a 50% reduction in recurrence of OM in those ears with the silver oxide–treated tubes. (Kelly, 1995)
- In a study of young twins with differing histories of OM, results of articulation, receptive, and expressive language tests were mixed. Across the group of five dyads, there were instances of similar performance, of OM-positive children scoring higher than their sibling, and of OM-positive children with lower scores than their sibling. (Hemmer and Ratner, 1994)

PROGNOSIS

One study has found that children with episodes of OM in childhood do not experience difficulties in the areas of intellectual performance, academic achievement, behavior, or attention during adolescence. (Trace, 1996)

REFERENCES

Abraham SS, IF Wallace, JS Gravel. Early otitis media and phonological development at age 2 years. *Laryngoscope.* 1996;106(6):727–32.

Dempster JH, GG Browning, SG Gatehouse. A randomized study of the surgical management of children with persistent otitis media with effusion associated with a hearing impairment. *Journal of Laryngology & Otology.* 1993;107(4):284–9.

Hemmer VH, NB Ratner. Communicative development in twins with discordant histories of recurrent otitis media. *Journal of Communication Disorders.* 1994;27:91–106.

Iskowitz M. Linking OME to gross motor deficits. *Advance for Speech-Language Pathologists & Audiologists.* 1997;7(24):7.

Kelly DA. Innovation decreases incidence of OM after PE tube insertion. *Advance for Speech-Language Pathologists & Audiologists.* 1995;5(27):8.

Layton RE. Considering allergies as cause of OM is food for thought. *Advance for Speech-Language Pathologists & Audiologists.* 1996;6(21):8.

Robert SE, MR Burchinal, LP Medley, SA Zeisel, M Mundy, J Roush, S Hooper, D Bryant, FW Henderson. Otitis media, hearing sensitivity, and maternal responsiveness in relation to language during infancy. *Journal of Pediatrics.* 1995;126(3):481–9.

Roberts JE, S Clarke-Klein. Otitis media. In: Bernthal JE, NW Bankson, eds. *Child Phonology: Characteristics, Assessment, and Intervention with Special Populations.* New York: Thieme Medical Publishers, Inc. 1994:182–98.

Roberts JE, IF Wallace, FW Henderson, eds. *Otitis Media in Young Children: Medical, Developmental, and Educational Considerations.* Baltimore: Paul H. Brookes Publishing Co. 1997.

Shoemaker A. Acute OME in infancy delays babbling. *Advance for Speech-Language Pathologists & Audiologists.* 1996;6(21):4.

Trace R. Researchers probe impact of OME-related hearing loss. *Advance for Speech-Language Pathologists & Audiologists.* 1996;6(21):6–7,38.

Vartiainen E, J Vartiainen. Age and hearing function in patients with chronic otitis media. *The Journal of Otolaryngology.* 1995;24(6):336–9.

Voice Disorders

DESCRIPTION

Persons engaged in some professions and avocations are more susceptible to vocal attrition due to the demands placed on their voice. Some of these include teachers, army instructors, cheerleaders, students who perform frequently in dramatic productions or choral groups, and voice students. Persons with adductor spastic dysphonia (SD) exhibit a strangled voice quality characterized by abrupt initiation and termination of voicing, reduction in volume, and monotone. Voice quality of those with abductor SD is breathy and effortful with abrupt termination of voicing. Intelligibility may be compromised in both types of SD. Most children with unilateral vocal cord paralysis (UVCP) have multiple congenital defects such as hydrocephalus, Arnold-Chiari malformation, or brain tumors.

ETIOLOGY

Vocal fold paralysis may result from lesions at the nucleus ambiguous, its supranuclear tracts, the main trunk of the vagus, or the recurrent laryngeal nerves. Other causes include intracranial neoplasms, vascular accidents, demyelinating diseases, neoplasms at the base of the skull, and neck trauma. Viral neuronitis likely accounts for most cases of idiopathic vocal cord paralysis.

There are a multitude of factors and conditions that can lead to vocal problems. Some of these include aging, accidental injuries, abusive injuries of the voice and vocal tract, infections, diseases, medication, respiratory problems, diseases that affect articulation and resonance, vibratory problems of the larynx, and genetic factors. (Mitchell, 1996)

Less commonly, voice disorders may be caused by papilloma (a benign tumor affecting the epithelium), laryngeal amyloidosis (deposition of acellular proteinaceous material in the tissues), laryngeal web (a band of tissues joining the two vocal folds), sulcus vocalis (furrows along the upper medial edge of the vocal folds), and granuloma (a result of intubation, a contact ulcer, gastroesophageal reflux, or Teflon injections). (Guteri, 1995)

SPEECH AND LANGUAGE DIFFICULTIES

- Impaired phonation.
- In cases of unilateral vocal cord paralysis, vocal quality is hoarse and breathy.
- In cases of bilateral vocal cord paralysis, voice quality is good but with limited intensity.
- Impaired respiration.
- Hoarseness.

- Vocal fatigue—characterized by changes in vocal quality, loudness, pitch, or effort. Symptoms increase as the day progresses and are generally absent by the next morning.
- Symptom of papilloma is a voice change.
- Symptoms of laryngeal amyloidosis include hoarseness and low-pitched voice. Pain, choking, or coughing may also be present.
- Symptoms of laryngeal web include high-pitched voice, hoarseness, and reduced range of pitch.
- Symptoms of sulcus vocalis include hoarseness, breathiness, low pitch, and reduced volume.

ASSOCIATED AND OTHER DIFFICULTIES

- Throat discomfort or pain.
- Benign mucosal lesions.
- Impaired ability to swallow.
- Aspiration may occur.
- Attacks of asthma may actually be all or partially vocal cord dysfunction (VCD).
- Dysphagia lasting as long as 7 days may occur following injection of botulinum toxin type A for the management of adductor spasmodic dysphonia.

ASSESSMENT

- Be present as otolaryngologist performs laryngovideostroboscopy (LVS). Instruct the client to perform vocal exercises, which can be observed during the procedure.
- Make use of videostroboscopy repeatedly for initial diagnosis as well as to assess changes.
- Work as a team member with otolaryngologists to evaluate clients preoperatively and postoperatively.
- Assess overall vocal production and vocal hygiene.

INTERVENTION TECHNIQUES

- For cases of spasmodic dysphonia (SD), provide injections of botulinum toxin type A (Botox®). Target the thyroarytenoid muscle in cases of adductor SD and the posterior cricoarytenoid muscle in cases of abductor SD.

- In addition to injections of Botox, therapy techniques for clients with SD include general body exercise to reduce strain, inhalation phonation, and slightly elevating pitch to increase or decrease loudness.
- Therapy for clients with vocal lesions includes counseling to avoid ingestion of substances that dehydrate and irritate the vocal tract (smoke, caffeine, alcohol, spicy foods).
- Assist clients in modifying their vocal habits, i.e., have clients brainstorm how to do less speaking or speaking with less strain. (Scott, 1998)
- Immediately following surgery for lesions, clients should adhere to complete vocal rest, followed by gradual and supervised voice use.
- Instruct performers in good vocal hygiene, i.e., avoiding stage dust and noxious environmental fumes as much as possible, refraining from vocal abuse at cast parties.
- Instruct in proper warm-up activities, proper breath support, etc.
- When working with children or adolescents, instruct all family members in proper vocal techniques. Any "rules" established for one member of the family should apply to all family members. (Shoemaker, 1997a)
- To enhance overall communication and to address specific vocal quality, use dramatic readings as a supplement to other therapy materials. (Shoemaker, 1997b)
- Instruct clients with rare voice disorders in techniques to reduce strain while speaking.

RESULTS OF RECENT STUDIES

- Three children with UVCP resulting in severe aspiration were treated with a vocal cord injection of an absorbable gelatin sponge. Aspiration in all three cases was resolved. (Levine, et al., 1995)
- In a questionnaire survey of female teachers, over half reported multiple symptoms of vocal attrition. Only 1% received speech and language therapy. (Sapir, et al., 1993)
- Reports of improved voice quality following injection of Botox in cases of SD indicate improvement in 95% to 100% of cases. The higher the dosage, the longer the recovery period. Very small doses can effect im-

provement lasting 4 to 5 months. Reported side effects include a breathy voice quality and mild dysphagia. (Iskowitz, 1998)

PROGNOSIS

Conventional voice therapy appears to be effective in reducing the recurrence of laryngeal lesions, in the treatment of vocal nodules, and in protecting against the early return of symptoms in SD following Botox injection. (Verdolini, et al., 1998)

REFERENCES

Brin MF, S Fahn, A Blitzer, LO Ramig, C Stewart. Movement disorders of the larynx. In: Blitzer A, ME Brin, CT Sasaki, S Fahn, KS Harris, eds. *Neurological Disorders of the Larynx.* New York: Thieme Medical Publishers, Inc. 1992:253–8.

Gottas C, CD Starr. Vocal fatigue among teachers. *Folia Phoniatrica & Logopedica.* 1993;45:120–9.

Guteri GO. Rare voice disorders: team approach enhances diagnosis and treatment. *Advance for Speech-Language Pathologists & Audiologists.* 1995;5(23):5.

Holzer SES, CL Ludlow. The swallowing side effects of botulinum toxin type A injection in spasmodic dysphonia. *Laryngoscope.* 1996;106:86–92.

Iskowitz M. New developments in treatment for spasmodic dysphonia. *Advance for Speech-Language Pathologists & Audiologists.* 1997;7(8):13,18.

Iskowitz M. Loosening SD's stranglehood on speech: voice improvement patterns following botulinum toxin injection. *Advance for Speech-Language Pathologists & Audiologists.* 1998;8(22):6–9,25.

Johnston RG, FG Umberger. Moving toward objective voice assessment and therapy. *Advance for Speech-Language Pathologists & Audiologists.* 1997;7(22):9.

Levine BA, IN Jacobs, RF Wetmore, SD Handler. Vocal cord injection in children with unilateral vocal cord paralysis. *Archives of Otolaryngology—Head & Neck Surgery.* 1995;121(1):116–9.

Mitchell SA. Medical problems of professional voice users. *Comprehensive Therapy.* 1996;22(4):231–8.

Sapir S, A Keidar, B Mathers-Schmidt. Vocal attrition in teachers: survey findings. *European Journal of Disorders of Communication.* 1993;28:177–85.

Scott A. Adults at risk. *Advance for Speech-Language Pathologists & Audiologists.* 1998;8(22):16–17.

Shoemaker A. Collaboration enhances voice care for children. *Advance for Speech-Language Pathologists & Audiologists.* 1997a;7(24):9,11.

Shoemaker A. Dramatic results: creativity in voice therapy. *Advance for Speech-Language Pathologists & Audiologists.* 1997b;7(22):11.

Trace R. Vocal health of stage performers requires special care. *Advance for Speech-Language Pathologists & Audiologists.* 1993;3(12):10.

Varnell M. Diagnosing VCD. *Advance for Speech-Language Pathologists & Audiologists.* 1998;8(13):32.

Verdolini K, L Ramig, B Jacobson. Outcomes measurement in voice disorders. In: Frattali CM, ed. *Measuring Outcomes in Speech-Language Pathology.* New York: Thieme. 1998:354–86.

Zarrella S. Voice team: a comprehensive approach to care. *Advance for Speech-Language Pathologists & Audiologists.* 1995;5(23):6–7.

Chapter 9

Infectious Disease

- AIDS (acquired immunodeficiency syndrome)
- Creutzfeldt-Jakob disease (CJD)

AIDS (Acquired Immunodeficiency Syndrome)

DESCRIPTION

A secondary syndrome resulting from human immunodeficiency virus (HIV) infection and characterized by infections, malignancies, neurologic dysfunction, and a variety of other syndromes. Pediatric AIDS is one of the 5 leading causes of death among children in the United States and accounts for 10% of American AIDS cases.

AIDS is the leading cause of death among men ages 25 to 44 years and is among the 10 leading causes of death in children between the ages of 1 and 4 years; 84% of children with AIDS in the United States are members of minorities. Pediatric AIDS shows a higher prevalence in the eastern third of the nation.

ETIOLOGY

A retrovirus becomes integrated with the host DNA and then duplicates with each cell division. T cells are infected, as are nonlymphoid cells, such as pulmonary macrophages and microglial cells of the brain, and dendritic cells in the skin and lymph nodes.

SPEECH AND LANGUAGE DIFFICULTIES

- In children, receptive and expressive language deficits, dysarthria, voice disorders, otitis media, dysphagia, and inadequate respiratory support for speech.
- Decreased volume.
- Speaking rate may increase or decrease.
- Dysarthria.
- Apraxia.

ASSOCIATED AND OTHER DIFFICULTIES

- In children, failure to thrive and general delays in development.
- Pulmonary involvement is common and is present in 80% of pediatric cases.

- AIDS encephalitis develops in 60% of pediatric cases.
- Otitis media may be chronic.
- Tuberculosis.
- Difficulties associated with neurologic disorders as a result of AIDS include headache, lethargy, confusion, seizures, and focal signs.
- A more serious neurologic complication, subacute encephalitis, may develop, with symptoms of memory loss, confusion, psychomotor retardation, seizures, and dementia.
- 79% of adults with AIDS have some auditory dysfunction, and 49% acquire a hearing loss greater than 25 dB. Losses may be conductive, as a result of eustachian tube dysfunction, or sensorineural, as a result of infections of the inner ear or central nervous system. (Zarella, 1995)
- Tinnitus.
- Dysphagia.
- Dementia.

ASSESSMENT

- Assess for dysphagia.
- In children, assess receptive and expressive language skills.
- Perform hearing screening and refer to audiologist as indicated.
- Assess for dysarthria. (See Appendix A.)
- Assess overall speech intelligibility.
- Perform all assessments repeatedly over time to document changes as the illness progresses.

INTERVENTION TECHNIQUES

- Consider some form of augmentative and alternative communication (AAC) if indicated.
- To treat flaccid dysarthria, work to increase support for speech breathing.
- Consider use of pacing device to decrease rate.
- Treat for dysphagia.

RESULTS OF RECENT STUDIES

No recent studies regarding communication skills were found in the literature.

PROGNOSIS

HIV is a progressive disease. New treatments are continuously being developed and length of survival is increasing in some cases.

REFERENCES

Bartlett CL. Communication disorders in adults with AIDS. In: Ratzan SC, ed. *AIDS: Effective Health Communication for the 90's*. Washington, DC: Taylor & Francis. 1993:189–202.

Miller T. Pediatric AIDS: treatment issues include developmental delays and dysphagia. *Advance for Speech-Language Pathologists & Audiologists*. 1996;6(30):10–11.

Scott GS, TL Layton. Epidemiologic principles in studies of infectious disease outcomes: pediatric HIV as a model. *Journal of Communication Disorders*. 1997;30:303–24.

Zarella S. Etiology of hearing loss varies in patients with AIDS. *Advance for Speech-Language Pathologists & Audiologists*. 1995;5(18):10.

Creutzfeldt-Jakob Disease (CJD)

DESCRIPTION

A rapidly progressive viral disease of the central nervous system characterized by progressive dementia and myoclonic seizures. Symptoms first appear in midlife and include memory failure, behavioral changes, difficulty with concentration and coordination, or visual disturbances.

ETIOLOGY

The etiologic agent is believed to be a protein infectious agent. Mode of transmission is unclear. About 10% of cases are familial.

SPEECH AND LANGUAGE DIFFICULTIES

- Aphasia.
- Apraxia.
- Mutism.

ASSOCIATED AND OTHER DIFFICULTIES

- Delusions and hallucinations.
- Dementia.
- Apathy.
- Self-neglect.
- Irritability.
- Dyslexia.
- Dysgraphia.
- Fatigue and sleep disorders.
- Disorientation.
- Rigidity and/or tremor.
- Progressive muscular atrophy.
- Visual field defects.
- Dysphagia in later stages.

ASSESSMENT

- Assess for dysphagia.
- Assess for aphasia.

INTERVENTION TECHNIQUES

- Treat for dysphagia.
- Encourage forms of nonverbal communication.

RESULTS OF RECENT STUDIES

No recent studies regarding communication skills were found in the literature.

PROGNOSIS

The disease is fatal and death generally occurs within 3 to 12 months; 5% to 10% of affected persons live 2 years or longer.

REFERENCES

Thoene JG, NP Coker, eds. *Physicians' Guide to Rare Diseases*. New York: Dowden Publishing Co. 1995:293–4.

Chapter 10

Burns

- Burns

Burns

DESCRIPTION

Burns are tissue injuries caused by thermal, chemical, or electrical contact.

ETIOLOGY

Inhalation of the incomplete products of combustion, such as steam and hot gases, causes respiratory tract ventilation injury. Electrical burns may cause immediate respiratory paralysis and/or ventricular fibrillation. Chemical burns are caused by strong acids and alkalies, phenols, cresols, mustard gas, or phosphorus.

SPEECH AND LANGUAGE DIFFICULTIES

- Aphonia may result.
- Inability to initiate swallow reflex may result in wet vocal quality.
- Breathy voice quality.

ASSOCIATED AND OTHER DIFFICULTIES

- Dysphagia. Buildup of facial scar tissue impedes ability to suck from a straw or to take food from a utensil; skin retraction also results in poor bilabial control, making it difficult to retain food in the mouth; tautness of the skin results in decreased jaw mobility. (Shoemaker, 1997)
- Ingestion of caustic substances may severely damage the larynx.
- Peripheral nerve damage may result following electrical injury.
- Immediately following electrical injury, loss of consciousness, confusion, and amnesia may occur.
- Sensorineural hearing loss may result from electrical injury.
- Impaired memory.
- Impaired motor skills.
- Impaired ability to concentrate.

ASSESSMENT

- Assess for dysphagia. Consider positioning problems, skin retraction, and tracheostomy and ventilator dependency.
- Assess voice quality.
- Assess oral motor skills—for speech production and for eating.
- Perform a hearing screening and refer to audiologist as indicated.
- Assess memory skills and ability to concentrate in both quiet and distracting environments.

INTERVENTION TECHNIQUES

- Provide therapy for management of pharyngeal dysphagia, including reducing latency of swallow reflex, modifying and improving respiration, and improving positioning. Instruct in techniques such as head/chin tuck, Mendelsohn maneuver, supraglottic swallow, effortful swallow, and volitional cough as appropriate. (Shikowitz, et al., 1996)
- Teach clients on ventilators to coordinate their swallow with the timing of the ventilator.
- Use a cold bolus to assist with localization in the mouth.
- Use oral motor exercises.
- Help the client to develop strategies to aid memory and concentration.

RESULTS OF RECENT STUDIES

- In a study of three clients recovering from caustic ingestion, improvements in voice quality were related to increasing swallowing efficiency. (Shikowitz, et al., 1996)

PROGNOSIS

Recovery is related to the severity of the injury.

REFERENCES

Grossman AR, CE Tempereau, MF Brones, HS Kulber, LJ Pembrook. Auditory and neuropsychiatric behavior patterns after electrical injury. *Journal of Burn Care & Rehabilitation*. 1993;(March/April):169–75.

Shikowitz MJ, J Levy, D Villano, LM Graver, R Pochaczevsky. Speech and swallowing rehabilitation following devastating caustic ingestion: techniques and indicators for success. *Laryngoscope*. 1996;106:1–12.

Shoemaker A. Treating dysphagia in patients with severe burns requires interdisciplinary approach. *Advance for Speech-Language Pathologists & Audiologists*. 1997;7(17):8,46.

Appendix A

Types of Dysarthria

Types of Dysarthria	Areas of Damage	Frequently Occurring In	Physiological Features	Speech Features
Ataxic	Cerebellum	Friedreich's ataxia; Shy-Drager syndrome; multiple sclerosis; encephalitis; congenital malformations of the cerebellum; gunshot wounds; transient ischmetic attacks; infarction; hemorrhage	Reduction in vital capacity and total lung capacity; discoordinated rib cage/abdomen movements; hypotonicity in speech musculature; asynchronization of muscle activation/suppression	Speech is slurred, irregular, labored, jerky, explosive, staccato, singsong; imprecise consonants; prolongation of vowels; harsh voice quality; reduced rate; poor volume control; poor pitch control; increased duration of syllables; loss of distinction between stressed and unstressed syllables
Flaccid	Cranial and peripheral nerves that support motor speech production; damage to Vagus nerve	Myasthenia gravis; Bell's palsy; brainstem stroke; postpolio syndrome; AIDS; Guillain-Barré syndrome; muscular dystrophy; polymyositis; progressive bulbar palsy; ALS; effects of postradiation	Muscle weakness, including muscles of respiration, facial muscles, tongue and lip muscles	Imprecise articulation; reduced rate and volume; difficulty controlling pitch; breathy voice quality; rapid, shallow breathing; hypernasality

continues

Hyperki-netic	Extrapyrami-dal system; lesions in the basal ganglia and their major path-ways	Huntington's disease; Tourette's syndrome and other tic disorders; athetoid cerebral palsy; dyskinesia and dystonia	Myoclonus (sudden unsustained muscle contractions) of the soft palate, larynx, and diaphragm	Variable imprecision of articulation; harsh/strained voice quality; variable rate; monopitch; intermittent voice arrest during contextual speech; lower habitual pitch; restricted pitch range; reduced maximum phonation time; involuntary disturbances of respiration and phonation
Hypokinetic	Basal ganglia	Parkinson's disease; progressive supranuclear palsy; Shy-Drager syndrome; Wilson's disease; closed head injury	Reduced vital capacity; vocal fold asymmetry and bowing; vocal fold paralysis; reduction in size and peak velocity of jaw movement during speech; decreased maximum voluntary lip closing force	Monopitch; reduced volume; breathiness; hoarseness; tremor; harsh voice quality; imprecise articulation of consonants; difficulty modifying rate

continues

Types of Dysarthria	Areas of Damage	Frequently Occurring In	Physiological Features	Speech Features
Spastic	Bilateral disruption of upper motor neuron connections in the corticobulbar tracts	Pseudobulbar palsy; progressive supranuclear palsy; traumatic brain injuries; brain tumors; multiple sclerosis; spastic cerebral palsy	Excessive muscle tone; weakness in muscles of the lips and tongue; drooling; restricted protrusion and lateral movement of tongue; compromise of velopharyngeal function; reduced abdominal contribution to speech breathing; difficulty inhibiting laughter and crying	Imprecise consonants; monopitch; slow rate; decreased volume variability; harsh/ strangled voice quality; pitch breaks; distorted vowels; increased duration of syllables; impaired respiratory support

Source: Data from J.R. Duffy, *Motor Speech Disorders: Substrates, Differential Diagnosis, and Management,* © 1995, Mosby Year-Book, Inc. and M.R. McNeil, *Clinical Management of Sensorimotor Speech Disorders,* © 1997, Thieme.

Appendix B

A Description of Pragmatic Skills

To be successful, communication must ultimately result in a meaningful transfer of information between two or more persons. Merely understanding the meanings of individual words, articulating sounds and words intelligibly, and using correct syntax are not enough. In addition, both listeners and speakers must be cognizant of the overall environment in which meaningful verbal exchanges occur. The combination of factors involved in creating and maintaining this environment has come to be known as pragmatics, and a description of these factors is given below.

Within this book, conditions in which difficulty with pragmatic skills, or some aspect of these skills, has been recognized include Asperger's disorder, attention deficit disorder, autism, cerebrovascular accident—right hemisphere damage, child abuse and neglect, developmental disabilities—adults, fetal alcohol syndrome, Fragile X syndrome, head injury—adult, learning disabilities—children and adolescents, mental retardation—children, pervasive developmental disorder, Prader-Willi syndrome, prenatal cocaine exposure, schizophrenia, specific language impairment, spina bifida, and Tourette syndrome.

FUNCTIONS OF COMMUNICATION

I. At the simplest level of pragmatic skills is the realization that speech can serve different purposes. These include requesting, naming, thanking, warning, congratulating, describing, refusing, and answering. Successful communication necessitates that the speaker have an understanding of the type of speech necessary to convey the intended message. The listener, in turn, must have an understanding of the type of response expected following any given type of speech act.

RESPONSIBILITIES OF SPEAKERS AND LISTENERS

II. In order for conversation to proceed smoothly, both speakers and listeners must assume some responsibilities. These responsibilities lie in the areas of initiation, topic maintenance, turn-taking, and repairing utterances. Each participant must understand and employ strategies for introducing a desired topic of conversation. Once a topic has been introduced there is an expectation that immediate responses will in some way relate to that topic. Expectations also exist regarding conversational turn-taking. It is not expected that one person will do all the talking. It becomes incumbent on the speaker to know when to finish speaking and wait for a response from others. Similarly, it is incumbent on a listener to know when a response is expected, and to provide it. Conversational repair becomes necessary when a message has not been understood or has been misunderstood. Again both speaker and listener must assume responsibility. The person who has uttered the message must be alert for signs from the listener, either verbal or nonverbal, that the message has not been understood. It is then incumbent on the speaker not to let the misunderstanding persist, but rather to do whatever may be necessary to convey the intended message. Listeners may signal a lack of understanding by directly questioning the speaker or through body language, such as assuming a questioning look or puzzled expression.

continues

GAUGING THE AUDIENCE

III. Speakers have a responsibility to gear their utterances to the specific audience they are addressing. Factors to be considered by speakers should include the overall setting of the conversational exchange as well as the chronological age and language age of the audience.

PRESUPPOSITIONS

IV. In order for conversations to proceed smoothly, speakers should be skilled at making some presuppositions—specifically, presuppositions regarding existing knowledge of the listener(s). Accurate presuppositions allow the speaker to give explanations when necessary while at the same time not giving redundant information that is already known by the listener(s).

Persons who have deficits in the area of pragmatic skills may exhibit difficulty in any or all of these areas. Often such persons show a limited repertoire in their use of language. In addition, difficulties in the areas of turn-taking, topic maintenance, responsibility for repairing utterances, and presuppositions of listener knowledge are often evident.

Appendix C

Factors in Assessment for Augmentative and Alternative Communication (AAC)

Providing a means of communication for those who cannot communicate verbally is the responsibility of the speech-language pathologist in conjunction with other team members. AAC may range from systems that are very simple, inexpensive, and "low-tech" to systems that are complex, expensive, and "high-tech." To be successful in evaluating a client for AAC, and in choosing and implementing an appropriate system, a myriad of factors must be considered. The factors given below are appropriate considerations in assessment for all types and levels of AAC.

I. Purpose of AAC
   A. Is AAC needed for short- or long-term use?
   B. Will the client be totally dependent on the AAC system or will it be used to supplement speech?
   C. Will AAC be used in all environments? If so, what are all the different environments in which a client will find himself or herself? Will different systems be necessary in different environments? Does the system(s) allow a way to signal for help in an emergency?
II. Desire for and willingness to use AAC
   A. Does the client show interest in using a system of AAC?
   B. Who are potential communication partners of the client? Which of these partners express an interest in having the client use a system of AAC? Which potential partners express a willingness to assist in some way?

III. Portability
   A. Will the communication system be used in one location only or in multiple locations?
   B. Is the client ambulatory?
   C. Whether ambulatory or in a wheelchair, is the client physically capable of transporting the communication device? Is she or he intellectually and emotionally able to assume this responsibility?
   D. If the client is not able to transport the device, by what means will it be transported?

IV. Durability
   A. How well will the device stand up over time, given the type and frequency of use expected by any given client?

V. Selection of symbol system
   A. How will messages be conveyed—through objects, gestures, photographs, pictures, symbols, traditional orthography, code?
   B. Will different symbol systems be used in different settings or with different communication partners?
   C. Does the client have, or can she or he be taught, a thorough knowledge of the chosen system(s)?
   D. Do communication partners understand the chosen system(s)? If not, can a clear explanation be provided as an integral part of the communication system?

VI. Method of symbol selection
   A. How will the client access the symbols?
      1. Direct selection
      2. Scanning
         a. circular scanning
         b. linear scanning
         c. group-item scanning
         d. row-column scanning
      3. Each method of scanning may be controlled through:
         a. directed scanning, in which the client activates a switch to start and stop the indicator, or,
         b. automatic scanning, in which the indicator moves continuously until a switch is activated to stop its movement

VII. Activation of the system
   A. How will the client activate the system?

1. Directly, through eye gaze, fingerpointing or use of a finger(s), headstick, chinstick, mouthstick, or use of some other body part to strike a key or touch a screen or,
2. Through use of a switching device. Commonly used switches include jelly bean, button, plate, leaf, pillow, rocker, infrared, proximity, and sip-and-puff

VIII. Client considerations
   A. Does the client have an understanding of the cause-effect nature of communication?
   B. What is the client's overall intellectual/cognitive level?
   C. What are the client's levels of receptive and expressive language skills?
   D. Is the client able to read? At what level?
   E. What are the client's visual skills?
      1. visual acuity?
      2. range of visual field?
      3. scanning ability
      4. visual perceptual skills
   F. What is the range of motion of the hand, arm, or body part to be used to activate the device?
   G. What is the optimal body positioning for the client?
   H. What is the rate of fatigue?
      1. General fatigue?
      2. Fatigue of the body part to be used for accessing the device?
   I. How accurately can the client indicate a choice?
   J. What is the speed of indication?
   K. How much pressure can/must be exerted to activate the device?
   L. Are interfering abnormal reflexes present?
   M. Are interfering tremors or involuntary movements present?

IX. Device considerations
   NOTE: Results of this assessment should be matched with the results of the assessment of client considerations.
   A. What are the overall size and weight of the device?
   B. What are the size and shape of the display area?
   C. What are the size and spacing of the individual display items?
   D. What is the placement of the individual items across the display area?

    E. How good is the clarity of the display?
       1. Visual display?
       2. Quality of voice output?
    F. What is the speed of the device?
       1. Speed of scanning, if applicable?
       2. Speed of item display?
       3. Duration of item display?
       4. Capability of the device for speed adjustment?
    G. What is the total capacity of the device? How much information can be stored and accessed?
    H. What is the positioning of the device in relation to the client?
    I. How easily can items be added, changed, and/or deleted?
X. Cost and funding considerations
    A. Consider whether the device is for short- or long-term use?
    B. Explore all possible funding sources
       1. Private funds
       2. Foundation grants
       3. Community service grants
       4. School districts
       5. Departments of Vocational Rehabilitation
       6. Private medical insurance
       7. Medicaid

Appendix D

Facilitated Communication (FC)

AUTISM

Bebko JM, A Perry, S Bryson. Multiple method validation study of facilitated communication: II. Individual differences and subgroup results. *Journal of Autism & Developmental Disorders*. 1996;26(1):19–42.

Beck AR, CM Pirovano. Facilitated communicators' performance on a task of receptive language. *Journal of Autism & Developmental Disorders*. 1996;26(5):497–512.

Bomba C, L O'Donnell, C Markowitz , DL Holmes. Evaluating the impact of facilitated communication on the communicative competence of fourteen students with autism. *Journal of Autism & Developmental Disorders*. 1996;26(1):43–58.

Braman BJ, MP Brady, SL Linehan, RE Williams. Facilitated communication for children with autism: an examination of face validity. *Behavioral Disorders*. 1995;21(1):110–8.

Crossley R, J Remington-Gurney. Getting the words out: facilitated communication training. *Topics in Language Disorders*. 1992;12(4):29–45. (Note: Discusses individuals with autism, Down syndrome, Rett's syndrome, and tuberous sclerosis)

Duchan JF. Issues raised by facilitated communication for theorizing and research on autism. *Journal of Speech & Hearing Research*. 1993; 36(6):1108–19.

Eliasoph E, AM Donnellan. A group therapy program for individuals identified as autistic who are without speech and use facilitated communication. *International Journal of Group Psychotherapy*. 1995;45(4):549–60.

Howlin P, DPH Jones. An assessment approach to abuse allegations made through facilitated communication. *Child Abuse & Neglect: The International Journal*. 1996;20(2):103–10.

335

Jones DP. Autism, facilitated communication and allegations of child abuse and neglect [editorial; comment]. *Child Abuse & Neglect.* 1994;18(6):491–3.

Myles BS, et al. Collateral behavioral and social effects of using facilitated communication with individuals with autism. *Focus on Autism & Other Developmental Disabilities.* 1996;11(3):63–69,90.

Myles BS, et al. Impact of facilitated communication combined with direct instruction on academic performance of individuals with autism. *Focus on Autism & Other Developmental Disabilities.* 1996;11(1):37–44.

Sheehan CM, RT Matuozzi. Investigation of the validity of facilitated communication through the disclosure of unknown information. *Mental Retardation.* 1996;34(2):94–107.

Szempruch J, JW Jacobson. Evaluating facilitated communications of people with developmental disabilities. *Research in Developmental Disabilities.* 1993;14(4):253–64.

Trace R. Research findings fail to support early claims by advocates of FC in autism. *Advance for Speech-Language Pathologists & Audiologists.* 1994;4(6):6–7,20–22.

Vazquez CA. Failure to confirm the word-retrieval problem hypothesis in facilitated communication. *Journal of Autism & Developmental Disorder.* 1995;25(6):597–610.

Weiss MJS, SH Wagner, ML Bauman. A validated case study of facilitated communication. *Mental Retardation.* 1996;34(4):220–30.

DEVELOPMENTAL DISABILITIES

Regal RA, JR Rooney, T Wandas. Facilitated communication: an experimental evaluation. *Journal of Autism & Developmental Disorders.* 1994;24(3):345–55.

Sheehan CM, RT Matuozzi. Investigation of the validity of facilitated communication through the disclosure of unknown information. *Mental Retardation.* 1996;34(2):94–107.

GENERAL

Jacobson JW, JA Mulick, AA Schwartz. A history of facilitated communication: science working group on facilitated communication. *American Psychologist.* 1995;50(9):750–65.

Sailor W. Science, ideology, and facilitated communication. *American Psychologist.* 1996;51(9):984–5.
See also other brief articles in *American Psychologist.* 1996;51(9):985–9.

LEARNING DISABILITIES

Crossley R. Remediation of communication problems through facilitated communication training: a case study. *European Journal of Disorders of Communication.* 1997;32:61–87.

MENTAL RETARDATION

Beck AR, CM Pirovano. Facilitated communicators' performance on a task of receptive language. *Journal of Autism & Developmental Disorder.* 1996;26(5):497–512.
Cardinal DN, D Hanson , J Wakeham. Investigation of authorship in facilitated communication. *Mental Retardation.* 1996;34(3):231–42.
Crews WD Jr, EC Sanders, LG Hensley, YM Johnson, S Bonaventura, RD Rhodes, MP Garren. An evaluation of facilitated communication in a group of nonverbal individuals with mental retardation. *Journal of Autism & Developmental Disorders.* 1995;25(2):205–13.
Ferguson DL, RH Horner. Negotiating the facilitated communication maze. *Mental Retardation.* 1994;32(4):305–7; discussion 1994;32(4):317–8.
Goode D. Defining facilitated communication in and out of existence: role of science in the facilitated communication controversy. *Mental Retardation.* 1994;32(4):307–11; discussion 1994;32(4):317–8.
Montee BB, RG Miltenberger, D Wittrock, N Watkins, A Rheinberger, J Stackhaus. An experimental analysis of facilitated communication. *Journal of Applied Behavior Analysis.* 1995;28(2):189–200.
Moore S. Facilitator-suggested conversational evaluation of facilitated communication. *Journal of Autism & Developmental Disorders.* 1993; 23(3):541–52.
Moore S, et al. Evaluation of eight case studies of facilitated communication. *Journal of Autism & Developmental Disorders.* 1993;23(3):531–39.
Simon EW, DM Toll, PM Whitehair. A naturalistic approach to the validation of facilitated communication. *Journal of Autism & Developmental Disorders.* 1994;24(5):647–57.

Simon EW, PM Whitehair, DM Toll. Keeping facilitated communication in perspective. *Mental Retardation.* 1995;33(5):338–9.

Szempruch J, JW Jacobson. Evaluating facilitated communications of people with developmental disabilities. *Research in Developmental Disabilities.* 1993;14(4):253–64.

Appendix E

Suggested Reading

AUGMENTATIVE AND ALTERNATIVE COMMUNICATION (AAC)

Beukelman DR, P Mirenda. *Augmentative and Alternative Communication: Management of Severe Communication Disorders in Children and Adults.* Baltimore: Paul H. Brookes Publishing Co. 1992.

Crane R. Incorporating critical thinking skills in AAC instruction. *Advance for Speech-Language Pathologists & Audiologists.* 1997;7 (11):18.

Crane R. Training staff to integrate AAC systems. *Advance for Speech-Language Pathologists & Audiologists.* 1997;7(15):19,21.

Crawford H. Tangible symbols: opening the lines of communication for children who are nonverbal. *Advance for Speech-Language Pathologists & Audiologists.* 1998;8(32):14–16.

Cummings F. AAC in the temple. *Advance for Speech-Language Pathologists & Audiologists.* 1997;7(30):5.

Iskowitz M. AAC strategies for preschoolers. *Advance for Speech-Language Pathologists & Audiologists.* 1997;7(30):8.

Iskowitz M. Augmenting language learning in toddlers with DD. *Advance for Speech-Language Pathologists & Audiologists.* 1997;7(30):10,18.

Iskowitz M. Setting realistic goals for AAC. *Advance for Speech-Language Pathologists & Audiologists.* 1997;7(30):7,18.

Lipner HS. Augmentative and alternative communication. In: Bain BK, D Leger. *Assistive Technology: An Interdisciplinary Approach.* New York: Churchill Livingstone. 1997:99–116.

McCloskey-Dale SR. The ABCs of AAC. *Advance for Speech-Language Pathologists & Audiologists.* 1997;7(47):22–23.

National Institute on Disability and Rehabilitation Research. Consensus statement: augmentative and alternative communication intervention.

1992. (Available from: The National Institute on Disability and Rehabilitation Research, 400 Maryland Avenue SW, Washington, DC 20202-2646. (202)205-9151.)

Rowland C, P Schweigert. Analyzing the communication environment to increase functional communication. *Journal of the Association for Persons with Severe Handicaps (JASH).* 1993;18(3):161–76.

Scherer MJ. Eye on outcomes. *Advance for Speech-Language Pathologists & Audiologists.* 1998;8(28):29.

Soto G, W Toro-Zambrana. Investigation of Blissymbol use from a language research paradigm. *AAC: Augmentative and Alternative Communication.* 1995;11(2):118–30.

Trace R. AAC camps augment learning with fun in alternative settings. *Advance for Speech-Language Pathologists & Audiologists.* 1993; 3(17):12–13.

Trace R. AAC research projects focus on literacy, symbols, artificial intelligence. *Advance for Speech-Language Pathologists & Audiologists.* 1993;3(17):7,15.

Trace R. Vocational specialists working to help AAC users overcome obstacles to employment. *Advance for Speech-Language Pathologists & Audiologists.* 1993;3(17):8.

Trace R. Building employee confidence in AAC interactions. *Advance for Speech-Language Pathologists & Audiologists.* 1995;5(45):11,17.

Trace R. Innovations in selecting and implementing AAC. *Advance for Speech-Language Pathologists & Audiologists.* 1995;5(37):6–7.

Trace R. Morse code applications in AAC and assistive technology. *Advance for Speech-Language Pathologists & Audiologists.* 1995;5(30): 14.

Young P. Implementing functional communication for DD. *Advance for Speech-Language Pathologists & Audiologists.* 1995;5(37):17.

Zarrella S. AAC in aphasia: evaluators must consider cognitive, linguistic skills. *Advance for Speech-Language Pathologists & Audiologists.* 1995;5(37):4,15.

Zarrella S. ECT approach merges AAC goals of educators, clinicians. *Advance for Speech-Language Pathologists & Audiologists.* 1995;5(37):5.

Zarrella S. Optimal AAC assessment takes time and expertise. *Advance for Speech-Language Pathologists & Audiologists.* 1995;5(37):3,8.

Zarrella S. Toward communicative competence: matching nonverbal clients with appropriate AAC. *Advance for Speech-Language Pathologists & Audiologists.* 1995;5(26):6.

DYSPHAGIA

Beecher R. Pediatric dysphagia treatment requires specialized knowledge, special caution. *Advance for Speech-Language Pathologists & Audiologists.* 1992;2(21):6.

Billeaud FP. The role of the SLP in the NICU: premies, micropremies, and medically fragile infants. In: Billeaud FP, ed. *Communication Disorders in Infants and Toddlers.* Woburn, Mass: Butterworth-Heinemann, Andover Medical Publishers. 1993:47–60.

Chalfon-Seedman J. 'New age' alternatives for dysphagia population in SNF. *Advance for Speech-Language Pathologists & Audiologists.* 1996;6(25):11,14.

Cherney LF. *Clinical Management of Dysphagia in Adults and Children,* 2nd ed. Gaithersburg, Md: Aspen Publishers, Inc. 1994.

Comrie JD, JM Helm. Common feeding problems in the intensive care nursery: maturation, organization, evaluation, and management strategies. *Seminars in Speech and Language.* 1997;18(3):239–61.

Fox S. EMG biofeedback accelerates dysphagia treatment. *Advance for Speech-Language Pathologists & Audiologists.* 1993;3(15):6.

Gelman J. Managing dysphagia in degenerative diseases. *Advance for Speech-Language Pathologists & Audiologists.* 1995;5(39):8,16.

Gelman J. Treating dysphagia across patient populations. *Advance for Speech-Language Pathologists & Audiologists.* 1995;5(39):6–7,17.

Groher ME, ed. *Dysphagia: Diagnosis and Management,* 2nd ed. Boston: Butterworth-Heinemann. 1992.

Hughes TAT, CM Wiles. Clinical measurement of swallowing in health and in neurogenic dysphagia. *Quarterly Journal of Medicine.* 1996; 89:109–116.

Iskowitz M. Premature infants at risk for feeding problems. *Advance for Speech-Language Pathologists & Audiologists.* 1996;6(41): 10,50.

Iskowitz M. Biomechanical assessment of the swallow: laryngeal measurements used in dysphagia diagnosis and treatment. *Advance for Speech-Language Pathologists & Audiologists.* 1997;7(41):6,54.

Iskowitz M. Esophageal dysphagia: looking at the total ingestion system. *Advance for Speech-Language Pathologists & Audiologists.* 1997; 7(41):5.

Iskowitz M. Evaluating the infant swallow. *Advance for Speech-Language Pathologists & Audiologists.* 1997;7(28):5,13.

Iskowitz M. Overcoming aversion problems in young patients. *Advance for Speech-Language Pathologists & Audiologists.* 1997;7(45):5–46.

Iskowitz M. Pathways help organize swallowing intervention for patients with trach, ventilator dependency. *Advance for Speech-Language Pathologists & Audiologists.* 1997;7(45):6,11.

Iskowitz M. Pediatrics and DD: airway issues and dysphagia. *Advance for Speech-Language Pathologists & Audiologists.* 1997;7(28):9,46.

Iskowitz M. Xerostomia impacts feeding, swallowing and voicing. *Advance for Speech-Language Pathologists & Audiologists.* 1997; 7(23): 7,16.

Kazandjan M, A Schwartz-Cohen. Team approach to dysphagia essential in long-term care. *Advance for Speech-Language Pathologists & Audiologists.* 1993;3(9):8.

Kerr T. An occupational approach to treating dysphagia. *Advance for Speech-Language Pathologists & Audiologists.* 1994;4(2):19.

Logemann JA. The dysphagia diagnostic procedure as a treatment efficacy trial. *Clinics in Communication Disorders.* 1993;3(4):1–10.

Rosenthal SR, JJ Sheppard, M Lotze, eds. *Dysphagia and the Child with Developmental Disabilities: Medical, Clinical, and Family Interventions.* San Diego, Calif: Singular Publishing Group, Inc. 1994.

Scott A. Modifying the clinical recipe to manage dysphagia. *Advance for Speech-Language Pathologists & Audiologists.* 1997;7(41):7.

Scott A. Better swallows through biofeedback. *Advance for Speech-Language Pathologists & Audiologists.* 1998;8(18):10–11.

Scott A. Preparing a feast for the senses. *Advance for Speech-Language Pathologists & Audiologists.* 1998;8(30):10–11.

Scott A. Step by step: school-based program transitions children from tube to oral feeding. *Advance for Speech-Language Pathologists & Audiologists.* 1998;8(26):22–23.

Shoemaker A. Decision-making in dysphagia. *Advance for Speech-Language Pathologists & Audiologists.* 1996;6(50):8,38.

Shoemaker A. Dysphagia in geriatrics: preserving quality of life for elderly patients. *Advance for Speech-Language Pathologists & Audiologists.* 1996;6(41):8,20.

Shoemaker A. Objective measure of liquid viscosity in dysphagia care. *Advance for Speech-Language Pathologists & Audiologists.* 1996;6 (41):15,17.

Shoemaker A. Monitoring swallowing function with CA. *Advance for Speech-Language Pathologists & Audiologists.* 1997;7(28):6.

Shoemaker A. Religious and cultural issues in dysphagia treatment. *Advance for Speech-Language Pathologists & Audiologists.* 1997;7(10): 10,19.

Trace R. Dysphagia: new directions in assessment and treatment. *Advance for Speech Language Pathologists & Audiologists.* 1992;2(21):10–11.

Trace R. Food for thought: cultural considerations in dysphagia treatment. *Advance for Speech-Language Pathologists & Audiologists.* 1992;2 (22):9,34.

Trace R. Formalizing a dysphagia program for nursing home residents. *Advance for Speech-Language Pathologists & Audiologists.* 1995;5 (50):10.

Trace R. Role of nutrition in interdisciplinary care. *Advance for Speech-Language Pathologists & Audiologists.* 1995;5(11):5,16.

Underdahl CW. Team approach to dysphagia treatment at home. *Advance for Speech-Language Pathologists & Audiologists.* 1996;6(41):21.

Willig TN, J Paulus, JL Saint Guily, C Béon, J Navarro. Swallowing problems in neuromuscular disorders. *Archives of Physical Medicine & Rehabilitation.* 1994;75:1175–81.

Zarrella S. Outcome measures prove efficacy of dysphagia intervention. *Advance for Speech-Language Pathologists & Audiologists.* 1995;5 (32):8.

Zarrella S. Specialized skills required for instrumental assessment. *Advance for Speech-Language Pathologists & Audiologists.* 1995;5(39):5.

Zarrella S. Studying the normal swallow with EMG biofeedback. *Advance for Speech-Language Pathologists & Audiologists.* 1995;5(39):9,14.

Appendix F

Bibliography of Authors

DAVID R. BEUKELMAN

Books

Beukelman DR, P Mirenda. *Augmentative and Alternative Communication: Management of Severe Communication Disorders in Children and Adults*, 2nd ed. Baltimore: Paul H. Brookes Publishing Co. 1998.

Beukelman DR, KM Yorkston. *Communication Disorders Following Traumatic Brain Injury: Management of Cognitive, Language, and Motor Impairments*. Austin, Tex: Pro-Ed. 1991.

Beukelman DR, KM Yorkston, PA Dowden. *Communication Augmentation: A Casebook of Clinical Management*. San Diego, Calif: College-Hill Press. 1985.

Cannito MP, KM Yorkston, DR Beukelman. *Neuromotor Speech Disorders: Nature, Assessment, and Management*. Baltimore: Paul H. Brookes Publishing Co. 1996.

Moore CA, KM Yorkston, DR Beukelman. *Dysarthria and Apraxia of Speech: Perspectives on Management*. Baltimore: Paul H. Brookes Publishing Co. 1991.

Robin DA, KA Yorkston, DR Beukelman. *Disorders of Motor Speech: Assessment, Treatment, and Clinical Characterization*. Baltimore: Paul H. Brookes Publishing Co. 1996.

Till JA, KM Yorkston, DR Beukelman. *Motor Speech Disorders: Advances in Assessment and Treatment*. Baltimore: Paul H. Brookes Publishing Co. 1994.

Yorkston KM, DR Beukelman, KR Bell. *Clinical Management of Dysarthric Speakers*. Austin, Tex: Pro-Ed. 1991.

Yorkston KM, DR Beukelman. *Recent Advances in Clinical Dysarthria*. Austin, Tex: Pro-Ed. 1991.

Articles

Beukelman DR, GH Kraft, J Freal. Expressive communication disorders in persons with multiple sclerosis: a survey. *Archives of Physical Medicine & Rehabilitation.* 1985;66(10):675–7.

Beukelman DR, KM Yorkston, SC Gorhoff, PM Mitsuda, VT Kenyon. Canon communicator use by adults: a retrospective study. *Journal of Speech & Hearing Disorders.* 1981;46(4):374–8.

Beukelman DR, KM Yorkston. Nonvocal communication: performance evaluation. *Archives of Physical Medicine & Rehabilitation.* 1980; 61(6):275–5.

Beukelman DR, CW Cummings, RA Dobie, EA Weymuller Jr. Objective assessment of laryngectomized patients with surgical reconstruction. *Archives of Otolaryngology.* 1980;106(11):715–8.

Beukelman DR, KM Yorkston, PF Waugh. Communication in severe aphasia: effectiveness of three instruction modalities. *Archives of Physical Medicine & Rehabilitation.* 1980;61(6):248–52.

Beukelman DR, KM Yorkston. Influence of passage familiarity on intelligibility estimates of dysarthric speech. *Journal of Communication Disorders.* 1980;13(1):33–41.

Beukelman DR, K Yorkston. Communication options for patients with brain stem lesions. *Archives of Physical Medicine & Rehabilitation.* 1978;59(7):337–40.

Mahanna GK, DR Beukelman, JA Marshall, CA Gaebler, M Sullivan. Obturator protheses after cancer surgery: an approach to speech outcome assessment. *Journal of Prosthetic Dentistry.* 1998;79(3):310–6.

Yorkston KM, VL Harmen, DR Beukelman, CD Traynor. The effect of rate control on the intelligibility and naturalness of dysarthric speech. *Journal of Speech & Hearing Disorders.* 1990;55(3):550–60.

Yorkston KM, DR Beukelman. Ataxic dysarthria: treatment sequences based on intelligibility and prosodic considerations. *Journal of Speech & Hearing Disorders.* 1998;46(4):398–404.

Yorkston KM, DR Beukelman. Communication efficiency of dysarthric speakers as measured by sentence intelligibility and speaking rate. *Journal of Speech & Hearing Disorders.* 1981;46(3):296–301.

Yorkston KM, DR Beukelman. A comparison of techniques for measuring intelligibility of dysarthric speech. *Journal of Communication Disorders.* 1978;11(6):499–512.

LOIS BLOOM

Book

Bloom L. *Language Development from Two to Three*. New York: Cambridge University Press. 1991.

Articles

Bloom L, C Margulis, E Tinker, N Fujita. Early conversations and word learning: contributions from child and adult. *Child Development.* 1996; 67(6):3154–75.

Bloom L, M Rispoli, B Gartner, J Hafitz. Acquisition of complementation. *Journal of Child Language.* 1989;6(1):101–20.

Bloom L, JB Capatides. Sources of meaning in the acquisition of complex syntax: the sample case of causality. *Journal of Experimental Child Psychology.* 1987;43(1):112–28.

Bloom L. Notes for a history of speech pathology. *Psychoanalytic Review.* 1978;65(3):432–63.

Bloom L. Why not pivot grammar? *Journal of Speech & Hearing Research.* 1971;36(1):40–50.

Hood L, L Bloom. What, when and how about why: a longitudinal study of early expressions of causality. *Monographs of the Society for Research in Child Development.* 1979;44(6):1–37.

LOIS BLOOM AND MARGARET LAHEY

Books

Lahey M, L Bloom. *Language Disorders and Language Development.* New York: Macmillan; London: Collier Macmillan.1988.

Articles

Bloom L, M Lahey, L Hood, K Lifter , K Fiess. Complex sentences: acquisition of syntactic connectives and the semantic relations they encode. *Journal of Child Language.* 1980;7(2):235–61.

Lahey M, L Bloom. Planning a first lexicon: which words to teach first. *Journal of Speech & Hearing Disorders.* 1977;42(3):340–50.

DANIEL R. BOONE

Books

Boone DR, SC McFarlane. *The Voice and Voice Therapy*, 5th ed. Englewood Cliffs, NJ: Prentice-Hall. 1994.

Boone DR. *Human Communication and Its Disorders*. Englewood Cliffs, NJ: Prentice-Hall. 1987.

Boone DR. *Voice Disorders in Children and Adults: Strategies of Management*. New York: Thieme-Stratton. 1983.

Boone DR. *Cerebral Palsy*. Indianapolis, In: Bobbs-Merrill. 1972.

Boone DR. *An Adult Has Aphasia*, 3rd ed. Danville, Ill: Interstate Printers & Publishers. 1965.

Plante E, P Beeson, DR Boone. *Communication and Communication Disorders: A Clinical Introduction*. Boston: Allyn and Bacon. 1998.

Articles

Bayles KA, DR Boone, CK Tomoeda, TJ Slauson, AW Kaszniak. Differentiating Alzheimer's patients from the normal elderly and stroke patients with aphasia. *Journal of Speech & Hearing Disorders*. 1989; 54(1):74–87.

Bayles KA, DR Boone. The potential of language tasks for identifying dementia. *Journal of Speech & Hearing Disorders*. 1982;47(2):210–7.

Boone DR, SC McFarlane. A critical view of the yawn-sigh as a voice therapy. *Journal of Voice*. 1993;7(1):75–80.

Boone DR. Dismissal criteria in voice therapy. *Journal of Speech & Hearing Disorders*. 1974;(39)2:133–9.

Davis PJ, DR Boone, RL Carroll, P Darveniza, GA Harrison. Adductor spastic dysphonia: heterogeneity of physiologic and phonatory characteristics. *Annals of Otology, Rhinology & Laryngology*. 1988;97(2 PT 1):179-85.

Tomoeda CK, KA Bayles, DR Boone, AW Kaszniak, TJ Slauson. Speech rate and syntactic complexity effects on the auditory comprehension of Alzheimer patients. *Journal of Communication Disorders*. 1990; 23(2):151–61.

Zraick RI, DR Boone. Spouse attitudes toward the person with aphasia. *Journal of Speech & Hearing Research*. 1991;34(1):123–8.

FREDERIC L. DARLEY

Books

Darley FL. *Aphasia*. Philadelphia: Saunders. 1982.

Darley FL, WH Fay. *Evaluation of Appraisal Techniques in Speech and Language Pathology*. Reading, Mass: Addison-Wesley. 1979.

Darley FL, DC Spriestersbach, W Johnson. *Diagnostic Methods in Speech Pathology*, 2nd ed. New York: Harper & Row. 1978.

Darley FL, JR Brown, AE Aronson. *Motor Speech Disorders*, 1st ed. Philadelphia: Saunders. 1975.

Darley FL. *Diagnosis and Appraisal of Communication Disorders*. Englewood Cliffs, NJ: Prentice-Hall. 1964.

Keith RL, FL Darley. *Laryngectomee Rehabilitation*, 3rd ed. Austin, Tex: Pro-Ed. 1994.

Articles

Aten JL, DF Johns, FL Darley. Auditory perception of sequenced words in apraxia of speech. *Journal of Speech & Hearing Research*. 1971; 14(1):131–43.

Berry WR, FL Darley, AE Aronson. Dysarthria in Wilson's disease. *Journal of Speech & Hearing Research*. 1974;17(2):169–83.

Brown JR, FL Darley, AR Aronson. Ataxic dysarthria. *International Journal of Neurology*. 1970;7(2):302–18.

Brown JR, FL Darley, AE Aronson. Deviant dimensions of motor speech in cerebellar ataxia. *Transactions of the American Neurological Association*. 1968;93:193–6.

Darley FL. A retrospective view: aphasia. *Journal of Speech & Hearing Disorders*. 1977;42(2):161–9.

Darley FL. Treatment of acquired aphasia [review]. *Advances in Neurology*. 1975;7:111–45.

Darley FL, JR Brown, WM Swenson. Language changes after surgery for Parkinsonism. *Brain & Language*. 1975;2(1):65–9.

Darley FL. The efficacy of language rehabilitation in aphasia. *Journal of Speech & Hearing Disorders*. 1972;37(1):3–21.

Darley FL, JR Brown, NP Goldstein. Dysarthria in multiple sclerosis. *Journal of Speech & Hearing Research*. 1972;15(2):229–45.

Darley FL, AE Aronson, JR Brown. Clusters of deviant speech in the dysarthrias. *Journal of Speech & Hearing Research.* 1969; 12(3): 462–96.

Darley FL, AE Aronson, JR Brown. Differential diagnostic patterns of dysarthria. *Journal of Speech & Hearing Research.* 1969;12(2): 246–69.

Darley FL, AE Aronson, JR Brown. Motor speech signs in neurologic disease. *Medical Clinics of North America.* 1968;52(4):835–44.

Disimoni FG, RL Keith, FL Darley. Prediction of PICA overall score by short versions of the test. *Journal of Speech & Hearing Research.* 1980;23(3):511–6.

DiSimoni FG, FL Darley, AE Aronson. Patterns of dysfunction in schizophrenic patients on an aphasia test battery. *Journal of Speech & Hearing Disorders.* 1977;42(4):498–513.

Gomez MR, SO Richardson, JA Dyer, FL Darley, M Kinsbourne, L Eisenberg, RE Saunders, H Sheridan. Questions people ask about dyslexia. *Pediatric Annals.* 1979;8(11):648–59.

Halpern H, FL Darley, JR Brown. Differential language and neurologic characteristics in cerebral involvement. *Journal of Speech & Hearing Disorders.* 1973;38(2):162–73.

Johns DF, FL Darley. Phonemic variability in apraxia of speech. *Journal of Speech & Hearing Research.* 1970;13(3):556–83.

Podraza BL, FL Darley. Effect of auditory prestimulation on naming in aphasia. *Journal of Speech & Hearing Research.* 1977;20(4): 669–83.

Rosenbek JC, RT Wertz, FL Darley. Oral sensation and perception in apraxia of speech and aphasia. *Journal of Speech & Hearing Research.* 1973;16(1):22–36.

Square-Storer P, FL Darley, RK Sommers. Nonspeech and speech processing skills in patients with aphasia and apraxia of speech. *Brain & Language.* 1988;33(1):65–85.

Waller MR, FL Darley. The influence of context on the auditory comprehension of paragraphs by aphasic subjects. *Journal of Speech & Hearing Research.* 1978;21(4):732–45.

Yoss KA, FL Darley. Developmental apraxia of speech in children with defective articulation. *Journal of Speech & Hearing Research.* 1974; 17(3):399–416.

NANCY HELM-ESTABROOKS

Books

Helm-Estabrooks N, AL Holland. *Approaches to the Treatment of Aphasia*. San Diego, Calif: Singular Publishing Group. 1998.

Helm-Estabrooks N, J Aten. *Difficult Diagnoses in Adult Communication Disorders*. Austin, Tex: Pro-Ed. 1991.

Helm-Estabrooks N, ML Albert. *Manual of Aphasia Therapy*. Austin, Tex: Pro-Ed. 1991.

Articles

Albert ML, RW Sparks, NA Helm. Melodic intonation therapy for aphasia. *Archives of Neurology*. 1973;29(2):130–1.

Helm NA. Management of palilalia with a pacing board. *Journal of Speech and Hearing Disorders*. 1978;44(3):50–53.

Helm NA, RB Butler, DF Benson. Acquired stuttering. *Neurology*. 1978; 28(11):1159–65.

Helm-Estabrooks NA, PM Fitzpatrick, B Barresi. Visual action therapy for global aphasia. *Journal of Speech and Hearing Disorders*. 1981;47: 385–9.

Helm-Estabrooks NA, PM Fitzpatrick, B Barresi. Response of an agrammatic patient to a syntax stimulation program for aphasia. *Journal of Speech & Hearing Disorders*. 1981;46:422–7.

AUDREY L. HOLLAND

Books

Costello JM, AL Holland. *Handbook of Speech and Language Disorders*. San Diego, Calif: College-Hill Press. 1986.

Holland AL, MM. Forbes. *Aphasia Treatment: World Perspectives*. San Diego, Calif: Singular Publishing Group. 1993.

Holland AL. *Language Disorders in Adults: Recent Advances*. Austin, Tex: Pro-Ed. 1991.

Holland AL. *Language Disorders in Children*. San Diego, Calif: College-Hill Press. 1984.

Holland AL. *CADL—Communicative Abilities in Daily Living: A Test of Functional Communication for Aphasic Adults*. Baltimore: University Park Press. 1980.

Articles

Becker JT, FJ Huff, RD Nebes, A Holland, F Boller. Neuropsychological function in Alzheimer's disease: pattern of impairment and rates of progression. *Archives of Neurology*. 1988;45(3):263–8.

Fromm D, A Holland. Functional communication in Alzheimer's disease. *Journal of Speech & Hearing Disorders*. 1989;54(4):535–40.

Holland AL, DS Fromm, F DeRuyter, M Stein. Treatment efficacy: aphasia. *Journal of Speech & Hearing Research*. 1996;39:S27–S36.

Holland A. Observing functional communication of aphasic adults. *Journal of Speech & Hearing Disorders*. 1982;47:50–56.

Nebes RD, F Boller , A Holland. Use of semantic context by patients with Alzheimer's disease. *Psychology & Aging*. 1986;1(3):261–9.

MARGARET LAHEY

Book

Lahey M. *Readings in Childhood Language Disorders*. New York: Wiley. 1978.

Articles

Lahey M. Who shall be called language disordered? Some reflections and one perspective. *Journal of Speech & Hearing Disorders*. 1990; 55(4):612–20.

Blau AF, M Lahey, A Oleksiuk-Velez. Planning goals for intervention: language testing or language sampling? *Exceptional Children*. 1984; 51(1):78–79.

Lahey M. Use of prosody and syntactic markers in children's comprehension of spoken sentences. *Journal of Speech & Hearing Research*. 1974;17(4):656–8.

Lahey M, J Edwards. Specific language impairment: preliminary investigation of factors associated with family history and with patterns of language performance. *Journal of Speech & Hearing Research*. 1995; 38(3):643–57.

Lahey M, CD Feier. The semantics of verbs in the dissolution and development of language. *Journal of Speech & Hearing Research.* 1982; 25(1):81–95.

JERI A. LOGEMANN

Books

Logemann JA. *Evaluation and Treatment of Swallowing Disorders,* 2nd ed. Austin, Tex: Pro-Ed. 1998.

Logemann JA. *Manual for the Videofluorographic Study of Swallowing,.* 2nd ed. Austin, Tex: Pro-Ed. 1993.

Logemann JA. Relationship between speech and swallowing. *Seminars in Speech and Language.* New York: Thieme. 1985;6(4):257-359.

Articles

Bisch EM, JA Logemann, AW Rademaker, PJ Kahrilas, CL Lazarus. Pharyngeal effects of bolus volume, viscosity, and temperature in patients with dysphagia resulting from neurologic impairment and in normal subjects. *Journal of Speech & Hearing Research.* 1994;37(5):1041–59.

Blonsky ER, JA Logemann, B Boshes, HB Fisher. Comparison of speech and swallowing function in patients with tremor disorders and in normal geriatric patients: a cinefluorographic study. *Journal of Gerontology.* 1975;30(3):299–303.

Colangelo LA, JA Logemann, BR Pauloski, JR Pelzer, AW Rademaker. T stage and functional outcome in oral and oropharyngeal cancer patients. *Head & Neck.* 1996;18(3):259–68.

Georgian DA, JA Logemann, HB Fisher. Compensatory articulation patterns of a surgically treated oral cancer patient. *Journal of Speech & Hearing Disorders.* 1982;47(2):154–9.

Kahrilas PJ, S Lin, AW Rademaker , JA Logemann. Impaired deglutitive airway protection: a videofluoroscopic analysis of severity and mechanism. *Gastroenterology.* 1997;113(5):1457–64.

Lazarus C, JA Logemann. Swallowing disorders in closed head trauma patients. *Archives of Physical Medicine & Rehabilitation.* 1987;68(2): 79–84.

Lazarus CL, JA Logemann, BR Pauloski, LA Colangelo, PJ Kahrilas, BB Mittal, M Pierce. Swallowing disorders in head and neck cancer patients treated with radiotherapy and adjuvant chemotherapy. *Laryngoscope.* 1996;106(9 Pt 1):1157–66.

List MA. CA Ritter-Sterr, TM Baker, LA Colangelo, G Matz, BR Pauloski, JA Logemann. Longitudinal assessment of quality of life in laryngeal cancer patients. *Head & Neck.* 1996;18(1):1–10.

Logemann JA, BR Pauloski, L Colangelo. Light digital occlusion of the tracheostomy tube: a pilot study of effects on aspiration and biomechanics of the swallow. *Head & Neck.* 1998;20(1):52–57.

Logemann JA. Role of the modified barium swallow in management of patients with dysphagia. *Otolaryngology—Head & Neck Surgery.* 1997; 116(3):335–8.

Logemann JA, BR Pauloski, AW Rademaker, LA Colangelo. Super-supraglottic swallow in irradiated head and neck cancer patients. *Head & Neck.* 1997;19(6):535–40.

Logemann JA, BR Pauloski, AW Rademaker, LA Colangelo. Speech and swallowing rehabilitation for head and neck cancer patients [review]. *Oncology.* 1997;11(5):651-66, 659; discussion 659, 663–4.

Logemann JA. Screening, diagnosis, and management of neurogenic dysphagia. [review]. *Seminars in Neurology.* 1996;16(4):319–27.

Logemann JA. Dysphagia: evaluation and treatment [review]. *Folia Phoniatrica et Logopedica.* 1995;47(3):140–64.

Logemann JA, HB Fisher. Vocal tract control in Parkinson's disease: phonetic feature analysis of misarticulations. *Journal of Speech & Hearing Disorders.* 1981;46(4):348–52.

Logemann JA, HB Fisher, B Boshes, ER Blonsky. Frequency and cooccurrence of vocal tract dysfunctions in the speech of a large sample of Parkinson patients. *Journal of Speech & Hearing Disorders.* 1978; 43(1):47–57.

Logemann JA, B Boshes, ER Blonsky, HB Fisher. Speech and swallowing evaluation in the differential diagnosis of neurologic diseases. *Neurologia-Neurocirugia-Psiquiatria.* 1977;18(2-3 Suppl):71–78.

Logemann JA, P Gibbons, AW Rademaker, BR Pauloski, PJ Kahrilas, M Bacon, J Bowman, E.McCracken. Mechanisms of recovery of swallow after supraglottic laryngectomy. *Journal of Speech and Hearing Research.* 1994;37(5):965–74.

Logemann JA. Rehabilitation of the head and neck cancer patient [review]. *Seminars in Oncology.* 1994;21(3):359–65.

Logemann JA, AW Rademaker, BR Pauloski, PJ Kahrilas. Effects of postural change on aspiration in head and neck surgical patients. *Otolaryngology—Head & Neck Surgery.* 1994;110(2):222–7.

Logemann JA. The dysphagic diagnostic procedure as a treatment efficacy trial. *Clinics in Communication Disorders.* 1993;3(4):1–10.

Logemann JA. Noninvasive approaches to deglutitive aspiration. *Dysphagia.* 1993;8(4):331–3.

Logemann JA, T Shanahan, AW Rademaker, PJ Kahrilas, R Lazar, A Halper. Oropharyngeal swallowing after stroke in the left basal ganglion/internal capsule. *Dysphagia.* 1993;8(3):230–4.

Logemann JA. Factors affecting ability to resume oral nutrition in the oropharyngeal dysphagic individual [review]. *Dysphagia.* 1990;4 (4):202–8.

Logemann JA. Effects of aging on the swallowing mechanism [review]. *Otolaryngologic Clinics of North America.* 1990;23(6):1045–56.

O'Gara MM, JA Logemann, AW Rademaker. Phonetic features in babies with unilateral cleft lip and palate. *Cleft Palate—Craniofacial Journal.* 1994;31(6):446–51.

OhmaeY, JA Logemann, P Kaiser, DG Hanson, PJ Kahrilas. Effects of two breath-holding maneuvers on oropharyngeal swallow. *Annals of Otology, Rhinology & Laryngology.* 1996;105(2):123–31.

Pauloski BR, ED Blom, JA Logemann, RC Hamaker. Functional outcome after surgery for prevention of pharyngospasms in tracheoesophageal speakers. Part II: Swallow characteristics. *Laryngoscope.* 1995;105(10): 1104–10.

Pauloski BR, JA Logemann, JC Fox, LA Colangelo. Biomechanical analysis of the pharyngeal swallow in postsurgical patients with anterior tongue and floor of mouth resection and distal flap reconstruction. *Journal of Speech and Hearing Research.* 1995;38(1):110–23.

Pauloski BR, J Logemann, AW Rademaker, FM McConnel, MA Heiser, S Cardinale, D Shedd, L Lewin, SR Baker, D Graner, et al. Speech and swallowing function after anterior tongue and floor of mouth resection with distal flap reconstruction. *Journal of Speech & Hearing Research.* 1993;36(2):267–76.

Robbins JA, JA Logemann, HS Kirshner. Swallowing and speech production in Parkinson's disease. *Annals of Neurology.* 1986;19(3): 283–7.

Shanahan TK, JA Logemann, AW Rademaker, BR Pauloski, PJ Kahrilas. Chin-down posture effect on aspiration in dysphagic patients. *Archives of Physical Medicine & Rehabilitation.* 1993;74(7):736–9.

Sharp H, J Logemann, L Brady, A Moss. What if a patient refuses treatment? *ASHA.* 1997;39(3):56,52.

Sisson GA, FM McConnel, JA Logemann, S Yeh Jr. Voice rehabilitation after laryngectomy: results with the use of a hypopharyngeal prothesis. *Archives of Otolaryngology.* 1975;101(3):178–81.

Smith CH, JA Logemann, WR Burghart, TD Carrell, SG Zecker. Oral sensory discrimination of fluid viscosity. *Dysphagia.* 1997;12(2):68–73.

Wheeler RL, JA Logemann, MS Rosen. Maxillary reshaping protheses: effectiveness in improving speech and swallowing of postsurgical oral cancer patients. *Journal of Prosthetic Dentistry.* 1980;43(3):313–9.

PAT MIRENDA

Articles

Mirenda P, PA Locke. A comparison of symbol transparency in nonspeaking persons with intellectual disabilities. *Journal of Speech & Hearing Disorders.* 1989;54(2):131–40.

Mirenda PL, AM Donnellan, DE Yoder. Gaze behavior: a new look at an old problem. *Journal of Autism and Developmental Disorders.* 1983; 13(4):397–409.

Rydell PJ, P Mirenda. Effects of high and low constraint utterances on the production of immediate and delayed echolalia in young children. *Journal of Autism & Developmental Disorders.*1994;24(6):719–35.

JOSEPH G. SHEEHAN

Book

Sheehan JG. *Stuttering: Research and Therapy.* New York: Harper & Row. 1970.

Articles

Biggs B, J Sheehan. Punishment or distraction? Operant stuttering revisited. *Journal of Abnormal Psychology.* 1969;74(2):256–62.

Delali ID, JG Sheehan. Stuttering and assertion training. *Journal of Communication Disorders*. 1974;7(2):97–111.

Gould E, J Sheehan. Effect of silence on stuttering. *Journal of Abnormal Psychology*. 1967;72(5):441–5.

Jensen PJ, JG Sheehan, WN Williams, LL LaPointe. Oral sensory-perceptual integrity of stutterers. *Folia Phoniatrica*. 1965;27(1):38–45.

Martyn MM, J Sheehan, K Slutz. Incidence of stuttering and other speech disorders among the retarded. *American Journal of Mental Deficiency*. 1969;74(2):206–11.

Sheehan JG, MS Costley. A reexamination of the role of heredity in stuttering. *Journal of Speech & Hearing Disorders*. 1977;42(1):47–59.

Sheehan JG. Stuttering behavior: a phonetic analysis. *Journal of Communication Disorders*. 1974;7(3):193–212.

Sheehan JG, MA Lyon. Role perception in stuttering. *Journal of Communication Disorders*. 1974;7(2):113–25.

Sheehan JG, MM Martyn. Therapy as seen by stutterers. *Journal of Speech & Hearing Research*. 1971;14(2):445–6.

Sheehan JG, MM Martyn. Stuttering and its disappearance. *Journal of Speech & Hearing Research*. 1970;13(2):279–89.

Sheehan J, MM Martyn. Methodology in studies of recovery from stuttering. *Journal of Speech & Hearing Research*. 1967;10(2):496–9.

Sheehan J, R Hadley, E Gould. Impact of authority on stuttering. *Journal of Abnormal Psychology*. 1967;72(3):290–3.

Sheehan JG, MM Martyn. Spontaneous recovery from stuttering. *Journal of Speech & Hearing Research*. 1966; 9(1):121–35.

ROBERT J. SHPRINTZEN

Books

Shprintzen RJ. *Genetics, Syndromes, and Communication Disorders*. San Diego, Calif: Singular Publishing Co. 1997.

Shprintzen RJ, J Bardach. *Cleft Palate Speech Management: A Multidisciplinary Approach*. St. Louis, Mo: Mosby. 1995.

Articles

Arvystas M, RJ Shprintzen. Craniofacial morphology in Treacher Collins Syndrome. *Cleft Palate-Craniofacial Journal*. 1991;28(2):230–1.

Arvystas M, RJ Shprintzen. Craniofacial morphology in the velo-cardio-facial syndrome. *Journal of Craniofacial Genetics & Developmental Biology.* 1984;4(1):39–45.

Croft CB, RJ Shprintzen, RJ Ruben. Hypernasal speech following adenotonsillectomy. *Otolaryngology—Head & Neck Surgery.* 1981;89 (2):179–88.

Croft CB, RJ Shprintzen, SJ Rakoff. Patterns of velopharyngeal valving in normal and cleft palate subjects: a multi-view videofluoroscopic and nasendoscopic study. *Laryngoscope.* 1981;91(2):265–71.

Mitnick RK. JA Bello, KJ Golding-Kushner, RV Argamaso, RJ Shprintzen. The use of magnetic resonance angiography prior to pharyngeal flap surgery in patients with velocardiofacial syndrome. *Plastic & Reconstructive Surgery.* 1996;97(5):908–19.

Pollack MA, RJ Shprintzen. Velopharyngeal insufficiency in neurofibromatosis. *International Journal of Pediatric Otorhinolaryngology.* 1981; 3(3):257–62.

Shprintzen RJ. The implications of the diagnosis of Robin sequence [review]. *Cleft Palate-Craniofacial Journal.* 1992;29(3):205–9.

Shprintzen RJ, L Singer, EJ Sidoti, RV Argamaso. Pharyngeal flap surgery: postoperative complications. *International Anesthesiology Clinics.* 1992;30(4):115–24.

Shprintzen RJ, L Singer. Upper airway obstruction and the Robin sequence [review]. *International Anesthesiology Clinics.* 1992;30(4): 109–14.

Shprintzen RJ. Fallibility of clinical research. *Cleft Palate-Craniofacial Journal.* 1991;28(2):136–40.

Shprintzen RJ. Pierre Robin, micrognathia, and airway obstruction: the dependency of treatment on accurate diagnosis. *International Anesthesiology Clinics.* 1988;26(1):64–71.

Shprintzen RJ. Palatal and pharyngeal anomalies in craniofacial syndromes. *Birth Defects: Original Article Series.* 1982;18(1):53–78.

Shprintzen RJ, RB Goldberg, D Young, L Wolford. The velo-cardio-facial syndrome: a clinical and genetic analysis. *Pediatrics.* 1981;67(2): 167–72.

Shprintzen RJ, CB Croft. Abnormalities of the Eustachian tube orifice in individuals with cleft palate. *International Journal of Pediatric Otorhinolaryngology.* 1981;3(1):15–23.

Siegel-Sadewitz V, RJ Shprintzen. The relationship of communication disorders to syndrome identification. *Journal of Speech & Hearing Disorders.* 1982;47(4):338–54.

CHARLES VAN RIPER

Books

Van Riper C, RL Erickson. *Speech Correction: An introduction to Speech Pathology and Audiology,* 9th ed. Boston: Allyn and Bacon. 1996.

Van Riper C. *The Nature of Stuttering,* 2nd ed. Englewood Cliffs, NJ: Prentice-Hall. 1982.

Van Riper C. *A Career in Speech Pathology.* Englewood Cliffs, NJ: Prentice-Hall. 1979.

Van Riper C. *Speech Correction: Principles and Methods,* 6th ed. Englewood Cliffs, NJ: Prentice-Hall. 1978.

Van Riper C. *The Treatment of Stuttering.* Englewood Cliffs, NJ: Prentice-Hall. 1973.

Van Riper C. *Your Child's Speech Problems,* 1st ed. New York: Harper. 1961.

Van Riper C. *Voice and Articulation.* Englewood Cliffs, NJ: Prentice Hall. 1958.

Van Riper C, L Gruber. *A Casebook in Stuttering.* New York: Harper. 1957.

Van Riper C. *A Case Book in Speech Therapy.* New York: Prentice-Hall. 1953.

Van Riper C. *Speech Therapy: A Book of Readings.* New York: Prentice-Hall. 1953.

Articles

Van Riper C. An early history of ASHA. *ASHA.* 1981;23(11):855–8.

Van Riper C. Stuttering: where and whither? *ASHA.* 1974;16(9):483–7.

Van Riper C. Stuttering and cluttering: the differential diagnosis. *Folia Phoniatrica.* 1970;22(4):347–53.

Van Riper C. Recollections from a pioneer. *ASHA.* 1989;31(6–7): 72–73.

DAVID E. YODER

Books

McLean BM, JE McLean, RL Schiefelbusch , DE Yoder, eds. *Language Intervention with the Retarded: Developing Strategies*. Baltimore: University Park Press. 1972.

Yoder DR, RD Kent. *Decision Making in Speech-Language Pathology*. Philadelphia: B.C. Decker. 1988.

Articles

Bailey DB Jr, RJ Simeonsson, DE Yoder, GS Huntington. Preparing professionals to serve infants and toddlers with handicaps and their families: an integrative analysis across eight disciplines. *Exceptional Children*. 1990;57(1):26–35.

Miller JF, DE Yoder. On developing the content for a language teaching program. *Mental Retardation*. 1972;10(2):9–11.

Yoder DE, S Calculator. Some perspectives on intervention strategies for persons with developmental disorders. *Journal of Autism and Developmental Disorders*. 1981;11(1):107–23.

Appendix G

Unpublished Tests

ALS SEVERITY SCALE

Hillel AD, RM Miller, K Yorkston, E McDonald, FH Norris, N Konikow. Amyotrophic lateral sclerosis severity scale. *Neuroepidemiology.* 1989;8:142–50. *Note:* Rates function in areas of speech, swallowing, lower extremities, and upper extremities.

AUTISM DIAGNOSTIC OBSERVATION SCHEDULE (ADOS)

Lord CM, M Rutter, S Goode, J Heemsbergen, H Jordan, L Mawhood, E Schopler. Autism Diagnostic Observation Schedule: a standardized observation of communicative and social behavior. *Journal of Autism and Developmental Disorders.* 1989;19:185–212.

BURKE DYSPHAGIA SCREENING TEST (BDST)

DePippo KL, MA Holas, MJ Reding. The Burke Dysphagia Screening Test: validation of its use in patients with stroke. *Archives of Physical Medicine & Rehabilitation.* 1994;75(12):1284–6.

BZOCH ERROR PATTERN DIAGNOSTIC ARTICULATION TEST

Bzoch KR. Clinical assessment, evaluation, and management of 11 categorical aspects of cleft palate speech disorders. In: Bzoch KR, ed. *Communicative Disorders Related to Cleft Lip and Palate,* 4th ed. Austin, Tex: Pro-Ed. 1997:261–311.

CLINICAL ASSESSMENT OF OROPHARYNGEAL MOTOR DEVELOPMENT IN YOUNG CHILDREN

Robbins J, T Klee. Clinical assessment of oropharyngeal motor development in young children. *Journal of Speech and Hearing Disorders.* 1987;52:271–7.

CLINICAL LINGUISTIC AND AUDITORY MILESTONE SCALE (CLAMS)

Capute AJ, FB Palmer, BK Shapiro, RC Wachtel, S Schmidt, A Ross. Clinical linguistic and auditory milestone scale: predictions of cognition in infancy. *Developmental Medicine & Child Neurology.* 1986;28:762–71.

FREIBURG QUESTIONNAIRE ON COPING WITH ILLNESS

Herrmann M, A Britz, C Bartels, C-W Wallesch. The impact of aphasia on the patient and family in the first year post stroke. *Topics in Stroke Rehabilitation.* 1995;2(3):5–19.

FUNCTIONAL OUTCOME MEASURES FOR LLD CHILDREN

Contact: Linda C. Badon, PhD, University of Southwestern Louisiana, Department of Communication Disorders, P.O. Box 43170, Lafayette, LA 70504; (318) 482–5241.

GLASCOW COMA SCALE

Berkow R, ed. *The Merck Manual of Diagnosis and Therapy,* 16th ed. Rahway, NJ: Merck & Co., Inc. 1992:1463.

IOWA PRESSURE ARTICULATION TEST

Morris HL, DC Spriesterbach, FL Darley. An articulation test for assessing competency of velopharyngeal closure. *Journal of Speech and Hearing Disorders.* 1961;4:48–57.

MINI-MENTAL STATE EXAMINATION

Folstein MF, SE Folstein, PR McHugh. Mini-Mental State: a practical method for grading the cognitive state of patients for the clinician. *Journal of Psychiatric Research.* 1975;12:189–98.

PRAGMATIC PROTOCOL

Prutting CA, DM Kirchner. A clinical appraisal of the pragmatic aspects of language. *Journal of Speech and Hearing Disorders.* 1981;52: 105–9.

PRE-LINGUISTIC AUTISM DIAGNOSTIC OBSERVATION SCHEDULE (PL-ADOS)

DiLavore PC, C Lord, M Rutter. The Pre-Linguistic Autism Diagnostic Observation Schedule. *Journal of Autism and Developmental Disorders.* 1995;25(4):355–79.

RIC EVALUATION OF COMMUNICATION PROBLEMS IN RIGHT HEMISPHERE DYSFUNCTION

Halper AS, LR Cherney, MS Burns. *Clinical Management of Right Hemisphere Dysfunction,* 2nd ed, Appendixes A and B. Gaithersburg, Md: Aspen Publishers, Inc. 1996.

SELF-EFFICACY SCALE OF ADULT STUTTERERS (SESAS) AND SELF-EFFICACY SCALE FOR ADOLESCENTS

Hillis J, W Manning. Multidimensional assessment of stuttering: a clinical perspective. Second World Conference on Fluency Disorders, San Francisco, CA. Aug. 19, 1997.

SEVERITY OF PSYCHOSOCIAL CHANGE

Herrmann M, A Britz, C Bartels, C-W Wallesch. The impact of aphasia on the patient and family in the first year post-stroke. *Topics in Stroke Rehabilitation.* 1995;2(3):5–19.

SPEECH PERFORMANCE QUESTIONNAIRE

Perkins WH. Measurement and maintenance of fluency. In: Boberg E, ed. *Maintenance of Fluency.* New York: Elsevier. 1981:147–78.

Appendix H

Assessment Instruments

ANALYSIS OF THE LANGUAGE OF LEARNING (ALL)

Copyright Date: 1987.
Intended Population: Children from 5 years to 9 years, 11 months.
Purpose: To assess a child's level of classroom language awareness.
Administration Time: 30 minutes.
Publisher: LinguiSystems.

ARIZONA BATTERY FOR COMMUNICATION DISORDERS OF DEMENTIA (ABCD)

Copyright Date: 1991.
Intended Population: Persons suspected of exhibiting Alzheimer's disease. The test is not age specific.
Purpose: To identify and quantify those linguistic deficits associated with Alzheimer's disease. Screening tests are in the areas of speech discrimination, visual perception and literacy, visual field, and visual agnosia.
Administration Time: 45 to 90 minutes.
Publisher: Communication Skill Builders (a division of The Psychological Corporation).

ASSESSING LINGUISTIC BEHAVIORS: ASSESSING PRELINGUISTIC AND EARLY LINGUISTIC BEHAVIORS IN DEVELOPMENTALLY YOUNG CHILDREN (ALB)

Copyright Date: 1987.
Intended Population: Children functioning below age 2 years.
Purpose: To assess performance in the areas of cognitive-social and linguistic development. Specific areas assessed include antecedents to

word meaning, play, communicative intention, language comprehension, and language production.
Administration Time: Variable.
Publisher: University of Washington Press.

ASSESSMENT LINK BETWEEN PHONOLOGY AND ARTICULATION—REVISED (ALPHA-R)

Copyright Date: 1995.
Intended Population: Phonologically disordered children from 3 years through 8 years, 11 months
Purpose: To assess phonetic repertoire through sound-in position analysis and to assess deviant use of phonological processes through phonological analysis.
Administration Time: 15 minutes.
Publisher: ALPHA.

ASSESSMENT OF CHILDREN'S LANGUAGE COMPREHENSION (ACLC)

Copyright Date: 1983.
Intended Population: Children from 3 years to 6 years, 11 months.
Purpose: To assess understanding of word classes in different combinations of length and complexity.
Administration Time: 20 minutes.
Publisher: Applied Symbolics.

ASSESSMENT OF INTELLIGIBILITY OF DYSARTHRIC SPEAKERS (AIDS)

Copyright Date: 1984.
Intended Population: Adolescent and adult dysarthric speakers. The instrument is not age specific.
Purpose: To provide a means of measuring single-word and sentence-level intelligibility and speaking rate of dysarthric speakers.
Administration Time: 40 minutes.
Publisher: Pro-Ed.

BANKSON-BERNTHAL TEST OF PHONOLOGY (BBTOP)

Copyright Date: 1990.

Intended Population: Phonologically disordered children between the ages of 3 years and 9 years, 11 months.

Purpose: To assess the phonology of preschool and school-aged children.

Administration Time: 20 to 30 minutes.

Publisher: Applied Symbolics.

BAYLEY SCALES OF INFANT DEVELOPMENT, 2ND ED. (BSID-II)

Copyright Date: 1993.

Intended Population: Children 1 month through 3 years, 6 months.

Purpose: To identify children with cognitive or motor delays.

Administration Time: Up to 60 minutes.

Publisher: The Psychological Corporation.

BEHAVIOURAL INATTENTION TEST (BIT)

Copyright Date: 1987.

Intended Population: Persons recovering from cerebrovascular accident, head injury, or cerebral tumors suspected of unilateral visual neglect.

Purpose: To assess for the presence of unilateral visual neglect.

Administration Time: 45 minutes.

Publisher: Western Psychological Services.

BIRTH TO THREE SCREENING TEST OF LEARNING AND LANGUAGE DEVELOPMENT

Copyright Date: 1986.

Intended Population: Children from birth to 36 months.

Purpose: To assist in identifying those children at risk for developmental delay in one or more of the following areas: language comprehension, language expression, avenues to learning (problem-solving), social/personal development, and motor development.

Administration Time: 25 minutes.

Publisher: Pro-Ed.

BOSTON DIAGNOSTIC APHASIA EXAMINATION, 2ND ED. (BDAE)

Copyright Date: 1983.
Intended Population: Individuals with aphasia. The test is not age specific.
Purpose: To assess levels of language function in persons with aphasia.
Administration Time: 1 to 1.5 hours.
Distributor: The Psychological Corporation.

BOSTON NAMING TEST (BNT)

Copyright Date: 1983.
Intended Population: Adults with aphasia.
Purpose: To detect mild word-fining deficits.
Administration Time: Untimed.
Distributor: The Psychological Corporation.

BRIEF TEST OF HEAD INJURY (BTHI)

Copyright Date: 1991.
Intended Population: Persons with acute and long-term head injuries, age 10 years or above.
Purpose: To identify and measure deficits in individuals with head injury in the areas of orientation/attention, following commands, linguistic organization, reading comprehension, naming, memory, and visual-spatial skills.
Administration Time: 45 minutes.
Publisher: Applied Symbolics.

BURNS/ROE INFORMAL READING INVENTORY: PREPRIMER TO 12TH GRADE, 3RD ED. (IRI)

Copyright Date: 1993.
Intended Population: Beginning readers to 12th grade level.
Purpose: To provide information regarding reading skills and abilities for the purpose of planning an appropriate program of reading instruction.
Administration Time: 40 to 50 minutes.
Publisher: Houghton Mifflin Co.

CALIFORNIA VERBAL LEARNING TEST—ADULT VERSION (CVLT)

Copyright Date: 1987.

Intended Population: Persons 17 years and older.

Purpose: To assess verbal learning and memory deficits in adults.

Administration Time: Approximately 30 minutes, plus 20-minute delay period.

Publisher: The Psychological Corporation.

CALIFORNIA VERBAL LEARNING TEST—CHILDREN'S VERSION (CVLT-C)

Copyright Date: 1994.

Intended Population: Children 5 years through 16 years, 11 months.

Purpose: To evaluate children and adolescents who have learning and memory impairments.

Administration Time: 15 to 20 minutes, plus a 20-minute interval.

Publisher: The Psychological Corporation.

CARROW ELICITED LANGUAGE INVENTORY (CELI)

Copyright Date: 1974.

Intended Population: Children 3 years to 7 years, 11 months.

Purpose: To measure a child's productive control of grammar based on a technique of eliciting imitation of a series of 52 sentences.

Administration Time: 15 to 20 minutes.

Publisher: Pro-Ed.

CLINICAL EVALUATION OF LANGUAGE FUNDAMENTALS, 3RD ED. (CELF-3)

Copyright Date: 1995.

Intended Population: Individuals from 6 years to 21 years, 11 months.

Purpose: To identify individuals who lack the basic foundations of content and form that characterize mature language use. Assessment is in the areas of semantics, morphology, syntax, and memory.

Administration Time: Minimum 30 to 45 minutes. The test may be administered in two sessions, but any subtest must be completed before a session is discontinued.

Publisher: The Psychological Corporation.

COMMUNICATION AND SYMBOLIC BEHAVIOR SCALE (CSBS)

Copyright Date: 1993.

Intended Population: Children from 8 months to 2 years. As appropriate, it may be used with children up to 6 years.

Purpose: To provide early identification of children at risk for having or developing communication impairment; to develop a profile of communicative, social-affective and symbolic functioning for the purposes of providing direction for intervention planning and to monitor changes.

Administration Time: 1 hour.

Publisher: Applied Symbolics.

COMMUNICATIVE ABILITIES IN DAILY LIVING (CADL)

Copyright Date: 1980.

Intended Population: Adults with aphasia.

Purpose: To assess functional communication skills in adults with aphasia.

Administration Time: 45 minutes.

Publisher: Pro-Ed.

DENVER II [A REVISION OF THE DENVER DEVELOPMENTAL SCREENING TEST (DDST)]

Copyright Date: 1990.

Intended Population: Children from birth to 6 years, 6 months.

Purpose: To screen a child's performance on various tasks in the areas of personal-social, fine motor-adaptive, language, and gross motor skills.

Administration Time: Variable up to 20 minutes.

Publisher: Denver Developmental Materials (DDM).

DIAGNOSTIC READING SCALES (DRS-81)

Copyright Date: 1963–1981.

Intended Population: Persons with reading skills at the first to seventh grade levels.

Purpose: To identify strengths and weaknesses that affect reading proficiency.

Administration Time: 60 minutes.

Publisher: CTB MacMillan/McGraw-Hill.

DISCOURSE COMPREHENSION TEST (DCT)

Copyright Date: 1993.

Intended Population: Adults who are aphasic, right-brain damaged, and/or traumatically head injured. The DCT is not age specific.

Purpose: To assess comprehension and retention of spoken narrative discourse for main ideas and detail. The test can also be used as an assessment of silent reading comprehension.

Publisher: Communication Skill Builders (a division of The Psychological Corporation).

EXPRESSIVE ONE-WORD PICTURE VOCABULARY TEST, REVISED (EOWPVT-R)

Copyright Date: 1990.

Intended Population: Children from 2 years to 11 years, 11 months.

Purpose: To obtain an estimate of expressive language development.

Administration Time: 7 to 15 minutes.

Publisher: Pro-Ed.

FISHER-LOGEMANN TEST OF ARTICULATION COMPETENCE

Copyright Date: 1974.

Intended Population: Any individual with articulation deficits.

Purpose: To assess an individual's phonological repertoire with analysis and categorization of errors.

Administration Time: 15 minutes.

Publisher: Pro-Ed.

FRENCHAY DYSARTHRIA ASSESSMENT

Copyright Date: 1983.
Intended Population: Adults with dysarthria.
Purpose: To diagnose dysarthria.
Administration Time: 30 minutes.
Publisher: Pro-Ed.

FULD OBJECT-MEMORY EVALUATION

Copyright Date: 1977.
Intended Population: Persons between the ages of 70 and 90 years regardless of language and sensory handicaps.
Purpose: To "evaluate memory and learning under conditions that virtually guarantee attention and minimize anxiety." Scores are in the areas of total recall, storage, consistency of retrieval, ability to benefit from reminding, and ability to say words in categories.
Administration Time: Not reported.
Publisher: Stoelting Company.

FUNCTIONAL ASSESSMENT OF COMMUNICATION SKILLS FOR ADULTS (ASHA FACS)

Copyright Date: 1995.
Intended Population: Adults with aphasia resulting from left hemisphere stroke and adults with communication disorders resulting from traumatic brain injury.
Purpose: To assess functional communication abilities in the areas of social communication; communication of basic needs; reading, writing, and number concepts; and daily planning.
Administration Time: Not given.
Publisher: American Speech-Language-Hearing Association (ASHA).

FUNCTIONAL COMMUNICATION PROFILE (FCP)

Copyright Date: 1953.
Intended Population: Clients with developmental delays.

Purpose: To assess communication skills in the areas of sensory/motor, attentiveness, receptive language, expressive language, pragmatic/social skills, speech development, voice, and fluency.
Administration Time: No suggested time given.
Publisher: AliMed, Inc.

GOLDMAN-FRISTOE TEST OF ARTICULATION (GFTA)

Copyright Date: 1972.
Intended Population: Children from 2 years to 16 years, 11 months.
Purpose: To assess all necessary phonemes under conditions ranging from imitative to conversational speech.
Administration Time: 20-45 minutes.
Publisher: American Guidance Service.

GRAY ORAL READING TEST, 3RD ED. (GORT-3)

Copyright Date: 1992.
Intended Population: Students from 7 years to 17 years.
Purpose: To provide a system for analyzing errors in the areas of meaning similarity, function similarity, graphic/phonemic similarity, and self-correction.
Administration Time: 45 minutes.
Publisher: Riverside Publishing Company.

HAWAII EARLY LEARNING PROFILE (HELP)

Copyright Date: 1994.
Intended Population: Children from birth to 3 years.
Purpose: To provide developmental assessment, intervention, planning, and instruction in the areas of cognition, language, gross motor, fine motor, social, and self-help skills.
Administration Time: N/A.
Publisher: VORT Corporation.

LANGUAGE PROCESSING TEST, REVISED (LPT-R)

Copyright Date: 1995.
Intended Population: Children from 5 years to 11 years, 11 months.
Purpose: To evaluate students at risk for language processing deficits.
Administration Time: 30 minutes.
Publisher: LinguiSystems.

MACARTHUR COMMUNICATIVE DEVELOPMENT INVENTORIES (CDI)

Copyright Date: 1993.
Intended Population: Children 8 months to 30 months.
Purpose: To assess early child language from first nonverbal gestural signals through expansion of early vocabulary and the beginning of grammar.
Administration Time: 20 to 40 minutes.
Publisher: Singular Publishing Group.

MCCARTHY SCALES OF CHILDREN'S ABILITIES

Copyright Date: 1972.
Intended Population: Children 2 years, 6 months through 8 years, 6 months.
Purpose: To measure cognitive and motor development; to determine general intellectual level as well as strengths and weaknesses in areas such as verbal ability and memory.
Administration Time: 45 minutes for children under age 5 years; 1 hour for older children.
Publisher: The Psychological Corporation.

MINI INVENTORY OF RIGHT BRAIN INJURY (MIRBI)

Copyright Date: 1989.
Intended Population: Adults between 20 and 80 years with right brain injury.
Purpose: To identify deficits in visual processing, language processing, emotion/affect processing, and general behavior associated with right brain injury.

Administration Time: 20 to 30 minutes.
Publisher: Pro-Ed.

MINNESOTA TEST FOR DIFFERENTIAL DIAGNOSIS OF APHASIA (MTDDA)

Copyright Date: 1972.
Intended Population: Adults with aphasia.
Purpose: To assess language function in aphasic individuals.
Administration Time: 1.5 to 2 hours.
Publisher: The Psychological Corporation.

MULTILINGUAL APHASIA EXAMINATION, 3RD ED. (MAE-3)

Copyright Date: 1994.
Intended Population: Adults who have aphasia.
Purpose: To assess oral expression, spelling, oral verbal understanding, reading, articulation and writing.
Administration Time: 45 to 60 minutes.
Publisher: The Psychological Corporation.

NATURAL PROCESS ANALYSIS (NPA)

Copyright Date: 1986.
Intended Population: Children with phonological disorders. The NPA is not age specific.
Purpose: To assess phonological development in children by evaluating eight natural phonological processes in spontaneous conversational speech.
Administration Time: About 3 hours.
Publisher: Macmillan.

NELSON-DENNY READING TEST

Copyright Date: 1993.
Intended Population: Adolescents and adults.
Purpose: To assess achievement and progress in vocabulary, comprehen-

sion, and reading rate.

Administration Time: 35 minutes. Time may be extended to meet the needs of special populations.

Publisher: Riverside Publishing Company.

NEUROPSYCHOLOGICAL INVESTIGATION OF CHILDREN (NEPSY)

Copyright Date: 1997.

Intended Population: Children from 3 years through 12 years, 11 months.

Purpose: To assess learning in the areas of executive functions (including attention, planning, and problem-solving), language and communication, sensorimotor functions, visuospatial functions, and learning and memory.

Administration Time: Full form: Less than 2.5 hours for older children, approximately 1 hour for younger children. Core form: Less than 1 hour.

Publisher: The Psychological Corporation.

ORAL MOTOR/FEEDING RATING SCALE

Copyright Date: 1990.

Intended Population: This instrument is not age specific.

Purpose: To assist with client management decisions regarding feeding.

Administration Time: 45 minutes (may be administered over multiple sessions).

Publisher: Communication Skill Builders (a division of The Psychological Corporation).

PEABODY PICTURE VOCABULARY TEST, REVISED (PPVT-R)

Copyright Date: 1981.

Intended Population: Individuals from 2 years, 6 months to 40 years, 11 months.

Purpose: To measure receptive (hearing) vocabulary for Standard American English. A Spanish version is also available.

Administration Time: 10 to 15 minutes.

Publisher: American Guidance Service.

PHONOLOGICAL ASSESSMENT OF CHILD SPEECH

Copyright Date: 1985.

Intended Population: Children with severe phonological deficits.

Purpose: To assess and analyze the sound system of children with severe phonological deficits; to compare phonology with that of normal developmental levels.

Administration Time: Variable.

Publisher: NFER-Nelson Publishing Co., Ltd.

Distributor: Stoelting & Co.

PORCH INDEX OF COMMUNICATIVE ABILITY, 3RD ED. (PICA)

Copyright Date: 1981.

Intended Population: Adults with aphasia. The PICA is not age specific.

Purpose: To evaluate an aphasic client's change in language skills over time. Note: Examiners must complete specific training before administering this test.

Administration Time: 1 hour.

Publisher: Pro-Ed.

PRESCHOOL LANGUAGE ASSESSMENT INSTRUMENT (PLAI)

Copyright Date: 1978.

Intended Population: Children from 3 years to 6 years, 11 months and older children with language problems.

Purpose: To assess young children's skills in coping with language demands of the learning environment.

Administration Time: 20 minutes.

Publisher: The Psychological Corporation.

PRESCHOOL LANGUAGE SCALE—3 (PLS-3)

Copyright Date: 1992.

Intended Population: Children from 2 weeks to 6 years, 11 months or older children who are functioning within this developmental range. The test is not recommended for use with adults who are functioning within this developmental range.

Purpose: To measure receptive and expressive language skills in young children in the areas of language precursors, vocabulary, concepts, morphology, syntax, and integrative thinking skills.
Administration Time: 30 minutes.
Publisher: The Psychological Corporation.

PREVERBAL ASSESSMENT INTERVENTION PROFILE (PAIP)

Copyright Date: 1984.
Intended Population: Severely, profoundly, and/or multihandicapped preverbal individuals. The PAIP is not age specific.
Purpose: To evaluate prelinguistic abilities.
Administration Time: 1 hour.
Publisher: Pro-Ed.

PRE-VERBAL COMMUNICATION SCHEDULE (PVCS)

Copyright Date: 1987.
Intended Population: Children, adolescents, and adults.
Purpose: To assess existing nonverbal and vocal communication skills.
Administration Time: 120 to 150 minutes.
Publisher: NFER-Nelson Publishing Co., Ltd.
Distributor: Stoelting & Co.

RATING SCALE OF COMMUNICATION IN COGNITIVE DECLINE (RSCCD)

Copyright Date: 1991.
Intended Population: Persons diagnosed with dementia.
Purpose: To assess the communication abilities of persons with progressive dementia.
Administration Time: Not reported.
Publisher: United/DOK Publishers.

READING COMPREHENSION BATTERY FOR APHASIA (RCBA)

Copyright Date: 1979.
Intended Population: Adults with aphasia. The RCBA is not age specific.

Purpose: To evaluate the nature and degree of reading impairment in adults who are aphasic.

Administration Time: 45 minutes.

Publisher: Pro-Ed.

RECEPTIVE-EXPRESSIVE EMERGENT LANGUAGE TEST, 2ND ED. (REEL-2)

Copyright Date: 1991.

Intended population: Infants and toddlers from birth to 3 years. Also appropriate for older preschoolers with obvious developmental delays.

Purpose: To identify major receptive and expressive language problems in infants and toddlers.

Administration Time: 20 to 30 minutes.

Publisher: Pro-Ed.

REHABILITATION INSTITUTE OF CHICAGO FUNCTIONAL ASSESSMENT SCALE, VERSION V (RIC-FAS)

Copyright Date: 1998.

Intended Population: Persons aged 16 years or older who have been hospitalized or in an inpatient rehabilitation setting and who are now transferring to a less restrictive environment.

Purpose: To assess levels of independence in the areas of self-help and care, mobility, communication and cognitive skills.

Administration Time: Not given.

Publisher: Rehabilitation Institute of Chicago.

REVISED TOKEN TEST (RTT)

Copyright Date: 1978.

Intended Population: Any individual having adequate peripheral hearing and who speaks the language in which the test is administered. The test has been standardized on normal and on right and left hemisphere brain-damaged adults.

Purpose: To assess auditory processing inefficiencies associated with brain damage, aphasia, and some language and learning disabilities.

Administration Time: 45 minutes.
Publisher: Pro-Ed.

ROSS INFORMATION PROCESSING ASSESSMENT—2 (RIPA-2)

Copyright Date: Date of first edition—1986.
Intended Population: Adolescents and adults with closed head injury.
Purpose: To assess cognitive functioning in the areas of immediate memory, recent memory, temporal orientation, spatial orientation, orientation to environment, recall of general information, problem-solving and abstract reasoning, organization, and auditory processing and retention.
Administration Time: 60 minutes.
Publisher: Pro-Ed.

ROSSETTI INFANT AND TODDLER LANGUAGE SCALE

Copyright Date: 1990.
Intended Population: Children from birth to 3 years.
Purpose: To assess preverbal and verbal communication and interaction.
Administration Time: Approximately 1 hour.
Publisher: LinguiSystems.

SCALE FOR ASSESSMENT OF THOUGHT, LANGUAGE, AND COMMUNICATION DISORDERS (TLC)

Copyright Date: 1980.
Intended Population: Manics, those with depression and those with schizophrenia.
Purpose: To assess clinical and pathological characteristics of language, including poverty of speech, poverty of content of speech, distractibility, tangentiality, derailment, incoherence, illogicality, neologisms, word approximations, circumstantiality, loss of goal, perseveration, echolalia, blocking, stilted speech, and self-reference.
Administration Time: 45–60 minutes.
Publisher: Nancy C. Andreasen.

SCALES OF COGNITIVE ABILITY FOR TRAUMATIC BRAIN INJURY (SCATBI)

Copyright Date: 1992.

Intended Population: Clients with head injuries.

Purpose: To assess cognitive and linguistic deficits associated with traumatic brain injury.

Administration Time: 45 minutes.

Publisher: AliMed Inc.

SCAN: A SCREENING TEST FOR AUDITORY PROCESSING DISORDERS (SCAN)

Copyright Date: 1986.

Intended Population: Children aged 3 years to 11 years, 11 months who have language disorders or difficulty achieving in academic settings.

Purpose: To identify children who may have language problems compounded by auditory processing disorders.

Administration Time: 20 minutes.

Publisher: The Psychological Corporation.

SCAN-A: A SCREENING TEST OF AUDITORY PROCESSING DISORDERS IN ADOLESCENTS AND ADULTS (SCAN-A)

Copyright Date: 1994.

Intended Population: Adolescents and adults from 12 years to 50 years, 11 months suspected of having auditory processing disorders.

Purpose: To describe auditory processing abilities and deficits.

Administration Time: 20 minutes.

Publisher: The Psychological Corporation.

SCREENING TEST FOR DEVELOPMENTAL APRAXIA OF SPEECH (STDAS)

Copyright Date: 1980.

Intended Population: Children from 4 years to 12 years, 11 months suspected of having developmental apraxia of speech.

Purpose: A screening instrument to assist in the differential diagnosis of developmental apraxia of speech. Areas assessed include expressive language discrepancy, vowels and diphthongs, oral motor skills, verbal sequencing, articulation, motorically complex words, transposition, and prosody.
Administration Time: 10 to 15 minutes.
Publisher: Pro-Ed.

SEQUENCED INVENTORY OF COMMUNICATION DEVELOPMENT, REVISED (SICD-R)

Copyright Date: 1984.
Intended Population: Children from 4 months to 4 years. The adapted version of the test, A-SICD, is developed for use with adolescents who are severely handicapped and with adults who have little or no speech or who are understood only by those closest to them.
Purpose: To evaluate the development of verbal and nonverbal communication in very young children and to estimate levels of receptive and expressive language functioning.
Administration Time: 30 to 90 minutes.
Publisher: University of Washington Press.

SLOSSON INTELLIGENCE TEST, REVISED (SIT-R)

Copyright Date: 1990.
Intended Population: Persons 4 years to 65 years.
Purpose: To provide a screening of intelligence in the areas of vocabulary, general information, similarities and differences, comprehension, quantitative, and auditory memory.
Administration time: 10 to 20 minutes.
Publisher: Slosson Educational Publications, Inc.

STROOP COLOR AND WORD TEST

Copyright Date: 1978.
Intended Population: Individuals from second grade through adult.
Purpose: To investigate personality, cognition, stress response, psychiatric disorders, and other psychological phenomena and to differentiate between normal, psychiatric, and brain-damaged persons.

Administration Time: 5 minutes.
Publisher: The Riverside Publishing Company.

STUTTERING PREDICTION INSTRUMENT FOR YOUNG CHILDREN (SPI)

Copyright Date: 1981.
Intended Population: Children from 3 years to 8 years.
Purpose: To assess the likelihood of a child continuing to stutter beyond the period of normal developmental dysfluency.
Administration Time: 20 minutes.
Publisher: Pro-Ed.

STUTTERING SEVERITY INSTRUMENT, 3RD ED. (SSI-3)

Copyright Date: 1994.
Intended Population: Children and adults suspected of being dysfluent. The SSI-3 is not age specific.
Purpose: To assess the severity of dysfluent speech behavior, including frequency, duration of longest stuttering block, and presence of accompanying physical behaviors.
Administration Time: 20 minutes.
Publisher: Pro-Ed.

TEST FOR AUDITORY COMPREHENSION OF LANGUAGE, REVISED (TACL-R)

Copyright Date: 1985.
Intended Population: Children from 3 years to 8 years, 11 months.
Purpose: To assess auditory comprehension of vocabulary and linguistic structures.
Administration Time: 10 to 20 minutes.
Publisher: Pro-Ed.

TEST OF ADOLESCENT AND ADULT LANGUAGE, 3RD ED. (TOAL-3)

Copyright Date: 1994.
Intended Population: Individuals between the ages of 12 years and 24 years, 11 months.

Purpose: To identify adolescents and adults in need of intervention to improve language proficiency; to determine areas of relative strengths and weaknesses; and to document overall progress as a result of intervention. Subtests include listening/vocabulary, listening/grammar, speaking/vocabulary, speaking/grammar, reading/vocabulary, reading/grammar, writing/vocabulary, and writing/grammar.

Administration Time: 1 hour, 45 minutes.

Publisher: Pro-Ed.

TEST OF LANGUAGE COMPETENCE, EXPANDED (TLC-E)

Copyright Date: 1989.

Intended Population: Children from 5 years to 9 years, 11 months (level 1) and from 9 years to 18 years, 11 months (level 2).

Purpose: To measure metalinguistic abilities and linguistic strategy acquisition in the areas of semantics, syntax, and pragmatics.

Administration Time: 1 hour.

Publisher: The Psychological Corporation.

TEST OF LANGUAGE DEVELOPMENT (INTERMEDIATE), 2ND ED. (TOLD-I:2)

Copyright Date: 1988.

Intended Population: Clients from 8 years, 6 months to 12 years, 11 months.

Purpose: To identify children below their peers in language proficiency, identify strengths and weaknesses in language abilities, document progress, and provide a research measurement.

Administration Time: 30 to 60 minutes.

Publisher: Pro-Ed.

TEST OF LANGUAGE DEVELOPMENT (PRIMARY), 2ND ED. (TOLD-P:2)

Copyright Date: 1988.

Intended Population: Children from 4 years to 8 years, 11 months.

Purpose: To identify children below their peers in language proficiency; identify strengths and weaknesses in language abilities; document progress; and provide a research measurement instrument.
Administration Time: 30 to 60 minutes.
Publisher: Pro-Ed.

TEST OF NONVERBAL INTELLIGENCE, 3RD ED. (TONI-3)

Copyright Date: 1997.
Intended Population: Persons from 6 years through 89 years.
Purpose: To assess intelligence, aptitude, abstract reasoning, and problem-solving without the use of language.
Administration Time: 15 to 20 minutes.
Publisher: Pro-Ed.

TEST OF PROBLEM SOLVING—ADOLESCENT (TOPS—ADOLESCENT)

Copyright Date: 1991.
Intended Population: Adolescents from 12 years to 17 years, 11 months and older clients whose overall functional language abilities are within the performance level of the test.
Purpose: To assess language-based critical thinking skills. Information is provided on how a student uses language to think, reason, and solve problems.
Administration Time: 40 minutes.
Publisher: LinguiSystems.

TEST OF PROBLEM SOLVING—ELEMENTARY, REVISED (TOPS—ELEMENTARY, REVISED)

Copyright Date: 1994.
Intended Population: Children from 6 years to 11 years, 11 months and older clients whose overall functional language abilities are within the performance level of the test.

Purpose: To assess critical thinking abilities based on the client's language strategies using logic and experience.
Administration Time: 35 to 40 minutes.
Publisher: LinguiSystems

WESTERN APHASIA BATTERY (WAB)

Copyright Date: 1982.
Intended Population: Adults who have aphasia. The WAB is not age specific.
Purpose: To evaluate verbal skills of content, fluency, auditory comprehension, repetition, naming, reading, writing, and calculation. Nonverbal skills of drawing, block design, and praxis also are assessed.
Administration Time: 1 to 1.5 hours.
Publisher: The Psychological Corporation.

WOODCOCK READING MASTERY TESTS, REVISED (WRMT-R)

Copyright Date: 1973–1987. Normative data updated in 1997.
Intended Population: Kindergarten through adult.
Purpose: To assess reading readiness and reading skills, including letter identification, word identification, word attack, word comprehension (antonyms, synonyms, analogies), and passage comprehension.
Administration Time: 10 to 30 minutes for each cluster of tests.
Publisher: American Guidance Service.

WORD TEST—ADOLESCENT

Copyright Date: 1989.
Intended Population: Individuals from 12 years to 17 years, 11 months.
Purpose: To assess expressive vocabulary and semantics in contexts that are reflective of school assignments and language usage in everyday life.
Administration Time: 25 minutes.
Publisher: LinguiSystems.

WORD TEST—ELEMENTARY (REVISED)

Copyright Date: 1990.

Intended Population: Children from 7 years to 11 years, 11 months.

Purpose: To assess expressive vocabulary and semantics. Tasks involve categorizing, defining, verbal reasoning, and choosing appropriate words.

Administration Time: 25 minutes.

Publisher: LinguiSystems.

REFERENCES

Conoley JC, JC Impara. *The Twelfth Mental Measurement Yearbook*. Lincoln, Neb: The University of Nebraska-Lincoln; The Buros Institute of Mental Measurements. 1995.

Harris LG, IS Shelton. *Desk Reference of Assessment Instruments in Speech and Language, Revised*. San Antonio, Tex: Communication Skill Builders. 1996.

Murphy LL, JC Conoley, JC Impara. *Tests in Print IV*. Lincoln, Neb: The University of Nebraska-Lincoln; The Buros Institute of Mental Measurements. 1994.

Appendix I

Publishers

ALIMED, INC.
297 High Street
Dedham, MA 02026-9135
(800) 225-2610
(800) 437-2966 (fax)

ALPHA
Speech & Language Resources
P.O. Box 322
Mifflinville, PA 18631
(717) 752-2166
(717) 752-8432 (fax)

AMERICAN GUIDANCE SERVICE
4201 Woodland Road
P.O. Box 99
Circle Pines, MN 55014-1796
(800) 328-2560
(612) 786-9077 (fax)

AMERICAN SPEECH-LANGUAGE-HEARING ASSOCIATION (ASHA)
10801 Rockville Pike
Rockville, MD 20852
(888) 498-6699

NANCY C. ANDREASEN
College of Medicine
University of Iowa
500 Newton Road
Iowa City, IA 52242
(319) 335-3500

APPLIED SYMBOLICS
16 West Erie Street, Suite 300
Chicago, IL 60610
(312) 787-3772
787-3828 (fax)

CBT MACMILLAN/ MCGRAW-HILL

20 Ryan Ranch Road
Monterey, CA 93940-5703
(831)393-0700

COMMUNICATION SKILL BUILDERS (A DIVISION OF THE PSYCHOLOGICAL CORPORATION)

555 Academic Court
San Antonio, TX 78204
(800) 228-0752
(800) 232-1223 (fax)
(800) 723-1318 (TTD)

DENVER DEVELOPMENTAL MATERIALS (DDM)

P.O. Box 6919
Denver, CO 80206-0919
(303) 355-4729
(303) 355-5622 (fax)

HOUGHTON MIFFLIN CO.

P.O. Box 7050
Wilmington, MA 01887-7050
(800) 733-1717

LINGUISYSTEMS, INC.

P.O. Box 747
3100 Fourth Avenue
East Moline, IL 61265
(800) 776-4332
(309) 755-2300 (in Illinois)

NFER-NELSON PUBLISHING COMPANY, LTD.

Darville House
208 Ford Road East
East Windsor
Berkshire SL4 1Df England

PRO-ED, INC.

8700 Shoal Creek Boulevard
Austin, TX 78758
(512) 451-3246
(800) 397-7633 (fax)

THE PSYCHOLOGICAL CORPORATION

555 Academic Court
San Antonio, TX 78204
(800) 228-0752
(800) 232-1223 (fax)
(800) 723-1318 (TTD)

REHABILITATION INSTITUTE OF CHICAGO

345 East Superior, Room 1671
Chicago, IL 60611
(312) 908-6000

THE RIVERSIDE PUBLISHING COMPANY

8420 Bryn Mawr Avenue
Chicago, IL 60631
(800) 767-8378
(312) 714-7000
(312) 693-0325 (fax)

SINGULAR PUBLISHING GROUP

4284 41st Street
San Diego, CA 92105-1197
(800) 521-8545
(619) 563-9008 (fax)

SLOSSON EDUCATIONAL PUBLICATIONS, INC.

P.O. Box 280
East Aurora, NY 14052-0280
(716) 652-0930
(716) 655-3840 (fax)

STOELTING & COMPANY

620 Wheat Lane
Wood Dale, IL 60191
(800) 860-9775
(630) 860-9775 (fax)

UNITED/DOK PUBLISHERS

P.O. Box 1099
Buffalo, NY 14224

UNIVERSITY OF WASHINGTON PRESS

P.O. Box 50096
Seattle, WA 98145
(800) 441-4115
(800) 669-7993 (fax)

VORT CORPORATION

P.O. Box 60132
Palo Alto, CA 94306
(650) 322-8282
(650) 327-0747 (fax)

WESTERN PSYCHOLOGICAL SERVICES

12031 Wilshire Boulevard
Los Angeles, CA 90025
(800) 648-8857
(310) 478-7838 (fax)

WILLIAMS AND WILKINS

P.O. Box 1496
Baltimore, MD 21298
(800) 638-0672
(800) 447-8438 (fax)

Index